WILLFUL IGNORANCE

WILLFUL IGNORANCE
The Mismeasure of Uncertainty

HERBERT I. WEISBERG
Correlation Research, Inc.
Needham, MA

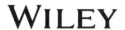

Published by John Wiley & Sons, Inc., Hoboken, New Jersey.
Published simultaneously in Canada.

For general information on our other products and services or for technical support, please contact our Customer Care Department within the United States at (800) 762-2974, outside the United States at (317) 572-3993 or fax (317) 572-4002.

Wiley also publishes its books in a variety of electronic formats. Some content that appears in print may not be available in electronic formats. For more information about Wiley products, visit our web site at www.wiley.com.

Library of Congress Cataloging-in-Publication Data

Weisberg, Herbert I., 1944- author.
  Willful ignorance : the mismeasure of uncertainty / Herbert I. Weisberg, Correlation Research, Inc., Needham, MA.
       pages cm
  Includes bibliographical references and index.
  ISBN 978-0-470-89044-8 (paperback)
 1. Research–Statistical methods.   2. Probabilities.   3. Research–Methodology.   I. Title.
   Q180.55.S7W45 2014
   001.4′22–dc23

                                                                              2014007297

Printed in the United States of America

ISBN: 9780470890448

10 9 8 7 6 5 4 3 2 1

I have known that thing the Greeks knew not—uncertainty. ... Mine is a dizzying country in which the Lottery is a major element of reality.

Jorge Luis Borges[1]

This fundamental requirement for the applicability to individual cases of the concept of classical probability shows clearly the role of subjective ignorance as well as that of objective knowledge in a typical probability statement.

Ronald Aylmer Fisher[2]

To a stranger, the probability that I shall send a letter to the post unstamped may be derived from the statistics of the Post Office; for me those figures would have but the slightest bearing on the question.

John Maynard Keynes[3]

CONTENTS

PREFACE   **xi**

ACKNOWLEDGMENTS   **xv**

1   THE OPPOSITE OF CERTAINTY   **1**

Two Dead Ends / 2
Analytical Engines / 4
What is Probability? / 6
Uncertainty / 9
Willful Ignorance / 12
Toward a New Science / 15

2   A QUIET REVOLUTION   **19**

Thinking the Unthinkable / 21
Inventing Probability / 24
Statistics / 27
The Taming of Chance / 31
The Ignorance Fallacy / 34
The Dilemma of Science / 35

3   A MATTER OF CHANCE   **41**

Origins / 43
Probability / 44
The Famous Correspondence / 56
What Did Not Happen Next / 60
Against The Odds / 64

4   HARDLY TOUCHED UPON   **71**

The Mathematics of Chance / 73
Empirical Frequencies / 82
A Quantum of Certainty / 100

5   A MATHEMATICIAN OF BASEL   **114**

Publication at Last / 116
The Art of Conjecturing / 117
A Tragic Ending / 142

6   A DEFECT OF CHARACTER   **147**

Man Without a Country / 150
A Fraction of Chances / 165

7   CLASSICAL PROBABILITY   **171**

Revolutionary Reverends / 173
From Chances to Probability / 194

8   BABEL   **213**

The Great Unraveling / 216
Probability as a Relative Frequency / 219
Probability as a Logical Relationship / 228
Probability as a Subjective Assessment / 239
Probability as a Propensity / 247

9 PROBABILITY AND REALITY   253

The Razor's Edge / 255
What Fisher Knew / 257
What Reference Class? / 262
A Postulate of Ignorance / 270
Laplace's Error / 279

10 THE DECISION FACTORY   283

Beyond Moral Certainty / 284
Decisions, Decisions / 298
Machine-Made Knowledge / 309

11 THE LOTTERY IN SCIENCE   312

Scientific Progress / 313
Fooled by Causality / 319
Statistics for Humans: Bias or Ambiguity? / 331
Regression toward the Mean / 339

12 TRUST, BUT VERIFY   346

A New Problem / 347
Trust, … / 354
… But Verify / 357
The Future / 363
Mindful Ignorance / 368

**APPENDIX: THE PASCAL–FERMAT
CORRESPONDENCE OF 1654**   373

NOTES   387

BIBLIOGRAPHY   415

INDEX   429

PREFACE

The History of Science has suffered greatly from the use by teachers of second-hand material, and the consequent obliteration of the circumstances and the intellectual atmosphere in which the great discoveries of the past were made.

R. A. Fisher[1]

Sir Ronald A. Fisher, the founder of modern statistics, was certainly correct to point out how much is lost by abstracting major scientific developments from the context in which they evolved. However, it is clearly impractical for all but a few specialists to delve into original source material, especially when it is technical (or in Latin). In this book, I have attempted to convey some of the "circumstances and intellectual atmosphere" that have led to our modern idea of probability. I believe this is important for two reasons. First, to really appreciate what probability is all about, we must understand the *process* by which it has come about. Second, to transcend the limitations our current conception imposes on us, we must demystify probability by recognizing its inadequacy as the sole yardstick of uncertainty.

Willful Ignorance: The Mismeasure of Uncertainty can be regarded as two books in one. On one hand, it is a history of a big idea: how we have come to *think* about uncertainty. On the other, it is a prescription for change, especially with regard to how we perform research in the biomedical and social sciences. Modern probability and statistics are the outgrowth of a convoluted process that began over three centuries ago. This evolution has sharpened, but also narrowed, how we have come to reason about uncertainty.

Willful ignorance entails simplifying our understanding in order to quantify our uncertainty as mathematical probability. Probability theory will no doubt continue to serve us well, but only when it satisfies Einstein's famous maxim to "make everything as simple as possible but not simpler." I believe that in many cases, we now deploy probability in a way that is simpler than it needs to be. The mesh through which probability often filters our knowledge may be too coarse. To reengineer probability for the future, we must account for at least some of the complexity that is now being ignored.

I have tried to tell the story of probability in 12 chapters. Chapter 1 presents the problem that needs to be addressed: the dilemma faced by modern research methodology. Chapter 2 is a whirlwind tour of the book's main themes. After these two introductory chapters, the next five are rich in historical detail, covering the period from 1654 to around 1800 during the time mathematical probability developed. Those readers who are more interested in current issues than history, might wish to skip ahead to read Chapter 12, in which I propose a "solution," before circling back to the historical chapters.

Chapter 8 is a mix of history and philosophy, sketching the diversity of interpretations that have been attached to the basic concept of probability. In Chapter 9, with help primarily from Fisher, I attempt to cut through the massive confusion that still exists about probability. Chapter 10 discusses the origins of modern statistical methodology in the twentieth century, and its impact on scientific research. In Chapter 11, I explore how mathematical probability has come to dominate and in certain respects limit our thinking about uncertainty. The final chapter offers a suggestion for adapting statistical methodology to a new world of greatly expanded data and computational resources.

Previous historical writing about probability has focused almost exclusively on the mathematical development of the subject. From this point of view, the story is one of steady progress leading to a mature intellectual achievement. The basic principles of probability and statistics are well established. Remaining advances will be mainly technical, extending applications by building on solid foundations. The fundamental *creative* work is behind us; the interesting times are over.

There is, however, an all but forgotten flip side of the story. This *non-*mathematical aspect pertains to a fundamental question: what is probability? If we interpret probability as a measure of uncertainty in its broadest sense, what do we really *mean* by probability? This conceptual, or philosophical, conundrum was effectively put aside many decades ago as an unnecessary distraction, or even impediment, to scientific progress. It was never resolved, leaving the future (us) with an intellectual debt that would eventually come due.

As a result, we have inherited a serious problem. The main symptoms of this problem are confusion and stagnation in the biomedical and social sciences. There is enormously more research than ever before, but precious little useful insight being generated. Most important, there is a serious disconnect between quantitative research methodology and clinical practice. I believe that our stunted understanding of uncertainty is in many ways responsible for this gap.

I have proposed that willful ignorance is the central concept that underlies mathematical probability. In a nutshell, the idea is to deal effectively with an uncertain situation, we must filter out, or ignore, much of what we know about it. In short, we must simplify our conceptions by reducing ambiguity. In fact, being able to frame a mathematical probability implies that we have found some way to resolve the ambiguity to our satisfaction. Attempting to resolve ambiguity fruitfully is an essential aspect of scientific research. However, it always comes at a cost: we purchase clarity and precision at the expense of creativity and possibility.

For most scientists today, ambiguity is regarded as the enemy, to be overcome at all cost. But remaining open-minded in the face of ambiguity can ultimately generate deeper insights, while *prematurely* eliminating ambiguity can lead to intellectual sterility. Mathematical probability as we know it is an *invention*, a device to aid our thinking. It is powerful, but not natural or inevitable, and did not even exist in finished form until the eighteenth century.

The evolution of probability involved contributions by many brilliant individuals. To aid in keeping track of the important historical figures and key events, I have provided a *timeline*. This timeline is introduced at the beginning, and lists all of the major "landmarks" (mostly important publications) in the development of the concept of probability. At several points in later chapters, a streamlined version of the timeline has been inserted to indicate exactly when the events described in the text occurred. Of course, the question of which landmarks to include in the timeline can be debated. Scholars who are knowledgeable about the history of probability may disagree with my selections, and indeed I have second-guessed myself.

Please keep in mind that my focus is not on the mathematics of probability theory, but on the *conception* of probability as the measure of our uncertainty. In this light, it is noteworthy that my timeline ends in 1959. Perhaps that is because I lack perspective on the more recent contributions of my contemporaries. However, I believe that it underscores the lack of any profound advances in thinking about the quantification of uncertainty. There have certainly been some impressive attempts to broaden the *mathematics* of probability (e.g., belief functions, fuzzy logic), but none of these has (yet) entered the mainstream of scientific thought.

Some readers may feel that I have given short shrift to certain important topics that would seem to be relevant. For example, I had originally intended to say much more about the early history of statistics. However, I found that broadening the scope to deal extensively with statistical developments was too daunting and not directly germane to my task. I have similarly chosen not to deal with the theory of risk and decision-making directly. Mathematical probability is central to these disciplines, but entails aspects of economics, finance, and psychology that lie outside my main concerns. I would be delighted if someone else deems it worthwhile to explore the implications of willful ignorance for decision-making.

The time is ripe for a renewal of interest in the philosophical and psychological aspects of uncertainty quantification. These have been virtually ignored for half a century in the mistaken belief that our current version of probability is a finished product that is fully adequate for every purpose. This may have been true in the relatively data-poor twentieth century, but no longer. We need to learn how willful ignorance can be better applied for a more data-rich world. If this book can help stimulate a much-needed conversation on this issue, I will consider the effort in writing it to have been very worthwhile.

ACKNOWLEDGMENTS

Researching and writing this book has been a long journey of exploration and self-discovery. It was on one hand a foray into the realm of historical research, which was new to me. On the other hand, it was a lengthy meditation on questions that had puzzled me throughout my career. I feel extremely fortunate to have had this opportunity. A major part of this good fortune is owed to many family members, friends, and colleagues who have made it possible by supporting me in various ways.

First I would like to thank my wife Nina, who has encouraged me to "follow my bliss" down whatever paths it might lead me. She gave me valuable feedback to help keep me on track when I needed a big-picture perspective. Finally, she has lifted from me the onerous administrative burden of obtaining permission when necessary for the numerous quotations included in the book. I would also like to thank my sons Alex and Dan Weisberg for their encouragement and feedback on various parts of earlier drafts.

Along the way, I have received helpful advice and suggestions from many colleagues and friends: Barbara Beatty, Art Dempster, Richard Derrig, Rich Goldstein, Jim Guszcza, Mike Meyer, Howard Morris, Jarvis Kellogg, Victor Pontes, Sam Ratick, Peter Rousmaniere, and Joel Salon. Dan, Mike, Howie, and Joel deserve special commendations for their thoughtful and diplomatic suggestions on the nearly complete manuscript.

For helping me to develop the general conception of this unusual book, and for his patience and many practical suggestions as this project evolved, I am grateful once again to Steve Quigley, my editor at Wiley. Robin Zucker, for all her talent, hard work, and patience in working with me on the graphics, deserves my sincere appreciation. In particular, her evocative cover design and the historical timelines truly reflect the spirit of the book and improve its quality. I would also like to pay homage to the memory of Stephen J. Gould, whose classic *The Mismeasure of Man* inspired my subtitle and was an examplar of what popular science writing can aspire to be.

Ten years ago, this book could not have been written (at least by me). The cost and effort involved in obtaining access to original source material would have been prohibitive. Today, thanks to the internet, these limitations have been largely alleviated. Two resources have been especially valuable to me in my research. One is Google Books, which allowed free access to photocopies of many original publications. The second is the incredibly useful and comprehensive website: *Sources on the History of Probability and Statistics*, maintained by Prof. Richard J. Pulskamp of Xavier University at http://www.cs.xu.edu/math/Sources/. He has assembled numerous original documents pertaining to the history of probability and statistics, including many of his own translations into English of documents originally in other languages.

Grateful acknowledgment is made to the American Philosophical Society for quotations from:

Gillispie, Charles Coulston (1972). Probability and politics: Laplace, Condorcet, and Turgot. *Proceedings of the American Philosophical Society*, 16: 1–20.

Grateful acknowledgment is made to the Oxford University Press on behalf of the British Society for the Philosophy of Science for the quotation from:

Popper, Karl R. (1959). The propensity interpretation of probability. *The British Journal for the Philosophy of Science*, 10: 25–42.

Grateful acknowledgment is made to Dover Publications, Inc. for the quotations from:

David, Florence N. (1962). *Games, Gods and Gambling: A History of Probability and Statistical Ideas*. London: Charles Griffin & Company.

Von Mises, Richard (1928). *Probability, Statistics, and Truth*. New York: Dover, 1981 [Translated by Hilda Geiringer from the 3rd edition of the German original].

Grateful acknowledgment is made to the Johns Hopkins University Press for the following material:

Bernoulli, Jacob (2006). Translated with an introduction and notes by Edith Dudley Sylla in 2006 as *The Art of Conjecturing, together with Letter to a Friend on Sets in Court Tennis*. Baltimore, MD: Johns Hopkins University Press. pp. 34, 37, 134, 139–140, 142, 193, 251, 305, 315–322, 325–330. Reprinted with permission from Johns Hopkins University Press.

Franklin, James (2001). *The Science of Conjecture: Evidence and Probability before Pascal*. Baltimore, MD: Johns Hopkins University Press. pp. 74–76, 234–235, 275, 366. Reprinted with permission from Johns Hopkins University Press.

I would particularly like to express my appreciation and admiration to Edith Dudley Sylla and James Franklin for their scholarship pertaining to the prehistory of modern probability. They have brought to light much previously obscure information that is essential for placing modern probability in perspective.

HERBERT I. WEISBERG

CHAPTER 1

THE OPPOSITE OF CERTAINTY

During the past century, research in the medical, social, and economic sciences has led to major improvements in longevity and living conditions. Statistical methods grounded in the mathematics of probability have played a major role in much of this progress. Our confidence in these quantitative tools has grown, along with our ability to wield them with great proficiency. We have an enormous investment of tangible and intellectual capital in scientific research that is predicated on this framework. We assume that the statistical methods as applied in the past so successfully will continue to be productive. Yet, something is amiss.

New findings often contradict previously accepted theories. Faith in the ability of science to provide reliable answers is being steadily eroded, as expert opinion on many critical issues flip-flops. Scientists in some fields seriously debate whether a majority of their published research findings are ultimately overturned[1]; the *decline effect* has been coined to describe how even strongly positive results often fade over time in the light of subsequent study[2]; revelations of errors in the findings published in prestigious scientific journals, and even fraud, are becoming more common.[3] Instead of achieving greater certainty, we seem to be moving backwards. What is going on?

Willful Ignorance: The Mismeasure of Uncertainty, First Edition. Herbert I. Weisberg.
© 2014 John Wiley & Sons, Inc. Published 2014 by John Wiley & Sons, Inc.

Consider efforts to help disadvantaged children through early childhood educational intervention. Beginning around 1970, the U.S. government sponsored several major programs to help overcome social and economic disadvantage. The most famous of these, Project Head Start, aimed to close the perceived gap in cognitive development between richer and poorer children that was already evident in kindergarten. The aims of this program were admirable and the rationale compelling. However, policy debates about the efficacy and cost of this initiative have gone on for four decades, with no resolution in sight. Research on the impact of Head Start has been extensive and costly, but answers are few and equivocal.

Medical research is often held up as the paragon of statistical research methodology. Evidence-based medicine, based on randomized clinical trials, can provide proof of the effectiveness and safety of various drugs and other therapies. But cracks are appearing even in this apparently solid foundation. Low dose aspirin for prevention of heart attacks was gospel for years but is now being questioned. Perhaps the benefits are less and the risks, more than we previously believed. Hormone replacement therapy for postmenopausal women was considered almost miraculous until a decade ago when a landmark study overturned previous findings. Not a year goes by without some new recommendation regarding whether, how, and by whom, hormone replacement should be used.

These are not isolated instances. The ideal of science is an evolution of useful theory coupled with improved practice, as new research builds upon and refines previous findings. Each individual study should be a piece of a larger puzzle to which it contributes. Instead, research in the biomedical and social sciences is rarely cumulative, and each research paper tends to stand alone. We fill millions of pages in scientific journals with "statistically significant" results that add little to our store of practical knowledge and often cannot be replicated. Practitioners, whose clinical judgment should be informed by hard data, gain little that is truly useful to them.

TWO DEAD ENDS

If I am correct in observing that scientific research has contributed so little to our understanding of "what works" in areas like education, health care, and economic development, it is important to ask why this is the case. I believe that much of the problem lies with our research methodology. At one end of the spectrum, we have what can be called the quantitative approach, grounded in modern probability-based statistical methods. At the other extreme are researchers who support a radically different paradigm, one that is primarily qualitative and more subjective. This school of thought emphasizes the use of case studies and in-depth participatory observation to understand the dynamics of complex causal processes.

Both statistical and qualitative approaches have important contributions to make. However, researchers in either of these traditions tend to view those in the other with suspicion, like warriors in two opposing camps peering across a great divide. Nowadays, the statistical types dominate, because methods based on probability and statistics virtually define our standard of what is deemed "scientific." The perspective of qualitative researchers is much closer to that of clinicians but lacks the authority that the objectivity of statistics seems to provide.

Sadly, each side in this fruitless debate is stuck in a mindset that is too restricted to address the kinds of problems we face. Conventional statistical methods make it difficult to think seriously about causal processes underlying observable data. Qualitative researchers, on the other hand, tend to underestimate the value of statistical generalizations based on patterns of data. One approach willfully ignores all salient distinctions among individuals, while the other drowns in infinite complexity.

The resulting intellectual gridlock is especially unfortunate as we enter an era in which the potential to organize and analyze data is expanding exponentially. We already have the ability to assemble databases in ways that could not even be imagined when the modern statistical paradigm was formulated. Innovative statistical analyses that transcend twentieth century data limitations are possible if we can summon the will and imagination to fully embrace the opportunities presented by new technology.

Unfortunately, as statistical methodology has matured, it has grown more timid. For many, the concept of scientific method has been restricted to a narrow range of approved techniques, often applied mechanically. The result is to limit the scope of individual creativity and inspiration in a futile attempt to attain virtual certainty. Already in 1962, the iconoclastic statistical genius John Tukey counseled that data analysts "must be willing to err moderately often in order that inadequate evidence shall more often *suggest* the right answer."[4]

Instead, to achieve an illusory pseudo-certainty, we dutifully perform the ritual of computing a significance level or confidence interval, having forgotten the original purposes and assumptions underlying such techniques. This "technology" for interpreting evidence and generating conclusions has come to replace expert judgment to a large extent. Scientists no longer trust their own intuition and judgment enough to risk modest failure in the quest for great success. As a result, we are raising a generation of young researchers who are highly adept technically but have, in many cases, forgotten how to think for themselves.

ANALYTICAL ENGINES

The dream of "automating" the human sciences by substituting calculation for intuition arose about two centuries ago. Adolphe Quetelet's famous treatise on his statistically based "social physics" was published in 1835, and Siméon Poisson's masterwork on probability theory and judgments in civil and criminal matters appeared in 1837.[5,6] It is perhaps not coincidental that in 1834 Charles Babbage first began to design a mechanical computer, which he called an *analytical engine*.[7] Optimism about the potential ability of mathematical analysis, and especially the theory of probability, to resolve various medical, social, and economic problems was at its zenith.

Shortly after this historical moment, the tide turned. The attempt to supplant human judgment by automated procedures was criticized as hopelessly naïve. Reliance on mathematical probability and statistical methods to deal with such subtle issues went out of favor. The philosopher John Stuart Mill termed such uses of mathematical probability "the real opprobrium of mathematics."[8] The famous physiologist Claude Bernard objected that "statistics teach absolutely nothing about the mode of action of medicine nor the mechanics of cure" in any particular patient.[9] Probability was again relegated to a modest supporting role, suitable for augmenting our reasoning. Acquiring and evaluating relevant information, and reaching final conclusions and decisions remained human prerogatives.

Early in the twentieth century, the balance between judgment and calculation began to shift once again. Gradually, mathematical probability and statistical methods based on it came to be regarded as more objective, reliable, and generally "scientific" than human theorizing and subjective weighing of evidence. Supported by rapidly developing computational capabilities, probability and statistics were increasingly viewed as methods to generate definitive solutions and decisions. Conversely, human intuition became seen as an outmoded and flawed aspect of scientific investigation.

Instead of serving as an adjunct to scientific reasoning, statistical methods today are widely perceived as a corrective to the many cognitive *biases* that often lead us astray. In particular, our naïve tendencies to misinterpret and overreact to limited data must be countered by a better understanding of probability and statistics. Thus, the genie that was put back in the bottle after 1837 has emerged in a new and more sophisticated guise. Poisson's ambition of rationalizing such activities as medical research and social policy development is alive and well. Mathematical probability, implemented by modern analytical engines, is widely perceived to be capable of providing scientific evidence-based answers to guide us in such matters.

Regrettably, modern science has bought into the misconception that probability and statistics can arbitrate truth. Evidence that is "tainted" by personal intuition and judgment is often denigrated as merely descriptive or "anecdotal." This radical change in perspective has come about because probability appears capable of objectively *quantifying* our uncertainty in the same unambiguous way as measurement techniques in the physical sciences. But this is illusory:

> Uncertain situations call for probability theory and statistics, the mathematics of uncertainty. Since it was precisely in those areas where uncertainty was greatest that the burden of judgment was heaviest, statistical tools seemed ideally suited to the task of ridding first the sciences and then daily life of personal discretion, with its pejorative associations of the arbitrary, the idiosyncratic, and the subjective. Our contemporary notion of objectivity, defined largely by the absence of these elements, owes a great deal to the dream of mechanized inference. It is therefore not surprising that the statistical techniques that aspire to mechanize inference should have taken on a normative character. Whereas probability theory once aimed to describe judgment, statistical inference now aims to replace it in the name of objectivity. ... Of course, this escape from judgment is an illusion. ... No amount of mathematical legerdemain can transform uncertainty into

certainty, although much of the appeal of statistical inference techniques stems from just such great expectations. These expectations are fed ... above all by the hope of avoiding the oppressive responsibilities that every exercise of personal judgment entails.[10]

Probability by its very nature entails ambiguity and subjectivity. Embedded within every probability statement are unexamined simplifications and assumptions. We can think of probability as a kind of devil's bargain. We gain practical advantages by accepting its terms but unwittingly cede control over something fundamental. What we obtain is a special kind of knowledge; what we give up is conceptual understanding. In short, by willingly remaining *ignorant*, in a particular sense, we may acquire a form of useful knowledge. This is the essential paradox of probability.

WHAT IS PROBABILITY?

Among practical scientists nowadays, the true *meaning* of probability is almost never discussed. This is really quite remarkable! The proper interpretation of mathematical probability within scientific discourse was a hotly debated topic for over two centuries. In particular, questions about the adequacy of mathematical probability to represent fully our uncertainty were deemed important. Recently, however, there has been virtually no serious consideration of this critical issue.

As late as the 1920s, a variety of philosophical ideas about probability and uncertainty were still in the air. The central importance of probability theory in a general sense was recognized by all. However, there was wide disagreement over how the basic concept of probability should be defined, interpreted, and applied. Most notably, in 1921 two famous economists independently published influential treatises that drew attention to an important theoretical distinction. Both suggested that the conventional concept of mathematical probability is incomplete.

In his classic, *Risk, Uncertainty and Profit*, economist Frank Knight described the kind of uncertainty associated with ordinary probability by the term *risk*.[11] The amount of risk can be deduced from mathematical theory (as in a game of chance) or calculated by observing many outcomes of similar events, as done, for example, by an insurance company. However, Knight was principally concerned with probabilities that pertain to another level of uncertainty. He had particularly in mind a typical business decision faced by an entrepreneur. The probability that a specified outcome will result from a certain action is ordinarily based on subjective judgment, taking into account all available evidence.

According to Knight, such a probability may be entirely intuitive. There may be no way, even in principle, to verify this probability by reference to a hypothetical reference class of similar situations. In this sense, the probability is completely subjective, an idea that was shared by some of his contemporaries. However, Knight went further by suggesting that this subjective probability also carries with it some sense of how much *confidence* in this estimate is actually entertained. So, in an imprecise but very important way, the numerical measure of probability is only a *part* of the full uncertainty assessment. "The action which follows upon an opinion depends as much upon the confidence in that opinion as upon the favorableness of the opinion itself." This broader but vaguer conception has come to be called Knightian uncertainty.

Knightian uncertainty was greeted by economists as a new and radical concept, but was in fact some very old wine being unwittingly rebottled. One of the few with even an inkling of probability's long and tortuous history was John Maynard Keynes. Long before he was a famous economist,[12] Keynes authored *A Treatise on Probability*, completed just before World War I, but not published until 1921. In this work, he probed the limits of ordinary probability theory as a vehicle for expressing our uncertainty. Like Knight, Keynes understood that some "probabilities" were of a different character from those assumed in the usual theory of probability. In fact, he conceived of probability quite generally as a measure of *rational belief* predicated on some particular *body of evidence*.

In this sense, there is no such thing as a unique probability, since the evidence available can vary over time or across individuals. Moreover, sometimes the evidence is too weak to support a firm numerical probability; our level of uncertainty may be better represented as entirely or partly *qualitative*. For example, my judgment about the outcome of the next U.S. presidential election might be that a Democrat is somewhat less likely than a Republican to win, but I cannot reduce this feeling to a single number between zero and one. Or, I may have no idea at all, so I may plead *complete ignorance*. Such notions of a non-numerical degree of belief, or even of complete ignorance (for lack of any relevant evidence), have no place in modern probability theory.

The mathematical probability of an event is often described in terms of the odds at which we should be willing to bet for or against its occurrence. For example, suppose my probability that the next president will be a Democrat is 40%, or 2/5. Then for me, the fair odds at which to bet on this outcome would be 3:2. So I will gain 3 dollars for every 2 dollars wagered if a Democrat actually wins, but lose my 2-dollar stake if a Republican wins. However, a full description of my uncertainty might also reflect how confident I would be about these odds. To force my expression of uncertainty into a precise specification of betting odds, as if I *must* lay a wager, may be artificially constraining.

Knight and Keynes were among a minority who perceived that uncertainty embodies something more than mere "risk." They understood that uncertainty is inherently *ambiguous* in ways that often preclude complete representation as a simple number between zero and one. William Byers eloquently articulates in *The Blind Spot* how such ambiguity can often prove highly generative and how attempts to resolve it completely or prematurely have costs.[13]

As a prime example, Byers discusses how the ancient proto-concept of "quantity" evolved over time into our current conception of numbers:

A unidirectional flow of ideas is at best a reconstruction. It is useful and interesting but it misses something. It inevitably takes the present situation to be definitive. It tends to show how our present knowledge is superior in every way to the knowledge of the Greeks, for example. In so doing, it ignores the possibility that the Greeks knew things we do not know, that we have forgotten or suppressed. It seems heretical to suggest, but is nevertheless conceivable, that the Greek conception of quantity was in a certain way richer than our own, that their conception of number was deeper than ours. It was richer in the sense that a metaphor can be rich—because it comes with a large set of connoted meanings. It may well be that historical progress in mathematics is in part due to the process of abstraction, which inevitably involves narrowing the focus of attention to precisely those properties of the situation that one finds most immediately relevant. This is the way I shall view the history of mathematics and science—as a process of continual development that involves gain and loss, not as the triumphant march toward some final and ultimate theory.

In very much the same way, our modern idea of probability emerged from earlier concepts that were in some respects richer, and perhaps deeper.[14]

When Knight and Keynes wrote, the modern interpretation of probability had already almost completely crystallized. Shortly afterwards, further "progress" took the form of "narrowing the focus" even more. Although the broader issues addressed by Knight and Keynes were ignored, there remained (and still remains) one significant philosophical issue. Should probability be construed as essentially *subjective* or *objective* in nature? Is probability purely an aspect of personal thought and belief *or* an aspect of the external world? I will suggest that this is a false dichotomy that must be transcended.

As statistical methods became more prominent in scientific investigations, objectivity became paramount. It became widely accepted that science must not reflect any subjective considerations. Rather, it must deal with things that we can measure and count objectively. Thus, mathematical probability, interpreted as the frequency with which observable events occur, became the yardstick for measurement in the context of scientific research. This link to empirical reality created a false sense of objectivity that continues to pervade our research methodology today, although a more subjective interpretation has recently made some limited inroads.

From our modern viewpoint, there appears to be a sharp distinction between the subjective and objective interpretations of probability. However, to the originators of mathematical probability, these two connotations were merged in a way that can seem rather muddled to us. Were they confused, or do we fail to grasp something meaningful for them now lost to us? Is there, as Byers intimates, a "transcendental" perspective from which this distinction would no longer seem meaningful? If so, it might point the way toward a resolution of the conflict between apparently opposing ways of thinking about science. That, in turn, could help bridge the gap between scientific research and clinical practice.

UNCERTAINTY

At the core of science is the desire for greater certainty in a highly unpredictable world. Probability is often defined as a measure of our degree of certainty, but what is certainty? If I am certain that a particular event will occur, what does that mean? For concreteness, suppose I have just enrolled in a course on a subject with which I am not very familiar. For the moment, let us assume I am absolutely *certain* of being able to pass this course.

Dictionary definitions of the word "certain" contain phrases like "completely confident" and "without any doubt." But what conditions would allow us to be in such a state of supreme confidence? Obviously, our knowledge of the situation or circumstances must be adequate for us to believe that the event *must* occur. My certainty about passing the course would rest on a matrix of information and beliefs that justify (for me) the necessary confidence.

Now, suppose that, on the contrary, I am *not certain* that I can pass this course. Clearly, this implies that I am lacking in certainty, but what does this mean? I would submit that uncertainty has two quite different connotations, or aspects. On one hand, my uncertainty can arise from *doubt*. So, the opposite of being sure of passing the course is being extremely doubtful. On the other hand, being uncertain could also mean that I just *do not know* whether I will be able to pass the course. I may suffer from confusion, because the situation facing me seems *ambiguous*. So the opposite of being highly confident would be something like having no idea, being literally "clueless."

The situation can be described graphically as in Figure 1.1. We can conceptualize our degree of uncertainty as the resultant of two psychological "forces." The horizontal axis represents our degree of *doubt* and the vertical axis, the degree of *ambiguity* we perceive. In general, certainty corresponds to the absence of *both* doubt and ambiguity. Our degree of uncertainty increases according to the "amounts" of doubt and ambiguity.

To be more specific, ambiguity pertains generally to the clarity with which the situation of interest is being conceptualized. How sure am I about the mental category, or classification, in which to place what I perceive to be happening? In order to exercise my judgment about what is likely to occur, I must have a sense of the relevant features of the situation. So, reducing uncertainty by resolving ambiguity, at least to some extent, seems to be a necessary prerequisite for assessing doubt. However, the relationship between ambiguity and doubt can be complex and dynamic. We certainly cannot expect to eliminate ambiguity completely before framing a probability.

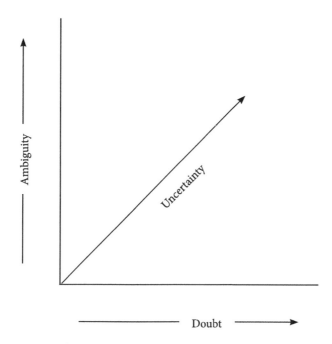

FIGURE 1.1   The two dimensions of uncertainty: ambiguity and doubt.

In relation to probability, there is an important difference between these two dimensions of uncertainty. It seems natural to think of a degree of doubt as a *quantity*. We can, for example, say that our doubt that the Chicago Cubs will win the World Series this year is greater than our doubt that the New York Yankees will be the champions. We may even be able to assign a numerical value to our degree of doubtfulness. Ambiguity, on the other hand, seems to be essentially *qualitative*. It is hard to articulate what might be meant by a "degree of ambiguity."

Probability in our modern mathematical sense is concerned exclusively with the doubt component of uncertainty. For us, the probability of a certain event is assigned a value of 1.0, or 100%. At the opposite end of the spectrum, an event that is deemed impossible, or virtually impossible, has a probability value of 0.0, or 0%. When we say that something, such as passing a course, has a probability of 95%, we mean that there exists a small degree of doubt that it will actually occur. Conversely, a probability of 5% implies a very strong doubt. In order to achieve such mathematical precision, we must suppress some subtlety or complexity that creates ambiguity. That way, our uncertainty can be ranged along a single dimension; our degree of confidence that the event *will* happen becomes identical to our lack of confidence that it *will not* happen.

As I will be explaining, this modern *mathematical* conception of probability emerged quite recently, about three centuries ago. Prior to its invention, there had existed for thousands of years earlier concepts of probability that were, indeed, "in a certain way richer than our own." Especially important, these archaic ideas about uncertainty encompassed *both* dimensions of uncertainty, often without clearly distinguishing between them. Dealing with uncertainty implicitly entailed two challenges: attempting to *resolve the ambiguity* and to *evaluate the doubtfulness* of what we know. By essentially ignoring ambiguity in order to quantify doubt, we have obtained the substantial benefits of mathematical probability.

Since the 1920s, the equally important issue of ambiguity has been left outside the pale of scientific (and most philosophical) thinking about probability. The concerns raised by Keynes, Knight, and others back then were never addressed. In essence, they perceived the dangers in reducing probability to a technology for measuring doubt that ignores ambiguity. Failing to address this issue has led to the moribund state in which many areas of science now find themselves.

WILLFUL IGNORANCE

Suppose you are an emergency-room physician confronted by a new patient who displays an unusual constellation of symptoms. Rapid action is required, as the patient's condition is life-threatening. You are uncertain about the appropriate course of treatment. Your task is twofold: resolve your confusion about what type of illness you are observing and decide on the optimal therapy to adopt.

The diagnosis aims to eliminate, or at least minimize, any ambiguity pertaining to the patient's condition and circumstances. The physician's methodology may include a patient history, a physical examination, and a variety of clinical testing procedures. All of the resulting information is evaluated and integrated subjectively by the physician and possibly other specialist colleagues. The usual outcome is a classification of the patient into a specific disease category, along with any qualifying details (e.g., disease duration and severity, concomitant medications, allergies) that may be relevant to various potential treatment options. The process of attempting to resolve ambiguity in this situation, or in general, draws mainly on the clinician's expertise and knowledge. It entails logic and judgment applied to the array of evidence available.

Once the diagnosis is determined, however, the situation changes. The focus shifts to the selection of a treatment approach. The ambiguity about what is happening has been largely resolved. The remaining task is to choose from among the different therapeutic candidates. Putting aside the issue of side effects, the therapy offering the best chance of a cure will be selected. Not that long ago, this too was settled mainly by appealing to the presumed clinical expertise of the clinician (doctor, psychiatrist, social worker, teacher, etc.). Not any longer.

Since the 1950s, research to evaluate alternative treatment modalities has become increasingly standardized and objective. So-called evidence-based medicine depends heavily on statistical theory for the design, conduct, and analysis of research. This technology appears to generate knowledge that is demonstrably reliable because human subjectivity and fallibility have been eliminated from the process. Central to the modern research enterprise is probability theory. Probability defines the terms within which questions and answers are framed. Moreover, rather than merely advising the clinician, evidence-based recommendations based on statistics are intended to represent the "optimal" decision.[15]

When these new statistical methods were originally introduced, they promised to ameliorate serious problems that were then widespread, such as exaggerated claims of efficacy and outright quackery. However, it could not be imagined to what extent these safeguards would eventually come to *define* our standard of what constitutes respectable science. Statistical methods are now virtually the *only* way to conduct research in many fields, especially those that study human beings. What has resulted is a profound *disconnect* between clinical and statistical perceptions in many instances.

Research focuses on what is likely to happen "on the average" in certain specified circumstances. What, for example, is the effect on the mortality rate for middle-aged men who adopt a low-dose aspirin regimen? However, the clinician's concern is her particular patient. What will happen to

Sam Smith if he starts on an aspirin regimen tomorrow? So, she may balk at mechanically following some general guidelines that are alleged to be statistically optimal:

> Each of us is unique in the interplay of genetic makeup and environment. The path to maintaining or regaining health is not the same for everyone. Choices in this gray zone are frequently not simple or obvious. For that reason, medicine involves personalized and nuanced decision making by both the patient and doctor. ... Although presented as scientific, formulas that reduce the experience of illness to numbers are flawed and artificial. Yet insurers and government officials are pressuring physicians and hospitals to standardize care using such formulas. Policy planners and even some doctors have declared that the art of medicine is passé, that care should be delivered in an industrialized fashion with nurses and doctors following operating manuals.[16]

In a real sense, clinicians and researchers tend to inhabit different conceptual worlds. The clinician is sensitive to the ambiguities of the "gray zone" in which difficult decisions must be made. She is in a land where the uncertainty is mainly of the "what is really going on here?" kind. For the researcher, on the other hand, the world must look black and white, so that the rules of probability math can be applied. This ambiguity blindness has become absolutely necessary. Without it, as we will see, the elaborate machinery of statistical methodology would come to a grinding halt. Consequently, there is no middle road between the clinical and statistical perspectives.

To be clearer on this point, let us hark back to our hypothetical problem of medical treatment. Suppose you have discovered the cause of the patient's symptoms, a rare type of virulent bacterial infection. Your problem now is to select which antibiotic to try first. There are three possibilities, each of which you have prescribed in the past many times. Your decision will hinge primarily on the probability of achieving a cure *for this patient*. We are accustomed to thinking that there actually exists, in some objective sense, a true probability that applies to this patient. In fact, there is no such probability out there!

A probability is a mental construct. In this sense, it is entirely subjective, or personal, in nature. However, probability must also have something to do with observations in the outside world. Indeed, an important (perhaps the only) relevant source of evidence may be a statistical rate of cure that you can find in the medical literature. Surely, these rates (percentages) can be interpreted as probabilities, or at least as approximations to them. Moreover, because these statistics are objective and precise, they are ordinarily expected to trump any subjective considerations.

The problem is that the "objective" probability may not be applicable to your particular patient. You may have specific knowledge and insight that influence your level of ambiguity or of doubt. For example, you might know that Sam Smith tends to comply poorly with complicated instructions for taking medicine properly. So, the statistically indicated treatment modality might not work as well for him as for the typical subject in the clinical studies. Ideally, you would possess some system for rationally taking account of all factors, both qualitative and quantitative, that seem relevant. However, the statistically based probability is not open to debate or refinement in any way. That is because probability by its very nature entails *willful ignorance*.

My term willful ignorance refers to the inescapable fact that probabilities are not geared directly to individuals. An assessment of probability can of course be *applied* to any particular individual, but that is a matter of judgment. By choosing a statistically based probability, you effectively regard this individual as a random member of the population upon which the statistics were derived. In other words, you *ignore* any distinguishing features of the individual or his circumstances that might modify the probability.

TOWARD A NEW SCIENCE

Relying uncritically on statistics for answers has become so second-nature to us that we have forgotten how recent and revolutionary this way of thinking really is. That is the crux of the problems we now face. Fortunately, there is a path out of the stagnation that plagues our research currently, and it is surprisingly simple, *in theory*. Unfortunately, practical implementation of this idea will require a seismic shift in behavior to achieve. In a nutshell, we must learn to become more *mindful* in applying probability-based statistical methods and criteria.

Mindfulness can be described as a way of perceiving and behaving that is characterized by openness, creativity, and flexibility. Psychologist Ellen

Langer has suggested several qualities that tend to characterize a mindful person.

- The ability to create new categories
- Openness to new information
- Awareness of multiple perspectives
- A focus on process more than outcome
- A basic respect for intuition.

These reflect precisely the attitude of a scientist who is motivated primarily by potential *opportunities* to advance human knowledge. Such an individual thrives on ambiguity, because it offers a wealth of *possibilities* to be explored.

In contrast, statistical methodology as it is applied today does not encourage these attributes. Rather, it has become *mindless* in its mechanical emphasis on prespecified hypotheses about average effects and formal testing procedures. It is no wonder that clinicians and qualitatively oriented researchers are uncomfortable with such unnatural modes of thinking:

> Just as mindlessness is the rigid reliance on old categories, mindfulness means the continual creation of new ones. Categorizing and recategorizing, labeling and relabeling as one masters the world are processes natural to children. They are an adaptive and necessary part of surviving in the world.

These dynamic processes are equally essential in scientific research to cope with and resolve ambiguity. By relying so heavily on statistical procedures based on probability theory, ambiguity is effectively swept under the rug. This is a *fundamental* problem, because the essence of probability is quantification of doubt, which requires ambiguity about categories and labels to be willfully ignored. So, the problem of ambiguity cannot truly be evaded within the framework of probability, only sidestepped. A better approach is to broaden our understanding of uncertainty in order to resolve ambiguity more productively.

Am I arguing that mathematical probability and statistical methods should be avoided? Far from it. We will need these tools to address the problems of a much more data-rich future. However, our research methodology needs somehow to make more room for mindfulness, even though that will entail confronting ambiguity as well as doubt. Doing so may require us to cultivate a greater degree of tolerance for error, but this is unavoidable. Being wrong, as Kathryn Schulz reminds us, is normal; the problem is how we deal with this ever-present possibility.[17]

We must avoid worrying about mistakes to the point of stifling creativity. After all, it took Einstein 10 years and countless false leads before coming up with the general theory of relativity.[18] It is OK to be wrong, as long as you are in the mode of continually testing and revising your theories in the light of evidence. In research that relies on the analysis of statistical data, that means placing more emphasis on successful *replication* of findings. By maintaining a balance between theoretical speculation and empirical evidence, we can increase the chances of generating knowledge that will make sense to both the researcher and the clinician.

Accomplishing this necessary evolution of methodology will entail both technical challenges and a major alteration of our scientific culture and incentives. Mathematical probability and statistical analysis will continue to play important roles in the future of research. But these tools must continue to develop in ways that take fuller advantage of the emerging opportunities. To conclude, I offer a personal anecdote that I have often used to exemplify the kind of mindful statistical analysis that will be necessary:

> The first legal case in which I provided statistical expertise was an employment discrimination lawsuit against a Boston-based Fortune 500 company. The plaintiffs were convinced that black workers were being systematically prevented from rising to higher-level positions within the manufacturing division of the company. … I dutifully subjected the data to various standard analyses, searching for an effect of race on promotion rates, but came up empty. Despite repeated failures, I harbored a nagging suspicion that something important had been overlooked.
>
> I began to scrutinize listings of the data, trying to discern some hidden pattern behind the numbers. Preliminary ideas led to further questions and to discussions with some of the plaintiffs. This interactive process yielded a more refined understanding of personnel decision-making at the company. Eventually, it became clear to me what was "really" going on.
>
> Up to a certain level in the hierarchy of positions, there was virtually no relationship between race and promotion. But for a particular level mid-way up the organizational ladder, very few workers were being promoted from within the company when openings arose. Rather, these particular jobs were being filled

primarily through outside hires, and almost always by white applicants. More-over, these external candidates were sometimes less qualified than the internally available workers. We came to call this peculiar dynamic "the bottleneck."

This subtle pattern, once recognized, was supported anecdotally in several ways. The statistical data, coupled with qualitative supporting information, was eventually presented to the defendant company's attorneys. The response to our demonstration of the bottleneck phenomenon was dramatic: a sudden interest in negotiation after many months of intransigence. Within weeks, a settlement of the case was forged.[19]

This unorthodox approach did not rely on any of the traditional statistical methods I had been taught, which made me somewhat uncomfortable. Throughout the subsequent 30 years, I have had a number of similar "out-of-the-box" experiences. Consequently, I have become much more confident that my approach in such cases was based on some kind of logic not encompassed in traditional methods. This book has resulted in part from my desire to understand and articulate what this logic might be.

CHAPTER 2

A QUIET REVOLUTION

In the last half of the seventeenth century, a revolution in science began, fueled by a radically new type of mathematics. This development occurred entirely in Western Europe, and was communicated mainly through a series of letters exchanged among a small network of highly gifted mathematicians and "natural philosophers." The impact of the novel ideas that originated during this period extended far beyond scientific thinking to alter our everyday understanding of reality. The Scientific Revolution led by Isaac Newton (1642–1727) and Gottfried Leibniz (1646–1716) would certainly fit this description. It has unquestionably had a profound impact on our basic interpretation of the world around us. But I am referring to a much less celebrated episode in the history of human thought that was also beginning to unfold at this time. The impact of this "quiet revolution" is highly visible today, but took a long and circuitous route before reaching popular awareness.

Beginning in the summer of 1654, an interchange of letters took place between two leading French mathematicians: Blaise Pascal (1623–1662) and Pierre de Fermat (1601–1665). One of the problems that occupied these savants had baffled the greatest mathematical minds for over 200 years. Indeed, it was not even clear that this problem even *had* a unique

Willful Ignorance: The Mismeasure of Uncertainty, First Edition. Herbert I. Weisberg.
© 2014 John Wiley & Sons, Inc. Published 2014 by John Wiley & Sons, Inc.

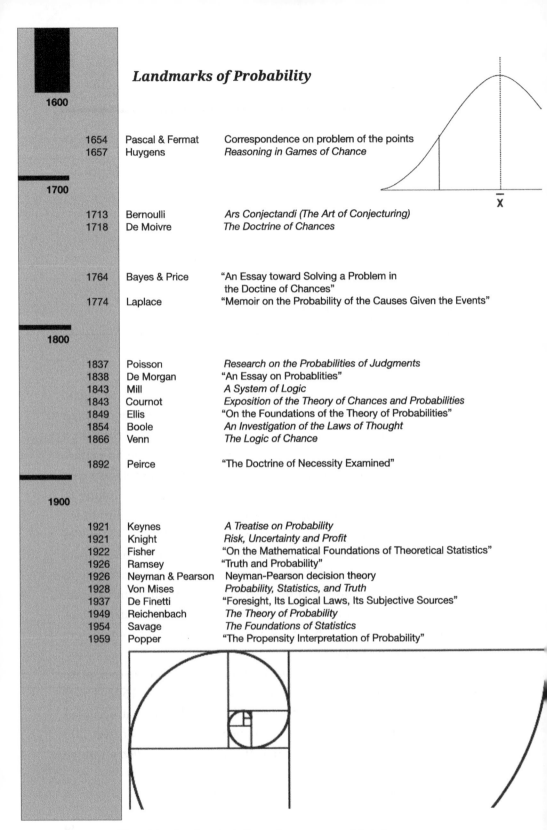

Landmarks of Probability

1654	Pascal & Fermat	Correspondence on problem of the points
1657	Huygens	*Reasoning in Games of Chance*
1713	Bernoulli	*Ars Conjectandi (The Art of Conjecturing)*
1718	De Moivre	*The Doctrine of Chances*
1764	Bayes & Price	"An Essay toward Solving a Problem in the Doctine of Chances"
1774	Laplace	"Memoir on the Probability of the Causes Given the Events"
1837	Poisson	*Research on the Probabilities of Judgments*
1838	De Morgan	"An Essay on Probablities"
1843	Mill	*A System of Logic*
1843	Cournot	*Exposition of the Theory of Chances and Probabilities*
1849	Ellis	"On the Foundations of the Theory of Probabilities"
1854	Boole	*An Investigation of the Laws of Thought*
1866	Venn	*The Logic of Chance*
1892	Peirce	"The Doctrine of Necessity Examined"
1921	Keynes	*A Treatise on Probability*
1921	Knight	*Risk, Uncertainty and Profit*
1922	Fisher	"On the Mathematical Foundations of Theoretical Statistics"
1926	Ramsey	"Truth and Probability"
1926	Neyman & Pearson	Neyman-Pearson decision theory
1928	Von Mises	*Probability, Statistics, and Truth*
1937	De Finetti	"Foresight, Its Logical Laws, Its Subjective Sources"
1949	Reichenbach	*The Theory of Probability*
1954	Savage	*The Foundations of Statistics*
1959	Popper	"The Propensity Interpretation of Probability"

Timeline markers: 1600, 1700, 1800, 1900

Note: A book title is in italics and a paper or article is in quotes.

solution! Known as the "problem of the points," this conundrum concerned the fair method of dividing the stakes when a game of chance was interrupted and could not be finished. If one of the two players was ahead on points, what share of the total stakes gambled should be returned to each?

In the course of their brief correspondence, the pair managed to derive not just one, but three distinct methods for solving this longstanding puzzle. The ways in which they conceived and solved this problem were new. Their seminal ideas soon led to an understanding of the basic principles applicable to all gambling-related problems. Thus began a chain of events whose impact would ultimately be second only to that initiated by Newton and Leibniz. Today, we refer to the ideas that grew from these roots as the *theory of probability*. The major landmarks in the evolution of modern probability are listed in the accompanying Timeline.

THINKING THE UNTHINKABLE

Newtonian physics proposed a set of universal laws that were believed to govern, in fact fully determine, the workings of the physical world. No object was exempt from these laws of nature, which could, in principle, be used to predict the state of the universe at any future moment, if only enough information were available. However, as a practical matter, the precise determination of this state could be obtained only in very simple and idealized situations. For example, in rolling a perfectly round and smooth ball down a frictionless surface, the transit time could be calculated exactly. But suppose that an archer was attempting to hit a bulls-eye on a target 100 paces distant. The exact point at which the arrow would strike the target could depend on many forces interacting in complex ways. So, the laws of physics could provide only a rough approximation.

The inevitable *uncertainty* in reasoning about complex situations was compounded enormously when it came to predictions related to such matters as health, economics, and social affairs. How might one determine a certain individual's life-expectancy in order to compute the correct price to charge for an annuity? What insurance premium should be charged to protect a merchant against the loss of his cargo on a long sea voyage? How could the initial signs of an incipient plague epidemic be flagged, so that appropriate preventive measures could be attempted? Such questions were of great practical importance in the 1600s, but were just beginning to be formulated, let alone answered. Today, we would immediately regard such questions as falling within the province of probability and statistics. In 1654, the very idea of framing such questions in any kind of quantitative terms was literally *unthinkable.*

Two significant events in 1654 planted the seeds of eventual change in this situation. First, the Pascal–Fermat correspondence broke a centuries-old intellectual logjam by solving the problem of the points. Second, Jacob Bernoulli (1654–1705) was born in Basel, Switzerland. Had these events not occurred, it is conceivable that a relationship between uncertainty and mathematics would never have evolved, or perhaps would have evolved more slowly, or into a form quite different from our modern notion of mathematical probability.

While this might seem a fantastic notion, consider this. Of the many past civilizations that managed to achieve a high level of cultural and scientific sophistication, not one of these ever hit upon the "obvious" idea of quantifying a degree of certainty. This truly novel idea began to develop only in Western Europe, and only in the wake of the mathematical analysis of gambling. Before mathematical probability could be conceived, a new mental model for uncertainty had to be devised. This model first became available when chance mechanisms, like dice and lotteries, came to be seen as subject to mathematical laws.

The realization that the whims of fortune were to some degree regulated and law-like in these games was a major revelation. Previously, throughout human history, risks could be managed only to the extent that expert knowledge and judgment were applicable. For example, a merchant in the 1600s who agreed to provide insurance for a ship's cargo would consider numerous factors in setting a price. He might examine the vessel, interview the captain, learn of the route that was planned, etc. In such a business transaction, it would be natural to find out as much as possible about the reasons *why* a particular event, such as a shipwreck, might occur. That way, a sound estimate of the risk might be made.

In many situations, however, our knowledge of the causal mechanisms underlying observed events is very limited. Moreover, even if known, the underlying process may be so complex that it is impossible to take adequate account of all the forces in operation. As examples, Jacob Bernoulli referred to the prediction of how long a particular person will live, the weather on a future specified date, and the winner in a certain game of tennis. Ironically, it is only by *ignoring* most of the details that potentially distinguish such individual events that we can hope to deduce meaningful information regarding what is likely to happen.

Bernoulli was the first to write that a kind of partial knowledge could be obtained that "differs from absolute certainty as a part differs from the whole." Furthermore, he proposed a method that could potentially be used in some situations to place a numerical value on this "probability." His approach depended on recognizing the futility in these circumstances of seeking to comprehend in fine detail the causes of observed events, and he made the radical proposal of essentially ignoring these specifics:

> In these and similar situations, since they may depend on causes that are completely hidden and that would forever mock our diligence by an innumerable variety of combinations, it would clearly be mad to want to learn anything in this way.

> Nonetheless, another way is open to us by which we may obtain what is sought. What cannot be ascertained a priori, may at least be found out a posteriori from the results many times observed in similar situations, since it should be presumed that something can happen or not to happen in the future in as many cases as it was observed to happen or not to happen in similar circumstances in the past.[1]

Here is a remarkably pregnant statement of the principle of willful ignorance and its potential utility.

Of course, like all truly big ideas, this one raised many subtle questions, some of which Jacob attempted to address and others that were not articulated until much later. Bernoulli's plan for making inductive inferences based on "many observed outcomes of similar events" was based on the new "combinatorial" mathematics first discovered by Pascal and Fermat in 1654 in their analyses of various gambling situations. He envisioned a way to ascertain probabilities applicable to "civil, moral and economic affairs" by viewing many natural and social processes as analogous to games of chance.

In this book I attempt to trace the history of willful ignorance from its first flickering to the point when it fully ignited. Unlike the Newtonian revolution, the initial sparks of the quiet revolution did not fall on dry tinder. It took a long time for the modern understanding of probability and statistics to gradually materialize. From our perspective, why these concepts should have taken so long to be discovered is mystifying. I believe that one particularly important source of this "delay" lies in the enigmatic nature of willful ignorance, upon which our notions of probability and statistics depend.

Willful ignorance was (and is) a very peculiar concept, something truly novel and without precedent. An eminent statistician observed that the appearance of statistical thinking based on mathematical probability represents a discontinuity in the arc of scientific history that simply cannot be explained as a natural extension of previously existing ideas:

> I conclude then that statistics in any sense akin to our own cannot be traced back before about A.D. 1660 ... such ideas were almost unknown ... There *are* new things under the sun and the attitude of mind towards experimental knowledge about natural and social phenomena which flourished after the Restoration is one of them.[2]

Why the modern concept of probability began to emerge just when it did and never before has puzzled many scholars. Probability for us seems almost self-evident. What we have forgotten is how great a departure from previously existing ideas about uncertainty our modern ideas represent.

Becoming comfortable with this novel idea and finding fruitful applications were not inevitable developments in the way that some other mathematical or scientific theories may have been. For instance, the basics of differential calculus were invented independently by Newton around 1666 and Leibniz less than a decade later, suggesting that circumstances were somehow ripe for this great leap forward. Their breakthroughs can be viewed as natural extensions of the analytic geometry introduced by René Descartes (1596–1650). In contrast, Jacob Bernoulli was virtually alone in appreciating the potential of what I am calling willful ignorance. Those who followed him perceived only dimly the full dimensions of his insight.

INVENTING PROBABILITY

Probability theory has become so second nature to us that it is viewed almost as a law of nature, or at least of logic, that was *discovered* in much the same way as Newton's inverse-square law of universal gravitation. However, probability theory is much more like an *invention* than a discovery.[3] Over the past century or so, probability has become ubiquitous and highly useful, helping us in a myriad of ways, ranging from ascertaining the political pulse of a nation to designing better products and even to measuring the performance of our favorite athletes.

Nassim Nicholas Taleb has dubbed unquestioning belief in the "laws" of classical probability theory the *ludic fallacy*.[4] The term is derived from the Latin word *ludus* (game). Taleb chose this term because the underlying metaphor of mathematical probability is the world as a huge casino, with rules like those in a game of chance. Ludic probability gradually supplanted an earlier usage of the word probability that reflected a qualitative analysis of uncertainty grounded in legal, ethical, and even religious considerations.

Slowly, a new *mathematical* probability took shape and was applied to a wide variety of practical problems that we would call statistical in nature. However, prior to the twentieth century, statistics in our modern sense did not exist as a separate discipline. Each statistical innovation was a byproduct of some attempt to deal with a specific scientific, commercial, or administrative problem. Eventually, statistics started to be recognized as a distinct *theoretical* discipline with many potential applications.

This development occurred as probability was acknowledged as a branch of theoretical mathematics, similar to geometry, algebra, number theory, etc. The merger of probability and statistics resulted in the new hybrid field of *mathematical statistics* around 1930. By this time, "probability and statistics" had come to connote a certain widely accepted set of core concepts. Moreover, the discipline of statistics after the 1930s came increasingly to be defined in terms of its mathematical character. Advances in probability and statistics tended to involve the derivation of mathematical formulas that were motivated more by abstract principles and hypothetical problems than by concrete practical concerns.

Throughout the eighteenth and nineteenth centuries, the topic of probability was understood to involve intertwined mathematical and philosophical aspects. In particular, probability was somehow related to *causation*. Beginning with Jacob Bernoulli, the mathematicians who advanced probability theory believed their work was a means of obtaining knowledge about complex causal processes. By the 1930s, discussion of causation was effectively banned from polite scientific society. In 1933, Andrei

Kolmogorov (1903–1987) published his landmark *Foundations of the Theory of Probability*.[5] This work represented the culmination of the trend toward viewing probability in purely mathematical terms.

Probability became defined as a "measure" that satisfied certain mathematical rules, or axioms. Games of chance became construed merely as convenient illustrative examples of this abstract theory, rather than as the mental model to which the axioms of probability owed their particular form. The logical implications of these axioms could be studied in the abstract, entirely divorced from any philosophical interpretation of what exactly the measure might be measuring.

Just as the physicist could theorize using concepts like mass and velocity without worrying about the specific details of particular objects that had these properties, so the mathematician or statistician could theorize about probability. Thus, probability became the mathematical backbone of virtually all thinking about uncertainty, and statistical inference was viewed as an application of the theory. Other ways of thinking about probability were relegated to a kind of philosophical shadowland and ignored.

As Kolmogorov's axioms rapidly became universally ratified by the scientific community, issues related to causation faded into the background. This development was consistent with a general trend in science to avoid metaphysical thinking and focus only on the observable surface of reality. The dominant philosophical attitude at the time was logical positivism. Bertrand Russell (1872–1970), perhaps its most famous exponent, argued that the notion of causes represented a kind of obsolete vestigial holdover: "The law of causality, I believe, like much that passes muster among philosophers, is a relic of a bygone age, surviving, like the monarchy, only because it is erroneously supposed to do no harm."[6]

By turning attention away from causal explanations, probability theory rejected any attempt to explain observed variability by reference to hypothetical causes. The axioms of probability formalized the rules operating in games of chance. In these games, an individual outcome is assumed completely unpredictable. That is to say, once the chance setup is defined (e.g., rolling a die), there is no information about the *particular* trial that could possibly improve our general prediction of the outcome. Nothing we might learn about the underlying causal structure of *this* toss would change our probability assessment (e.g., that a six will occur with probability 1/6).

STATISTICS

By the late 1800s, the field of statistics seemed to have reached intellectual maturity. The basic technical and philosophical issues had apparently been addressed. New discoveries seemed more like incremental refinements than significant breakthroughs. As in the apocryphal story about the U.S. patent office, everything important was thought to have already been invented. Suddenly, around the year 1890, that all began to change.

Like 1654, that year marked a major conceptual breakthrough (this time in the environs of London instead of Paris) and also the birth of the person who would build upon it to create an entirely new conceptual framework for statistics. Actually, the genesis of this breakthrough had been percolating quietly for about 20 years, through the efforts of a remarkable English gent by the name of Francis Galton (1822–1911). By 1890, Galton had fully developed his major statistical innovation. Equally important, Galton's work inspired Karl Pearson (1857–1936), who would go on to dominate statistical research for the next three decades.[7] Pearson's enormous influence would ultimately wane, but his work would lay the foundation for the next great leap forward.

The breakthrough achieved by Galton was not the solution of a purely mathematical problem, but rather of a conceptual riddle. For two decades, Galton had labored over the statistical evidence related to his primary area of interest, the transmission of exceptional talent from one generation to the next. Galton was fascinated by this topic and had authored a book on *Hereditary Genius* in 1869.[8] In it he had traced the lineages of notable families in which multiple "geniuses" over several generations were spawned, such families as the Bachs, the Darwins, and the Bernoullis (Jacob and his brother Johann, along with many of their descendants).

Galton was a data analyst *extraordinaire*, a man who could wax poetic over tables of numbers and graphical displays. Over the course of two decades, Galton gradually arrived at a new way to organize data about the diversity of human characteristics and capabilities, both physical and mental. The paradox he confronted related to two apparently irreconcilable findings. On the one hand, Galton confirmed that highly accomplished individuals tended to produce gifted offsprings, so that talents really did appear to run in families (as did lack of talent at the other end of the human spectrum). Therefore, he expected to find that the amount of diversity in a population would be increasing over time. On the other hand, the actual amount of variability he observed on every characteristic measured was fairly constant across generations.

How was this stability possible in a "smart get smarter" world? Galton eventually discovered that this apparent steady state was being maintained by a tendency for the sons of extremely accomplished fathers to "regress" partially toward the overall population mean (average). For example, the son of a genius such as Galton's cousin Charles Darwin, would also tend to be gifted, but "on average" less so than his father. But why should this be so? Was there some mystical force of nature pulling talent levels back toward mediocrity? Galton eventually worked out the answer: regression was the result not of any cause, but of a subtle aspect of randomness.

In 1890, Galton expressed his growing conviction of having stumbled upon a kind of methodological Rosetta stone. Galton at first called this statistical marvel the "co-relation" coefficient, but it soon morphed into the *correlation coefficient.* It was a numerical measure of the degree of relationship between two quantities, such as the heights of a father and son. Galton believed that the child's regression resulted from the fact that his level of talent was partially, but not entirely, determined by his parents' levels of talent. The correlation coefficient, in this context, provided a natural measure of the degree to which a particular ability tended to be inherited, rather than acquired, in a given population.

By 1890, Galton had become convinced that his solution to the regression problem might have very general applicability beyond the field of genetics: "I can only say that there is a vast field of topics that fall under the laws of correlation, which lies open to the research of any competent person who cares to investigate it."[9] Karl Pearson, who turned 33 in March of 1890, had previously been trained as a lawyer, physicist, and philosopher. He explained much later how Galton's breakthrough had struck him as revolutionary, destined to usher in a new era for the sciences:

> Henceforward the physical view of the universe was to be that of a correlated system of variates, approaching but by no means reaching perfect correlation, i.e. absolute causality, even in the group of phenomena termed physical. Biological phenomena in their numerous phases, economic and social, were seen to be differentiated from the physical by the intensity of their correlations. The idea Galton placed before himself was to represent by a single numerical quantity, the degree of relationship, or of partial causality between the different variables of our ever-changing universe.[10]

Pearson turned his attention to statistics, his perceived golden key to the science of the future. One of his principal early preoccupations was to place Galton's somewhat intuitive concepts on a firmer mathematical footing.

Pearson interpreted the correlation as a measure of "partial causality," in contrast with the "absolute causality" approached in the physical sciences. For him, correlations had the advantage of being based on observable (measurable) variables. They represented an indication that some sort of causal association existed. However, it was not necessary to delineate explicitly the underlying causes, which were for the most part metaphysical abstractions that could not be perceived directly. For Pearson, and many who followed in his tracks, correlations and related statistical concepts such as *regression coefficients* came to represent the proper tools to use for the biological and social sciences.

While the correlation coefficient and its statistical cousins held great promise, there were some difficulties to be overcome. For one thing, a correlation coefficient did not necessarily indicate that one of the two variables was a direct cause of the other. Does poverty lead to lack of education or vice versa? Perhaps the association between two variables might be attributable to some third factor, either known or not. In Galton's original context of genetics, the direction of causation was clear, but not so in many subsequent applications. The implications of such issues remain subject to confusion and controversy to the present day.

Pearson and his colleagues wrestled with the mathematics of these statistical measures for the next 30 years, making considerable progress. Unfortunately for them, however, their efforts were directed along an evolutionary branch that was ultimately doomed to extinction. The eventual future of statistics was first charted by Ronald Aylmer (R. A.) Fisher (1890–1962), beginning in the 1920s. Fisher's impact on the field of statistics, and indirectly on the many disciplines that came to depend on statistical methods, would turn out to be unparalleled. A giant of twentieth century science (he was also a co-founder of population genetics), Fisher remains virtually unknown to the general public.[11] Like Jacob Bernoulli, Fisher approached the analysis of data from a completely new vantage point. He drew upon, integrated and extended earlier ideas, placing statistics on a solid conceptual and mathematical foundation.

Like Bernoulli, Fisher labored essentially alone and in obscurity for many years, and his ideas went far beyond what his contemporaries could at first comprehend.[12] Unlike Bernoulli, Fisher lived long enough to see many of his innovations eventually acclaimed and widely adopted. However, his ideas, like Jacob's, were often misunderstood and (in his eyes at least) distorted by others, embroiling him in several famous long-running, and sometimes acrimonious, disputes.

Like Jacob Bernoulli, Fisher combined philosophical depth with a unique endowment of mathematical virtuosity. One important difference between Bernoulli and Fisher, however, was that the former was widely regarded as an excellent teacher who always expressed himself with great clarity, while the latter was a notoriously poor communicator. Fisher's logic and arguments were often difficult for others to follow. Many of his mathematical results were based on a unique way of envisioning data in a geometrical form.

His uncanny geometrical intuition is sometimes attributed to extremely poor eyesight. As a child he experienced great difficulty reading in artificial light, which forced him to learn complex mathematics largely by being tutored orally. To compensate, he cultivated a remarkable ability to visualize mathematical relationships in his head. This capacity often revealed insights that were obvious to Fisher, but difficult to re-express in more conventional algebraic terms. Some of his pronouncements had an oracular quality that could both awe and confuse his colleagues.

Fisher shared some similarities with Pierre-Simon Laplace, the greatest contributor to the mathematics of probability and statistics before him. Fisher and Laplace were eminently practical, regarding complex mathematical derivations as primarily a means of solving concrete scientific problems. They saw themselves primarily as scientists, not mathematicians. Both possessed supreme self-assurance regarding their fundamental philosophical and scientific intuitions. Finally, each of them rigidly espoused certain ideas that ultimately fell out of favor, somewhat tarnishing their legacies.[13]

In the late 1930s, when Fisher's new approach was first becoming widely appreciated, an alternative philosophical outlook on the function and methodology of statistical inference was evolving. Led by a Polish émigré named Jerzy Neyman (1894–1981) in collaboration with Karl Pearson's son, Egon Pearson (1895–1980), a new formulation of statistics as primarily an instrument for reaching rational *decisions* was being introduced. This meant that a statistical analysis should directly indicate a specific course of action, rather than just provide relevant evidence to be applied in some unspecified manner.

The Neyman–Pearson theory became widely regarded as an important refinement of Fisher's ideas and was incorporated into standard statistical practice and teaching. The decision-theoretic framework proved highly useful during World War II and in the great industrial expansion of the 1950s. Then it was extended into the important arena of medical research, especially in controlled experiments to "prove" whether a medical drug or device was safe and effective.[14] Finally, beginning around 1970, attempts to apply similar approaches in the context of economic, educational, and social policy research were introduced. In these more recent applications, the Neyman–Pearson perspective has become the foundation of the *evidence-based* approach to medical and policy research.

THE TAMING OF CHANCE

The rise of modern probability and statistics has been described as the taming of chance.[15] For millennia, the realm of chance had been conceived as completely wild and unmanageable, the province of the capricious goddess *Fortuna*. A *theory* of chance would have seemed an oxymoron. The Scientific Revolution redefined chance. Its great legacy was a conception of the universe as a giant mechanism subject to iron laws of causation. This notion of causality made it possible to imagine its opposite: pure *randomness*, the complete absence of causality.

Laplace famously asserted that probability was merely a measure of our ignorance regarding the true causes of complex phenomena. From this perspective, observed *variability* in biological and social phenomena was actually generated by a plethora of interlocking causes whose workings eluded our understanding. The appearance of chance was an illusion. However, from our limited human perspective, there was no hope of reducing this apparent chance to its "real" component causes. So, what could not be attributed to deterministic causation was regarded for all practical purposes as random.

Whatever randomness may be, it is certainly at the heart of mathematical probability. The taming of chance refers to the way in which our uncertainty has now been cut to the mold of probability's laws. This "good behavior" has become possible because we divide the world neatly into conceptual categories of causality and randomness. Everything that does not conform to strict causal regularities must be construed as completely random. In this way, we eliminate ambiguity and permit the mathematical laws of probability to govern.

For many practical purposes, this concept of randomness is invaluable. Not only does it serve as the basis of modern statistical methodology, but also as a conceptual tool in everyday life. However, the nature of randomness and the resulting implications are frequently misunderstood, leading us into poor choices and decisions. For example, we may overreact to risks that are in reality extremely rare, such as airplane crashes or tornados, while overlooking more common threats like vehicular accidents. A slew of popular books and an entire subfield of psychology have recently been devoted to pointing out these foibles, and teaching us how to avoid such "irrational" behavior.[16]

Many studies have revealed how we often unwittingly violate the laws of probability. Even experts in statistics can sometimes be tripped up by various forms of *bias*. Constant vigilance is necessary to guard against these flaws that seem built into our cognitive processing machinery. These cautions are valuable and should be taken to heart. However, in the rush to avoid being fooled by randomness, we may fall into another trap.

Variability and randomness are not identical. Sometimes the stories we tell really *do* capture some important elements of reality. What looks like randomness from one vantage point may actually be predictable from another perspective. Failure to perceive hidden regularities can hurt us in two ways. First, we may forego opportunities to benefit by understanding and capitalizing on how things really work. Second, *we* may be exploited by others who have such insight. It is certainly true that being fooled by randomness is quite common and can be costly. Being "fooled by causation" may be much less common, but sometimes have even more serious consequences.

To illustrate what I have in mind, let us imagine that Random Enterprises, Inc. operates a large casino in Las Vegas. In this casino are many standard-issue roulette wheels. A Las Vegas roulette wheel contains 38 compartments, or slots, into which a ball may roll, and is designed so that each of the 38 possible outcomes is equally likely to occur on any spin. Thirty-six of these outcomes are the numbers from 1 to 36 (half are red and half are black); the remaining two green slots on the wheel are labeled 0 and 00. The simplest way to bet is to select a particular number. Assume that the stake is one dollar. If the ball lands in the slot chosen, the player receives $36 ($35 plus the dollar staked). Since the probability of winning is 1/38, and the return is $36, the "expected" return on each such wager is 36/38, or about 94.7 cents. Thus, the amount actually taken in by the casino over the course of a large number of bets will be very close to 5.3% of the total amount wagered.

Random Enterprises reposes complete confidence in this long-run rate of return because of what is known to statisticians as the *law of large numbers*, although it is more popularly called the law of averages. It is the law of large numbers that allows casino owners (and insurance companies) to sleep soundly at night. But, suppose that George, an enterprising croupier in our casino, happens to be a brilliant MIT mechanical engineering dropout who has developed a tiny device that can control precisely where the ball will land. George decides to test this marvelous invention, but of course in secret.

While working the midnight shift, he manages to slip in, every now and then, a "controlled" spin among the many ordinary ones. To avoid detection, George tries to vary the compartment he selects for the ball's destination. In fact, having taken statistics while at MIT, he cleverly generates random numbers for scheduling exactly when to intervene, and which slot to select. He does this in a way that each of the 38 slots on the wheel will have the same chance of being selected, just as if the wheel were being spun in the usual manner.

Clearly, the underlying *causal process* has been dramatically altered. However, George's scheme will have absolutely *no impact* on the probability distribution of outcomes. The standard probability laws will remain in force despite the new causal process he has created. Each of the 38 possible outcomes still has a probability of 1/38 occurring on each spin. So, there is no way anyone could ever detect the change from the pattern of outcomes, no matter how many spins of George's wheel are observed. Furthermore, the casino's owners would have no reason (so far) to care that George had tampered with the system. The owners could remain blissfully ignorant, but still reap exactly the same profits as before. So, why would they lose sleep over George's experiment, even if they knew about it?

The answer is obvious. George could make use of his insider knowledge. For instance, he might arrange with a confederate to place large bets on the predestined numbers when he is using his nifty device. Rather than a 5.3% loss, George and his accomplice would enjoy a guaranteed 3500% profit. Now, although the distribution of winning numbers still conforms to the standard probability model, the distribution of *payoffs* most certainly does not.

THE IGNORANCE FALLACY

The common human tendency to discern patterns in what is actually random variation and to invent causal explanations has been termed the *narrative fallacy*. For example, if a baseball player manages to get a hit in each of many consecutive games, he may be said to be "swinging a hot bat." Baseball icon Joe DiMaggio of the 1941 New York Yankees holds the record for such a hot streak, hitting safely in a remarkable 56 straight games.

Batting streaks of this kind and similar "hot hands" in other sports and games are often attributed to various causes. However, extensive research has proved that such hot streaks are nearly always consistent with what probability theory would predict to occur by chance.[17] What appears to be a highly unusual occurrence is bound to occur once in a while; that is the nature of randomness. We just do not know ahead of time when and where such an apparent anomaly will happen. Avoiding the narrative fallacy requires us to be skeptical of an "unlikely" occurrence *unless* it can be shown that the probability of observing such an occurrence was actually very small. Long hitting streaks, it turns out, are to be expected from time to time, and even DiMaggio's famous achievement may one day be surpassed. So, it appears that streakiness is just a myth. Or is it?

Let us accept for the moment the hypothesis that pure randomness can plausibly explain almost any hot-hand streak in sports or games. Does that necessarily imply that such streaks do not really exist? Consider that there are a great many factors, most not measurable, that might influence any individual outcome, such as one particular game or at bat. Therefore, it might be possible, in principle, to detect the existence of such factors. Like George, a person with special insight, or inside information, might be able to profit handsomely by acting on it. What the research certainly tells us is that *if* such factors exist, they must be haphazard enough to *appear* essentially random. Thus, they will be very difficult to uncover and may require a large body of data and investment of effort to tease out.

The narrative fallacy refers to the folly of seeking causal explanations for phenomena that are essentially random in nature. However, the converse of the narrative fallacy is what I call the *ignorance fallacy*. When there *are* causal factors that *could* be exploited to great advantage, it is foolish to ignore them. By regarding chance as the most plausible explanation, just because the data appear consistent with randomness, we may remain (willfully) ignorant of potentially important discoveries. A more mindful approach that entertains such possibilities can avoid the ignorance fallacy. However, we must recognize that, as in the case of batting streaks, deviations from randomness may be very hard to detect.

THE DILEMMA OF SCIENCE

For over a quarter century, the two giants of statistical theory, Fisher and Neyman, argued about the function of statistical methods in scientific research. Their dispute was not primarily technical in nature; rather, it concerned philosophical issues regarding the nature of statistical inference. Fisher believed that statistical methods could provide useful evidence to inform the scientist's process of reasoning. Probability theory could be useful by identifying patterns in data that were unusual enough to be worthy of serious consideration. Neyman conceived the role of statistics as providing direct guidance about an optimal decision. Probability, he believed, could be used to calculate whether or not to "accept" or "reject" a given scientific hypothesis.

Fisher understood that scientific uncertainty embodied substantial ambiguity. Clarifying the ambiguity was mostly the scientist's responsibility. The statistician's work was dependent on the scientist's knowledge and theoretical framework. As I explained in Chapter 1, relying on mathematical probability is tantamount to assuming that there is no substantial remaining ambiguity. That way, only the more quantifiable dimension of doubtfulness need be considered. Neyman, on the other hand, could not appreciate the significance of ambiguity at all. For him, the laws of mathematical probability were absolute and unambiguous. Thus, scientific uncertainty could be reduced to a straightforward application of these laws.

One of Fisher's misunderstood insights was that probabilities were not absolute.[18] A probability statement was meaningful in the context of some particular scientific theory. Therefore, the quality of a probability statement depended on the degree of refinement of the theory. In particular, a more refined theory could allow specification of subpopulations whose probabilities might vary from those applicable to the overall population. Such "recognizable" subsets represent potential opportunities for more effective decision-making and action.

As a prime example, much of applied scientific research is aimed at improving some product or process. In this context, the central statistical problem is to predict the *effect* of some intervention, such as a new policy or procedure. In the simplest case, we may have data about outcomes under two different conditions, such as a standard policy and a new proposed alternative. Suppose the outcome is measured on a numerical scale. Typically, the research will compare the average outcome values under the two conditions. The difference between these two averages is interpreted as the effect of the intervention.

Unfortunately, there is an important ambiguity that is generally overlooked. The difference between the group averages can arise in two possible ways. One possibility is that the real causal effect is *uniform*. Under this scenario, the actual effect for each individual is composed of this systematic effect plus some random "noise." For example, a new educational program may raise every student's true knowledge level by some constant amount on a certain scale. This uniform-effect model underlies the usual applications of statistical methods.

Alternatively, it is possible that the real causal effect can vary to some extent, depending on a variety of individual circumstances and characteristics. In that case, the average effect may not apply to any particular individual. As an extreme example, suppose the new program is better for half of the students and worse for the other half. In that case, the average effect would be zero. However, focusing on the average would be irrelevant and misleading. Ideally, our objective should be to identify which program is best for each individual student.

Can we find ways to distinguish among individuals, in order to better match treatment options to individuals?[19] For example, given recent advances in such fields as information processing, genetics, and neuro-science, can we really maintain that estimating an average effect is still the best we can do? Certainly, in the commercial arena, individualized predic-tive modeling is exploding under the rubric of Big Data. The advantages of exploiting identifiable factors that distinguish individuals are becoming increasingly evident. There are still, thankfully, many differences between the scientific and business contexts of research. However, in one very important respect, science needs to become more like business.

Innovative business solutions are generated by entrepreneurs who seek advantages by applying their unique insight and risking the consequences. The odds may be against them, but the potential rewards are great. Their payoff is conferred by the marketplace in exchange for whatever value they manage to generate. In contrast, most researchers today operate within a system that insulates them from personal risk by substituting "fool-proof" statistical tests in place of scientific creativity and insight. These statistical procedures have become a universally established standard of scientific behavior. They are also believed capable of providing objective criteria for separating the wheat of valid findings from the chaff of false leads.

The problem is that the conditions under which such statistical criteria were developed no longer pertain. Hence, the sacrifices in terms of creativ-ity and individual initiative that seem to assure that scientific findings are credible and generalizable no longer do so. Yet, we have no way to know this, because our mechanisms for reality-testing have broken down. We have become so reliant on our probability-based technology that we have failed to develop methods for validation that can inform us about what *really* works and, equally important, why. Unlike the entrepreneur, the scientist is judged by standards that have, to a certain extent, lost touch with reality.

It has long been conventional in statistical analyses to concentrate pri-marily on the average effects for broad populations, which are referred to as the *main effects*. Only after establishing the existence of these main effects can more subtle *interactions* with individual factors be considered. This approach accords well with the probability models underlying statis-tical methodology but its logic is backwards. In studies of human popu-lations, at least, interaction effects should be presumed the rule, and uni-formity an exception. To insist on the reverse is to be like the proverbial drunk looking for his car keys under the lamppost because that is where there is light. Two important examples illustrate the consequences of the *main-effect fallacy*. In both cases, the search for simple solutions that work well on average have led us astray.

Back around 1970 there was considerable optimism about the potential to overcome social and economic disadvantage through educational supplementation in the preschool and early school years. One of the major programs introduced was Project Head Start, an effort to enrich the experiences of children from low income families. The aim was to close the perceived gap in cognitive development between richer and poorer children that was evident already by the time of entry into kindergarten. The pioneering studies that motivated the program appeared promising, and early evaluations by educational researchers were generally positive as well. I was personally involved in several of these studies, and remember well the sense of optimism that prevailed.[20]

Unfortunately, continued research over the ensuing decades has yielded mixed results. In the 1998 reauthorization of Head Start, the U.S. Congress mandated that a large and definitive evaluation should be performed. In 2010 the long-awaited and monumental Head Start Impact Study report was finally published.[21] Its main message landed with a thud.

> In sum, this report finds that providing access to Head Start has benefits for both 3-year-olds and 4-year-olds in the cognitive, health, and parenting domains, and for 3-year-olds in the social-emotional domain. However, the benefits of access to Head Start at age four are largely absent by 1st grade for the program population as a whole. For 3-year-olds, there are few sustained benefits, although access to the program may lead to improved parent–child relationships through 1st grade, a potentially important finding for children's longer term development.

A recent follow-up analysis that tracked the participants through third grade confirmed these disappointing findings.[22] After 40 years, is it not time to consider whether the kinds of questions being asked in all this research are the right ones?

My second exhibit concerns a medical issue that affects primarily older individuals. Prior to 1970, research on the use of aspirin for prevention of myocardial infarctions (heart attacks) had yielded some positive indications but was far from definitive. In the 1980s, two major studies involving physicians as subjects, one in England and one in the United States, seemed to confirm this effect. A number of follow-up studies were subsequently undertaken.[23]

Those studies that enrolled only patients with prior heart attacks or other heart disease (so-called secondary prevention studies) showed clear benefit. However, primary prevention studies (analyses of people without such a history) were more equivocal. Moreover, daily aspirin use was also associated with a slightly increased risk of serious bleeding, because of aspirin's "blood-thinning" effect. Nonetheless, the evidence until recently appeared on balance to be quite favorable, so millions of people, especially middle-aged men, have been strongly encouraged by their physicians to adopt a low-dose aspirin regimen.

Alas, two major reviews of the research, intended to increase our certainty about aspirin's benefits, have had just the opposite effect. In March of 2009, the U.S. Preventive Services Task Force (USPSTF) issued a set of official recommendations.[24] For example, the USPSTF strongly advised physicians to "encourage men age 45 to 79 years to use aspirin when the potential reduction in myocardial infarctions outweighs the potential harm of an increase in gastrointestinal hemorrhage." Based on the statistical evidence about benefits and risks, the great majority of middle-aged men would qualify for low-dose aspirin therapy under this guideline.

Two months after the USPSTF recommendations were promulgated, they were controverted by another equally authoritative opinion. In the prestigious medical journal, *Lancet*, the Antithrombotic Trialists' Collaboration (ATT) reported on a large "meta-analysis" of all the major clinical trials for aspirin prevention. A meta-analysis is a kind of statistical summarization that averages across a set of individual studies in order to reach an overall conclusion regarding some important issue. The ATT conclusion was far less sanguine than that of the USPSTF. The potential benefits of aspirin therapy for primary prevention of myocardial infarctions and other cardiovascular events turned out to be more modest than previously thought.

The ATT's guarded conclusion was that broad-based recommendations were not warranted.

Hence, although the currently available trial results could well help inform appropriate judgments by individuals ... they do not seem to justify general guidelines advocating the routine use of aspirin in all apparently healthy individuals above a moderate level of risk of coronary heart disease.[25]

The catch-22 in this carefully worded statement is that the major random-ized clinical trials in fact do not focus on individual differences in any meaningful way. So, it is extremely difficult for a physician, let alone a typical individual, to see how to use the "available trial results" to "inform appropriate judgments by individuals." Moreover, to further complicate matters, substantial evidence is piling up to indicate that aspirin may be protective against several types of cancer. This finding, if confirmed, will further modify the cost–benefit calculation.

In retrospect, over 40 years of effort have yielded meager knowledge gains with respect to the use of aspirin for prevention and the potential value of early childhood intervention. Are the hardworking researchers who have conducted this research to blame? No. By and large, they have diligently carried out first-rate studies according to current best practices. The way to do better is not, as some have counseled, to keep trying harder using the same tools. Rather it is to develop new methods that are more suitable.

Mathematical probability is one of the principal tools at our disposal. However, it would be a mistake to regard our current conceptions of prob-ability and its uses as graven in stone. Like all great ideas, the concept of probability has evolved over time and been adapted to changing circum-stances. At present, the rapidly developing technology for collecting, pro-cessing, and analyzing data is dramatically altering the world of science in many ways. The potential implications of this information revolution are being widely discussed. However, for the most part, probability is under-stood and presented as a technology, a branch of applied mathematics. Its basic principles are assumed to be known, permanent, and beyond question.

This attitude presents a dilemma. I believe that the emerging reality will require some radically new thinking about uncertainty and data anal-ysis. By holding fast to our current limited conceptions of probability and statistics, as if they were handed down from the mount, we are in danger of missing out on great opportunities. In particular, possibilities for bridg-ing the divide between methodologists and practitioners may be missed. It is my hope that tracing the evolution of thinking about scientific uncer-tainty can help place mathematical probability in a broader perspective that is more likely to foster the creative solutions that will be needed.

CHAPTER 3

A MATTER OF CHANCE

It is a sultry evening, the 28th of July in 1654 in Paris. Blaise Pascal has risen from his sickbed to await the arrival of his friend Pierre de Carcavi (1600–1684).[1] Carcavi is a fellow member of the Mersenne circle, a coterie of leading French intellectuals. Pascal awaits the latest news of recent scientific developments that Carcavi has gleaned from his contacts among the group. Recently turned 31, Pascal has always been frail and in precarious health, but his mental powers are legendary. A child prodigy, he published his first original mathematical paper on conic sections at age 16.

At 20, motivated by the desire to assist his father, then a tax collector in the city of Rouen, he began work on a mechanical calculator he dubbed the Pascaline, which he subsequently perfected and sold. Pascal has also studied physics and at the age of 24 authored a book about his experiments with vacuums that led to a famous dispute with René Descartes, the most celebrated French scientist and geometer of the era. Pascal argued that vacuums actually exist, an idea that Descartes scoffed at, quipping that the only vacuum in nature resided inside Pascal's head.

Pascal sometimes finds travel difficult and is grateful for the more mobile Carcavi's efforts to keep him current on the commerce of ideas.

Willful Ignorance: The Mismeasure of Uncertainty, First Edition. Herbert I. Weisberg.
© 2014 John Wiley & Sons, Inc. Published 2014 by John Wiley & Sons, Inc.

At last, his friend arrives and after a few comments about the weather and Pascal's health, the two begin to discuss what Carcavi has learned. Pascal is especially delighted to discover a letter from Pierre de Fermat continuing their discussion of some problems related to games of chance. Pascal has limited personal experience of gambling though he did experience a brief period of debauchery shortly after his father's death 3 years ago. Recently, he has become intrigued by certain mathematical puzzles introduced to him by Antoine Gombaud (1607–1684), the self-styled Chevalier de Méré, a true *bon vivant*. Unable to answer a particularly difficult question, Méré, who loves the gaming table and dabbles in mathematics, appealed to Pascal for assistance.

Fermat, nearing 53 years of age, is an attorney and prominent citizen in Toulouse, about 350 miles away, but also a world-renowned "geometer." He enjoys tantalizing fellow mathematicians by presenting solutions to very difficult problems, challenging them to find out how he has obtained his result. Carcavi, a close friend and noted geometer himself, has sometimes been the victim in these parlor games. Pascal eagerly skims through Fermat's reply, seems at first somewhat nonplussed, then nods toward Carcavi, smiling slowly as he grasps Fermat's characteristically elegant logic. Still, while Pascal admires the older man's cleverness, he is not accustomed to being upstaged.

Rising early the next morning, Pascal hurriedly pens a response for Carcavi to take back to Fermat. His missive begins with lavish praise for Fermat's brilliance, but offers an alternative method that draws on some related mathematical research of his own, for which he claims certain merits. Thus begins a cordial interchange that concludes with Pascal's letter of October 27, in which he states happily that he and Fermat are now in complete agreement.

Pascal is shortly to enter a period of religious crisis and turn his attention completely away from mathematics and science. This retreat from the world will last for the remainder of his tragically short life, with only a couple of brief "lapses." Fermat, the ultimate pure mathematician, has never had any real interest in gambling problems *per se*, other than as a vehicle for displaying his genius. So, late in 1654, it is entirely possible that the methods they have developed together will lie dormant, perhaps for centuries, rather than leading to our modern ideas of probability and statistics. That this did not happen was in some respects truly "a matter of chance."

ORIGINS

Much has been written about why the modern notion of probability, and statistical thinking conjoined with it, began to develop in the 1650s, *and not before.*[2] This question has many aspects to it and can be viewed from several different perspectives. All commentators agree that *something* very important was born in the Pascal–Fermat correspondence and contemporaneous developments, but reading the philosophical and historical analyses on this topic can be confusing. It is not clear *why* exactly these events were significant and *how* they engendered a revolution in thought.

To simplify, I will highlight two important philosophical themes with ancient roots. The first pertains to the issue of *uncertainty* and especially the concept of "chance" events. The second relates to the issue of *induction*, the problem of learning from limited experience to reach general conclusions. In particular, how can valid inferences about the future be derived from previous experience? Thinking about both uncertainty and induction began to undergo a radical and unexpected twist as a result of the unlikely attention focused on gambling by a few of the most brilliant minds in Europe.

Eventually, uncertainty would become measured quantitatively, as a fraction between zero and one, and the idea of systematically counting outcomes to determine a future expectation would begin to take hold. Both of these developments would be made possible because the ideas that emerged in the context of gambling provided a new conceptual *model* that had never before existed. In this sense, the connection between the discovery of probability and gambling is far from accidental.

Games of chance are not simply a convenient application of a natural concept that had been latent for centuries, waiting like America to be discovered someday. Rather, I believe, modern probability is in essence nothing but a way to calibrate uncertainty that is *patterned on* games of chance. When we think about a numerical probability, we are in effect making an analogy between the event of interest and an observed outcome of a random mechanism, such as the spinning of a wheel of fortune. Our notion of probability may have other connotations as well, but it is fundamentally this analogy with an idealized random mechanism that shapes our thought processes. Before mathematicians began to think seriously about games of chance, probability in this sense could not exist.

Much confusion about the genesis of probability arises because the usage of this word changed radically during the eighteenth century. Before our modern mathematical version of probability began to emerge, a qualitative concept of probability had long prevailed. Throughout this book, I will sometimes be referring to "probability" in this archaic sense, and sometimes in its modern connotation. I originally considered trying to distinguish this older use of probability from its modern namesake by representing the former as 𝔭𝔯𝔬𝔟𝔞𝔟𝔦𝔩𝔦𝔱𝔶 and the latter as probability. I will occasionally do so for special emphasis but will usually refer simply to probability. When needing to make clear that I am referring to modern probability, I often use "mathematical probability."

To minimize confusion, try to keep in mind the following rough chronological evolution of the word probability. Prior to around 1700, probability was almost entirely qualitative, referring to the strength of logical support for a statement or proposition. Between 1700 and 1750, a transition occurred; probability retained much of this traditional connotation, but started to assume as well a quantitative aspect. *Mathematical* probability emerged, measured on a scale between zero and one, with laws based on the mathematics of gambling. After approximately 1750, the word "probability" was applied almost exclusively to represent this new mathematical measure of certainty, or belief. Referring to the Timeline may help to place the discussion of probability in this chapter in perspective.

𝔓𝔯𝔬𝔟𝔞𝔟𝔦𝔩𝔦𝔱𝔶

What in many old texts is usually translated as probability is the Latin word *probabilitas*, whose etymological source was the Latin root for verbs related to proving, or proof. So, probability conveyed the sense of a degree to which a proposition was (or could be) *proved*. We might think of this concept as "prove-ability." Put differently, a person's probability

Landmarks of Probability

1600	
1654	**Pascal & Fermat**
1657	**Huygens**
1700	
1713	Bernoulli
1718	De Moivre
1764	Bayes & Price
1774	Laplace
1800	
1837	Poisson
1838	De Morgan
1843	Mill
1843	Cournot
1849	Ellis
1854	Boole
1866	Venn
1892	Peirce
1900	
1921	Keynes
1921	Knight
1922	Fisher
1926	Ramsey
1926	Neyman & Pearson
1928	Von Mises
1937	De Finetti
1949	Reichenbach
1954	Savage
1959	Popper

Pierre de Fermat

Christiaan Huygens

Blaise Pascal

regarding a statement was his level of *justification* for believing in it, based on all the available evidence.

A philosopher would say that probability had an *epistemic* quality; it referred to belief in a proposition or assertion, rather than to the occurrence of an event. The proposition at issue could sometimes be the statement that a certain event has occurred or will occur in future. Often, however, it would concern whether a particular course of action was morally correct. There was even in Catholicism a school of philosophy known as "probabilism."[3] In a legal context, probability might pertain to matters like the guilt or innocence of an accused person, or to the validity of competing claims in a dispute over inheritance.

The kind of justification supporting a statement of probability was quite different from what would generally be considered legitimate today. The relevant evidence might be an argument from logic and experience, from an appeal to the authority of a learned "doctor" (expert), or from a well-accepted written text. An argument derived from direct observation or logical reasoning was called *intrinsic*, and an argument derived from expert opinion or testimony was termed *extrinsic*.

Probability dealt with situations in which there was uncertainty about the actual circumstances or moral imperatives involved. It often entailed a marshaling of several arguments and/or pieces of evidence. The number and weight of the arguments taken together would then somehow determine the subjective probability. This concept of probability as employed in medieval texts is confusing for us because of its ambiguity:

> Attribution of probability to an opinion has several connotations. In the first place, it refers to the authority of those who accept the given opinion, ... In the second place, 'probability' refers to the arguments which are presented in favor of the opinion in question; and from this point of view it suggests *provability*, ... In the third place 'probability' takes on a somewhat pejorative connotation precisely insofar as the proposition in question is *merely* probable ...[4]

Probability was sometimes expressed in terms of degrees. For instance, one opinion might be deemed more probable than another, or an event might simply be considered "probable," meaning at least as likely to occur as not. However, it was never expressed as a number, let alone as a fraction between 0 and 1. In the case of conflicting assertions, say those put forward by a defendant and her accuser, a separate probability appraisal for each would be obtained. Then the relative probabilities of these opposing positions would be compared.

As I mentioned in Chapter 1, this sort of probability encompassed both doubtfulness and ambiguity. So, there was not necessarily a common understanding or agreement about the relevant evidence. Therefore, it would have seemed strange in the 1600s to combine all the arguments on both sides of a proposition into a single probability assessment. Rather, the separate qualitative probability evaluations (pro and con) would have been developed independently. This approach seems similar to the way many judges and juries still weigh legal evidence and arguments in a court of law today. Our legal system may thus retain, at least partially, an older and richer approach to decision-making that is not fully compatible with modern probabilistic analysis.

This holdover can be confusing when legal disputes are interpreted narrowly as problems in modern decision theory, which is based on mathematical probability. "Even in the United States, where quantification and experts are most welcome, the inroads of mathematical probability into law have been minimal."[5] This situation is often misinterpreted today by failing to appreciate that probability (whatever it might mean) in the law "is certainly different from the mathematical concept; indeed, it is rare to find a situation in which the two usages coexist."[6]

Risky Business

The archaic philosophical interpretation of probability just described was essentially irrelevant to the questions considered by Blaise Pascal and Pierre de Fermat. Their conceptual framework for analyzing games of chance derived mainly from notions of fairness in legal and business transactions. In medieval and Renaissance Europe, business transactions were interpreted in the light of religious authority and examined through the lens of morality. Realizing an exorbitant profit or interest rate (usury) was widely condemned as illicit behavior. It was deemed critical that the gains be in some way proportionate to the expenditure of capital or labor. The practical problem was how to apply these principles of equity to specific situations.

Business dealings in which chance played an important part posed a special challenge to these ethical and legal maxims. Such transactions involved so-called *aleatory contracts*, stemming from the Latin word "alea," meaning a die or set of dice. This terminology tacitly recognized the analogy between a risky business venture and a game of chance. For example, transporting merchandise over long distances, especially by sea, was a hazardous enterprise. To reduce the risk of major loss, insurance mechanisms of various sorts were devised. These arrangements often became rather convoluted, so as to circumvent the religious prohibitions pertaining to usury. After all, the economic risk paled in comparison with the perceived risk of eternal punishment.

By the fourteenth century, maritime insurance in essentially the modern form had been established.[7] In 1389, a Genoese merchant entered into a contract that stipulated:

> I insure you for 200 ducats in gold, of good and fair weight, for your part of the cargo existing on said ship ... And for this insurance, according to our agreement, I have received from you 25 gold ducats.

In this instance, the "insurance" was against the rumored possibility that the ship in question had already sunk. The underwriter was wagering that the reports would turn out to be false. Insurance premiums were generally determined by the circumstances of the particular situation as understood by the parties involved and negotiated between them. There was no empirical basis for setting premiums other than the experience and informed judgment of experts.

Besides insurance, many other types of commercial dealings required some sort of accounting for risk in specifying prices and terms.[8] These included annuities on single or multiple lives, investments in partnerships to fund risky ventures, public lotteries for government financing, rights to shares in an inheritance, and sales of commodities to be delivered at some future specified date. In appraising the fair value of an asset whose value was somewhat uncertain, an important concept was the *expectation* of gain or loss. This notion of expectation had roots in Roman legal doctrine and could loosely be interpreted as a *reasonable hope*.

This rather vague concept of expectation has now been replaced by the precisely defined *mathematical expectation*. This expectation, or *expected value*, is the product obtained by multiplying the *value* of the thing hoped for by the *probability* of attaining it. Before the modern concept of probability existed, however, the expectation had a less specific meaning. The expectation of a commercial venture might be interpreted as its true worth, somehow balancing the possible rewards and the known risks. This older idea of expectation provided a conceptual yardstick by which fairness could be measured, although its application required experience and judgment rather than calculation.

Expectation was meaningful as an ideal but often difficult to define precisely. Detailed consideration of circumstances and precedents, as in a legal context, could be important in evaluating an expectation, which was firmly embedded in the raw material of concrete circumstances. In this light, what transpired in 1654 was the start of a distillation process that yielded first the mathematical expectation and eventually the abstraction we understand as mathematical probability.

Games, Odds, and Gambling

Games of chance have a long history, stretching back into antiquity.[9] The outcomes were thought to be determined by the whims of the gods. The Roman goddess *Fortuna* was the patron of good luck. Games that involved an early type of dice known as *astralagi* were popular in Roman times. Such "randomizing" devices were sometimes used for divination. Therefore, it might have seemed impious to attempt to submit the frequencies of possible outcomes to mathematical analysis.

While these religious superstitions may have continued to prevail during the Middle Ages, gambling was widespread throughout Europe during that period. It can be assumed that experienced gamblers possessed certain unwritten lore about the approximate frequencies of various outcomes. However, serious discussion of any general "theory" related to gambling appears practically nonexistent before the Italian Renaissance.

By around 1500, the basic facts regarding what is now called the "fundamental probability set" for games that involved dice were probably known, at least to a few. This set consists of all the possible outcomes that can result from the throws made in the game. For example, a simple game might involve a wager that a particular point (say, obtaining a 6) would be obtained in a given number of throws. With two throws, there are 36 possible ways that the dice can fall, as shown in Table 3.1. With three throws there would be 216 (= 6 × 6 × 6).

TABLE 3.1   Possible Distinct Outcomes for Two Rolls of a Die

First Roll	Second Roll					
	1	2	3	4	5	6
1	(1,1)	(1,2)	(1,3)	(1,4)	(1,5)	(1,6)
2	(2,1)	(2,2)	(2,3)	(2,4)	(2,5)	(2,6)
3	(3,1)	(3,2)	(3,3)	(3,4)	(3,5)	(3,6)
4	(4,1)	(4,2)	(4,3)	(4,4)	(4,5)	(4,6)
5	(5,1)	(5,2)	(5,3)	(5,4)	(5,5)	(5,6)
6	(6,1)	(6,2)	(6,3)	(6,4)	(6,5)	(6,6)

To us, it is self-evident that the 36 possibilities for two dice, or 216 for three, are distinct and that each is "equally likely" in some sense. However, before there was any concept akin to probability, it was not even obvious why enumerating these 36 possibilities might be useful. For example, rolling a 1 and a 2 could be considered one distinct possibility, and rolling two 1s another. It was not obvious that obtaining a 1 and 2 was more likely than getting two 1s. So, perhaps there were really 21 possibilities to count, as displayed in Table 3.2.

Counting the number of distinct ways in which an event of interest can occur is central to the mathematical analysis of chance. For example, suppose we are betting that we will obtain a 7 as the total of points on two dice. This can occur in six different ways out of the 36 possibilities, as can be seen in Table 3.3. So, the odds against us are 30:6, or 5:1.

If we believed, on the contrary, that the 21 possible outcomes shown in Table 3.2 were equally likely, we would (incorrectly) place the odds at 18:3, or 6:1 (See Table 3.4).

The branch of mathematics that deals with such counting problems is known as *combinatorics*, because it concerns the number of ways in

TABLE 3.2   Possible Distinct Pair Values for Two Rolls

(1,1)	(1,2)	(1,3)	(1,4)	(1,5)	(1,6)
	(2,2)	(2,3)	(2,4)	(2,5)	(2,6)
		(3,3)	(3,4)	(3,5)	(3,6)
			(4,4)	(4,5)	(4,6)
				(5,5)	(5,6)
					(6,6)

TABLE 3.3   Possible Distinct Outcomes for Two Rolls in which Total = 7

First Roll	Second Roll					
	1	2	3	4	5	6
1	(1,1)	(1,2)	(1,3)	(1,4)	(1,5)	**(1,6)**
2	(2,1)	(2,2)	(2,3)	(2,4)	**(2,5)**	(2,6)
3	(3,1)	(3,2)	(3,3)	**(3,4)**	(3,5)	(3,6)
4	(4,1)	(4,2)	**(4,3)**	(4,4)	(4,5)	(4,6)
5	(5,1)	**(5,2)**	(5,3)	(5,4)	(5,5)	(5,6)
6	**(6,1)**	(6,2)	(6,3)	(6,4)	(6,5)	(6,6)

which certain things (such as the outcomes for rolls of two dice) can be combined. From what little evidence we have, it seems that some general knowledge existed that certain outcomes could happen "more easily" than others, because there were more "chances" for them to occur. However, there was apparently little awareness of how to apply this knowledge to the complex situations arising in actual games.

Even if some gamblers did possess such arcane knowledge, how would we know? On the one hand, a shrewd gamester who happened to know the correct odds would presumably keep this information to himself. Serious mathematicians, on the other hand, would ordinarily have disdained such a mundane and perhaps disreputable pastime as gambling. One flamboyant exception, however,[10] was the Italian physician and mathematician Gerolamo Cardano (1501–1576).

Born out of wedlock to a Milanese attorney, Cardano was a real rarity—a compulsive gambler and a brilliant mathematician. To top it off, he was an extraordinarily prolific writer, publishing over 100 books on topics as diverse as astrology, psychology and the occult, as well as

TABLE 3.4   Possible Distinct Pair Values for Two Rolls in which Total = 7

(1,1)	(1,2)	(1,3)	(1,4)	(1,5)	**(1,6)**
	(2,2)	(2,3)	(2,4)	**(2,5)**	(2,6)
		(3,3)	**(3,4)**	(3,5)	(3,6)
			(4,4)	(4,5)	(4,6)
				(5,5)	(5,6)
					(6,6)

mathematics, physics, and medicine. His candor about personal struggles and triumphs, which were many and exceptional, made colorful reading. He was a flawed genius who reached the pinnacle of fame and fortune, several times over, only to sink repeatedly into Lear-like tragedy, often of his own making.

One of Cardano's many treatises was *De Ludo Aleae* (*On Games of Chance*). It is thought to have been completed by around 1563 but was lost to posterity until 1663, when Cardano's collected works resurfaced in Lyon, France. This little book appears to be intended as a kind of handbook for the gamester. It is chock full of practical information, including tips on cheating and tales of Cardano's personal philosophy and exploits, along with the most sophisticated mathematical treatment of gambling prior to 1654. It provides a fascinating, if somewhat idiosyncratic, window on the kinds of games being played with dice and cards and the level of knowledge that existed. Cardano anticipated some basic mathematical results by almost a century and is acknowledged by some as the true father of probability. However, since his work was unknown until 9 years after the Pascal–Fermat discoveries, which superseded Cardano's, he had no influence on later developments.

It seems likely, though not certain, that Cardano's discoveries represent the high-water mark in thinking about the mathematics of gambling before 1654. As such, his manner of framing the questions is quite enlightening. First, it is clear that Cardano was very concerned with the question of *equity* in determining the amounts to be staked by the players. He discusses gambling in games of pure chance, games that involve a mixture of skill and chance (backgammon, card games), and games of pure skill (chess). In all these games, the critical issue is the determination of the correct *odds* to assure a fair game.

The concept of odds has a very long, if obscure, history. The basic notion is that a future event will result from a preponderance of forces, or causes, for and against its occurrence. These underlying causes translate into a number of *chances* for and against. The metaphysical concept of chances was intuitively understood. We can think of chances as the number of distinct possible ways in which the outcome of a particular situation could occur "equally easily." However, except possibly in certain games of chance, these underlying chances could never be identified or enumerated.

Calculating the odds in most practical situations was a matter of judgment. Odds were the first way of representing uncertainty *numerically*, albeit informally. They may have been used quite commonly as a figure of speech, especially to express the idea that something was not very likely. In Shakespeare's plays, the expression "ten to one" was often used to indicate an event whose occurrence would be quite doubtful, though not impossible. For example, in Henry IV, Part II we find:

We all that are engaged to this loss

Knew that we ventured on such dangerous seas

That if we wrought out life, 'twas ten to one.[11]

In a game of skill like chess, on which wagers were often made the odds would be negotiated between the two opponents. (Cardano was a master chess player who supported himself for years in this way.) To be equitable, the odds for an individual's wager would ideally reflect his chances of winning. For example, suppose that an opponent of Cardano received odds of three to one (3:1). We would automatically translate this into a probability of 1/4 that the weaker player would win. In the sixteenth century, there was no concept of probability in this sense. Rather, the weaker player was imagined to have only one "chance" against three "chances" for the master.

The odds of 3:1 would mean that out of every four games, Cardano would normally win about three and his opponent one. So, the 30 ducats staked by Cardano versus 10 for his adversary would level the playing field (or board). In four games, Cardano's expectation would be to win three times, thus gaining him 30 ducats, and to lose once, costing him 30. In this way, the odds would presumably even out the contest.

In games that involved chance, the odds must have been based upon a crude understanding of the relative frequencies of the different possible outcomes. Suppose that someone was wagering on the outcomes of three successive throws of a pair of dice. The bet would be won if a 1, 2, or 3 happened to appear on at least one die for all three of these throws. Without complex calculations based on probability theory, the chances of such an occurrence are far from obvious. It is conceivable that a regular dice-player would have acquired some approximate estimate based on experience. Remarkably, Cardano understood clearly the essential basis for calculations of fair odds in such circumstances and made considerable progress in applying this insight.

Cardano called the fundamental probability set (the set of all possible outcomes) the "circuit" and stated a general rule of wagering:

> So there is one general rule, namely, that we should consider the whole circuit and the number of those casts which represent how many ways the favorable result can occur and compare that number to the remainder of the circuit, and according to that proportion should the mutual wagers be laid so that one may contend on equal terms.[12]

He illustrates this method with the problem mentioned above. Today, we might solve this problem as follows. On a single roll of a die, the probability is 1/2 of obtaining a 1, 2, or 3, and the probability of failing is also 1/2. Therefore, with a pair of dice, the probability of failing on both is 1/4, and the probability of succeeding 3/4. To find the probability of success three times in a row, we multiply 3/4 × 3/4 × 3/4 to obtain 27/64. In terms of odds, this result can be restated as 37:27.

Cardano, of course, had no concept of mathematical probability, and attacked the problem of calculating the odds more directly. By enumeration of the "circuit" he determined that for a single cast of two dice, there are 36 possibilities. Of these, 27 contain a 1, 2, or 3 (refer to Table 3.1). He reasoned that the total circuit for all three casts must contain 36 × 36 × 36 outcomes, or 46,656. Similarly the tally of "favorable" outcomes is 27 × 27 × 27, or 19,683. Thus, the number of unfavorable outcomes is the difference between these, or 26,973. So the true odds against the desired result would be 26,973 to 19,683, or roughly 7:5.

Cardano's logic is sophisticated, but his calculation is quite cumbersome. In his biography of Cardano, mathematician Oystein Ore wondered why "in performing these calculations Cardano does not make use of the reduced form of the probability fraction but takes the cube of the numbers 27 and 36." Ore assumed that the simpler modern calculation I described above would have been evident to Cardano.[13] That Cardano did *not* take this route is revealing. From his vantage point, the "probability fraction" would have had no meaning whatsoever; his focus was exclusively on the odds. He had no way to foresee the enormous advantages that would accrue in the future, when probability would come to be expressed as a fraction. The ingenious Cardano, despite his solid grasp of combinatorial mathematics, failed to see what seems so obvious to us now.

This "paradox" is a testament to the gap between the mathematics of chance *per se* and our modern notion of probability. I mentioned previously that this modern idea entails the measurement of uncertainty in terms of a fraction between zero and one and systematically tallying outcomes to derive inductive inferences. Nothing that Cardano or any of his contemporaries (as far as we know) thought about games of chance even remotely foreshadowed these modern conceptions. Modern probability, as I have emphasized, is by no means a natural or inevitable vehicle for reasoning about uncertainty.

A half-century later, the great Galileo Galilei (1564–1642) wrote on the mathematics of gambling, revealing that no advances had been made. Galileo had reluctantly agreed to indulge his patron, the Grand Duke of Tuscany, by penning some *Thoughts about Dice Games*.[14] This short essay suggests that the basic facts regarding the fundamental probability set were known, but little else. Galileo begins by describing the common misconception about how to count equally likely cases. He observes that in rolling three dice, a total of 9 or 12 "can be made up in as many ways" as a 10 or 11. Each can be composed in six different ways. For instance, one way that a 9 can occur is by getting a 1, 2, and 6 in any order. Thus, the six ways to obtain a 9 in total are (1,2,6), (1,3,5), (1,4,4), (2,3,4), (2,2,5), (3,3,3). A 10 can occur as (1,3,6), (1,4,5), (2,2,6), (2,3,5), (2,4,4), (3,3,4). This might lead one to infer that a 9, for example, is "of equal utility" to a 10. However, it is known "that long observation has made dice-players consider 10 and 11 more advantageous than 9 and 12."

Galileo then proceeds to spell out clearly the correct analysis, noting that for two dice there are 36 different possibilities and for three dice there are 216. Galileo explains in pedantic detail why we must consider all 216 possible "throws" as distinct:

> I will begin by considering how, when a die has six faces, and when thrown it can equally well fall on any one of these, only six throws can be made with it, each different from all the others. But if together with the first die we throw a second, which also has six faces, we can make 36 throws each different from all

the others, since each face of the first can be combined with each of the second, and in consequence can make six different throws, whence it is clear that such combinations are 6 times 6, i.e., 36. And if we add a third die, since each one of its six faces can be combined with each one of the 36 combinations of the other two dice we shall find that the combinations of three dice is 6 times 36, i.e. 216, each different from the others.

He then demonstrates how 27 of these 216 chances can result in a 10 (or an 11), but only 25 can result in a 9 (or a 12).

Galileo had no real interest in the mathematics of gambling and never pursued this topic seriously. Despite his broad and profound interest in scientific matters, his knowledge about the mathematics of gambling actually fell short of Cardano's 50 years earlier. (Of course, Cardano had a much more practical motivation to pursue this subject.) Like Cardano, Galileo failed to perceive any connection between games of chance and problems of science or commerce.

THE FAMOUS CORRESPONDENCE

When Pascal and Fermat began their momentous correspondence, the main problem of interest in games of chance was how to determine the correct odds. The odds were conceived as the ratio of the number of chances for the players. If two opponents started out on equal terms, the odds would technically be "one-to-one" (1:1), although this situation might be described colloquially as an "even chance," an "even lay," or even as the oxymoronic "even odds." So, if the total amount staked on the outcome of a game was 1000 pounds, say, each player would stake 500.

If the players did not start out on an equal footing, the odds would be established based on the ratio of chances that was believed to exist. Suppose that Peter was betting against Paul that a number less than 4 (i.e., 1, 2, or 3) would be obtained on each of three tosses of a pair of dice. I explained above that the correct odds against achieving this result would be 37:27. So a fair bet would entail a stake of 27 ducats from Peter and 37 from Paul. However, the odds would have been based on the gamblers' personal acumen and experience rather than such a mathematical analysis.

Breaking the Symmetry Barrier

Before 1654, the only theoretical method of determining odds was based on enumerating the favorable and unfavorable outcomes that could occur. Each of these outcomes was deemed equally likely to occur because of the *symmetry* of the gambling apparatus. That is, there was no reason to expect one particular outcome more than any of the others. So, in principle, it would have been possible to calculate the odds by applying Cardano's "general rule of wagering." However, this approach was severely limited; it could only be applied in games with a fixed number of "trials" (e.g., rolls of a die) specified in advance.

In some games, the actual duration of play (number of trials) could depend on when in a series of trials some particular event happened to occur. The game would continue only until the event occurred, which might happen before the stated maximum possible number of throws was reached. For example, a player might bet that with eight potential throws, a 6 would come up. What are the odds that the player would "make the point" specified? In this case, the 6 could occur on any of the trials, and the game would be terminated. So, the outcomes (winning on trial 1, winning on trial 2, etc.) were not symmetrical. It was obvious, for example, that a priori the outcome of winning on the first throw was more likely than winning on the eighth throw (which might never be reached).

Such a problem could not be solved straightforwardly by enumeration of equally likely possibilities. However, it could be attacked indirectly by first considering the reverse problem—finding the number of possible ways of *failing* to make the point. Then this number could be subtracted from the total number of chances. The resulting odds turn out to be approximately 77:23 in favor of the player. So, for a wager in which the total pot would be 100 coins, the player betting on this outcome would theoretically stake 77 coins against his opponent's 23.

The cagey Cardano never mentioned this clever stratagem and was apparently unaware of it. However, in the first extant letter from Fermat to Pascal, it is clear that the two Frenchmen have previously considered this very problem. Fermat clears up a subtle issue that has apparently confused Pascal, and the discussion then turns to the "problem of the points." The various convoluted and clever ways they develop to solve this age-old puzzle reveal just how far we have come, both conceptually and mathematically.

Their methods were much more complicated than ours, because the theory of mathematical probability did not yet exist. Indeed, differential and integral calculus did not yet exist. Thus, it required two mathematical geniuses to work out solutions from first principles. In this light, their methods were extremely clever, although not depending on any advanced mathematics. For readers interested in a more complete understanding of these solutions, I have included more detail in the Appendix. This material provides deeper insight into the intellectual breakthrough they achieved.

The Interrupted Game

The bulk of the correspondence between Pascal and Fermat concerned the *problem of the points*. Suppose that two equally matched opponents enter a contest that consists of a series of individual games. For example, a game might be as complex as a chess game or as simple as heads-or-tales with a fair coin. A point is awarded for each game won. The stakes are set equal, and the first player to win a given number of points collects the entire amount staked by both parties.

Now imagine that the match is interrupted at some stage, and the players wish to divide the stakes in a fair manner. If each player has won the same number of points, there is no problem; the stakes are divided equally. However, suppose that one player is ahead at the time. How should the stakes be divided? This conundrum, known as the problem of the points, or the *division problem*, had been rattling around for a very long time before it was finally solved by Pascal and Fermat.

The problem was mentioned by Luca Pacioli (1446–1517), the originator of double-entry bookkeeping, in his textbook in 1494.[15] Pacioli proposed to divide the stakes in proportion to the number of games previously won by each player. For example, if I had won two games and you had won three, I would receive 2/5 of the pot. Tallying up past successes in this manner certainly seems to fit the mindset of an accountant, but is clearly unsatisfactory.

The problem was pointed out by Niccolo Tartaglia (1500?–1557), a one-time nemesis of Cardano, a few decades later. He observed that if discontinuation occurred after a single game, the entire pot would go to the winner, which seemed unfair. Tartaglia believed that the division should depend on how close each competitor was to the goal. This was insightful (and essentially correct), but his specific proposal turned out to be somewhat arbitrary. Tartaglia later conceded that his method was flawed, and he expressed doubt that a definitive answer was even possible. Cardano also tilted at this windmill without success.

By 1654, it was generally conceded that the division of stakes should reflect the relative *expectations* of the contestants at the point when the match was broken off. How much was each player's position at that moment *worth?* To answer this question, it was necessary to determine the true odds at that point. The expectation of each player should be proportionate to these odds. But at the time, the only known way to calculate odds (and hence expectations) depended on enumeration of favorable and unfavorable equally possible outcomes. The problem then was either to translate the problem into an equivalent one in which a set of symmetrical (equally likely) outcomes could be specified or to find an alternative approach based on some other reasonable principle.

I have explained in the Appendix how Pascal and Fermat successfully pursued both of these strategies. In different ways, their solutions both foreshadowed and laid the groundwork for subsequent developments. Pascal's approach, and one of Fermat's two methods, essentially divided the total expectation into component parts that could be evaluated separately. The total could then be obtained by summing up the expectations for the parts. Implicit in these approaches was what would soon after be defined as a *mathematical expectation*. Both methods broke new ground in moving beyond Cardano's general rule, which could only deal with situations that involved a fixed number of equally likely cases.

One of Fermat's methods, however, managed to extend the equally likely case approach to deal with the division problem. In a practical sense, his method was less general than the other two, but also more insightful:

> Fermat's approach is undoubtedly more pedestrian, requiring only that you list all possibilities and then simply count them. But by penetrating to the heart of the problem and doing *just what is required* to get the answer, Fermat's approach shows true genius.[16]

Not only did Fermat discover a clever trick to obtain a simple solution, but he also achieved a remarkable *conceptual* breakthrough that ultimately became the foundation of mathematical probability.

Fermat realized that the player's expectation depended on the *fraction of chances* favoring a particular event (e.g., obtaining a given number of points). However, he perceived that these future chances were hypothetical. The game might *actually* be stopped at any time, and for any reason. But the stopping rule (whatever it might be) was irrelevant to the a priori chances. Thus, he suggested, we must count chances *as if* any of the possible future cases might occur.

This may seem paradoxical, but as we shall see, it is in fact the essential basis of mathematical probability. For example, suppose we are tossing two coins, each of which can land on heads (H) or tails (T). You will win the game as soon as H appears, and lose if H does not occur on either toss. There are four equally likely cases a priori: HH, HT, TH, TT. Therefore, prior to playing, you have three chances out of four to win, despite the fact that HH can never actually occur!

Fermat's thought-process seems to have been something like the following. The player might win either on toss 1 or on toss 2. A priori, he has one chance in two of winning on coin 1, and one chance in four of winning on coin 2. However, one chance out of two is mathematically equivalent to two chances out of four. So, his total expectation must be just the same as if he has three chances out of four. In effect, he is reducing the two possibilities to a "common denominator."

Fermat must have realized that this logic could be generalized to solve the problem of the points. In our simple example, two tosses at most would be needed to determine the outcome. In general, it would be necessary to determine the maximum duration of the game (number of trials) necessary to settle the outcome. Then all possible sequences (chances) of this duration could be listed. The winner corresponding to each sequence could easily be determined and each player's number of chances counted. It took a bit of convincing by Fermat to win Pascal over to this strange idea of hypothetical chances. Even today, this metaphorical concept strikes me as a bit enigmatic, but it is important to realize that our "obvious" ideas about probability depend on it.

WHAT DID NOT HAPPEN NEXT

As mentioned earlier, Pascal turned away from mathematics, except for a few short interludes. Religious philosophy had throughout his adult life held a strong competing attraction for him. On November 23, 1654, after a traumatic incident involving a harrowing carriage ride in which run-away horses nearly killed him, he experienced a mystical awakening that resolved this internal battle. Henceforth, he would devote himself entirely to asceticism and to the defense of Jansenist philosophy.

Like everything else about Blaise Pascal, his epiphany was far from ordinary, and it resulted in some classic philosophical writing.[17] In 1656, he published *Provincial Letters*, in which he defended the Jansenist views of Antoine Arnaud (1612–1694), who was then being persecuted by orthodox Catholicism and the Jesuits. Arnaud was the leader of the Port-Royal monastery, a Jansenist hotbed in the suburbs of Paris, and a close friend of Pascal. Some of the philosophical issues in the controversy between Port-Royal and the Church involved moral behavior under uncertainty. The idea of probability (i.e., prove-ability) was central to the debate. The Jansenists were strongly opposed to the use of arguments based on probability as a justification for liberalized religious practices.

In 1662, the year in which Pascal died, Arnaud and Pierre Nicole (1625–1695) published a treatise called in Latin the *Ars Cogitandi*, but known widely as the Port-Royal *Logic, or the Art of Thinking*.[18] This work is sometimes cited as the first book to deal quantitatively with "probability" as a quantitative measure of uncertainty. It contains little that we would recognize as formal probabilistic analysis, although Pascal is thought to have advised Arnaud. It does, however, include prudent advice about weighing the probability along with the potential consequences. For example, Arnaud and Nicole admonish us not to overreact to frightening possibilities that have only a remote chance of occurrence, such as being struck and killed by lightning.

In the spiritual sphere, a similar idea presented in the *Logic* is Pascal's Wager. Pascal offers a logical rationale for belief. He imagines that in deciding whether or not to be devout, one is wagering whether or not God exists. He points out that in betting that God exists, a person risks only a finite amount of inconvenience and discomfort, but stands to gain "an infinity of infinitely happy life" if God does exist. Thus, regardless of the perceived odds against the proposition of divine existence, one cannot (rationally) refuse to bet that God does exist.

It is sometimes suggested that Pascal's famous wager was an early example of the use of mathematical probability in our modern sense. Pascal may have been making a gambling analogy, but the nascent mathematics of chance had not yet been connected to the idea of probability. The *Logic* did not refer to any concept of probability that entailed *measuring* a degree of uncertainty as a number. Nor did it suggest making inductive inferences by counting the number or rate of actual past events, except in the traditional sense that observed frequencies could provide some relevant information to be considered in some unspecified manner.

It seems that the mathematics of gambling and matters of belief occupied two different, and even competing, compartments in Pascal's mind. At most, games provided him with a metaphor for the operations of chance but had no direct application to the practical or philosophical challenges posed by uncertainty. As mentioned above, probability was associated at the time with legal or moral questions that involved the careful weighing of arguments.

Ironically, this connotation may have militated against any usage of the term in relation to gambling. After all, Pascal was a strong opponent of what he considered the abuses of probabilism to justify immoral behavior. So, even had his life not been cut short at the age of 39, it is doubtful that Pascal would have pioneered a new concept of probability that linked uncertainty and empirical frequencies or was in any way connected with games of chance. That development would not occur for another couple of decades.

As for the mathematics of chance itself, we know of only one brief foray back to the issues of the famous correspondence. Sometime in 1656, Pascal wrote to Fermat, challenging him to solve a problem he believed was even more difficult than the problem of points.[19] This problem was a special case of what has come to be known as the "gambler's ruin" problem. Fermat returned the correct answer forthwith, but (of course) without any discussion of his method.

There is no other evidence of any interest in such matters on Pascal's part after 1654. In 1660, Fermat found himself in the vicinity of Paris and wrote to Pascal to propose a meeting, but Pascal declined, mentioning his ill-health. The two never actually met in person, and we can only wonder what more would have been accomplished had they been able to spend some time together.

As for Fermat, there is no evidence that he pursued the study of gambling problems any further on his own initiative. He did, however, respond to several inquiries from others who had become interested in these matters. Indirectly, as we will see, he played a role in the future development of probability. However, Fermat was basically reactive, and did not engage in any efforts to extend the methods systematically. He also did not try to link the purely mathematical exercises to any broader problems of real-world uncertainty. In his avocation as a mathematician, Fermat would gladly rise to the bait of solving a difficult puzzle posed to him, but for him it was merely a hobby. In her biographical sketch of Fermat, F. N. David, statistician and historian, perhaps summed up his contribution best:

> For although Fermat, if provoked, could have done as much and more than his successors, yet the fact remains that his contribution was in effect the extension of the idea of the exhaustive enumeration of the fundamental probability set, which had already been given by Galileo.[20]

Presumably, he was never "provoked" by anyone in his own time.

The Pascal–Fermat correspondence is generally considered to be the initial step in the formulation, or discovery, of mathematical probability. However, there is nothing in the Pascal–Fermat letters that comes close to the notion of probability in the modern sense. Neither is there any mention that observations can provide the raw material for inductive inference. Indeed, the idea of verifying their mathematical results by performing experiments apparently never occurred to them. I would submit that seeking an explanation for the emergence of probability around 1660 is barking up the wrong tree. Fermat may have grasped the essence of mathematical probability, but like Cardano, he was an isolated figure who did not directly influence the future course of events.

What did emerge in 1654 was a quantum leap in technical sophistication regarding the mathematics of gambling. In effect, Pascal and Fermat had effectively introduced the concept of a *mathematical expectation*, although they did not employ this term. Within a few years, this powerful new idea would turn out to be a critical way station on the road toward mathematical probability.

Why did this important step occur at this juncture and not before? I do not believe that any deep philosophical or historical explanations are necessary. Prior to this point, it seems that circumstances in which serious mathematicians had occasion to think much about games of chance were literally few and far between. So, there was no critical mass of talent and interest trained in this direction. Finally, in France in 1654, the circumstances were propitious.

At least one serious gambler, Antoine Gombaud, aka the Chevalier de Méré, had considerable mathematical ability and was well acquainted with several of France's finest mathematicians. Such a confluence of motivation and talent to address the problems raised by games of chance was probably unprecedented. What a perfect example of the fortuitous meeting of great minds with fertile conditions described so well by Malcolm Gladwell as an *outlier!*[21]

However, by itself, the technical breakthrough achieved by the group was far from sufficient to bring about probability as we know it. In fact, with the notable exception of Jacob Bernoulli, no one had a well-elaborated conception of quantitative degrees of belief until about a century later. It is by no means obvious that the events of 1654 would inevitably have led to the ideas of probability as a measure of belief or as an idealized frequency of occurrence. Indeed, except for a fortuitous occurrence, the breakthroughs that occurred in France that year might have become a mere historical footnote, much like the earlier efforts of Cardano and Galileo.

AGAINST THE ODDS

By the end of 1654, the smoldering embers of the mathematics of gambling were perilously close to dying out. Nowhere outside of France had any similar advances been made. In France, neither Pascal nor Fermat had any great desire to pursue these matters further. The handful of other mathematicians with any knowledge of their correspondence lacked the ability to carry it forward. Things did not look promising for the fledgling calculus of chance when something truly remarkable transpired. *Mirabile dictu*, perhaps the only man in Europe capable of appreciating and extending what Pascal and Fermat had begun just happened to be passing through Paris the very next summer. What are the odds?

A Fateful Journey

In July 1655, Christiaan Huygens (1629–1695) was traveling back to his home in The Hague in the company of his younger brother Ludwig (1631–1699) and a cousin.[22] The three were returning from the Protestant University at Angers, where they had all received law degrees. Christiaan, then 26 years of age and Ludwig, just 24, were scions of a powerful Dutch family. Their father was a political leader of the Dutch Republic and their mother a member of one of the most distinguished families in the Netherlands. The two brothers had been bred to play prominent roles in the halls of power and society, and were being trained accordingly. A few months in the City of Light would have been considered a valuable educational experience.

Christiaan Huygens would go on to an illustrious career in scientific research. He would become famous throughout Europe for his many contributions to physical science. These include the invention of the pendulum clock and substantial improvements in the design of telescopes, in addition to numerous theoretical discoveries. He would spend much of his life in France, under Royal auspices and with the full financial support of Louis XIV. He would become a founding member of the French Academy of Sciences and one of the earliest members of the Royal Society of London. This fame was achieved despite Huygens's notorious lack of interest in self-promotion; he rarely published his research, except when prodded by others, and could afford the luxury of pursuing his intellectual interests on his own terms.

When he reached Paris in 1655, however, all this still lay in the future. As part of his broad educational background, Christiaan had spent some time as a student of the mathematician Frans van Schooten (1615–1660), with whom he had developed a close relationship. By all accounts, van Schooten was quite personable as well as a talented teacher and had attracted a wide circle of students and disciples from among the Dutch nobility. He was a follower of René Descartes and successfully expounded Cartesian methods in his teaching and publications.

Huygens was able to establish contact with leading French intellectuals, including Pascal's friend Pierre de Carcavi. Through Carcavi he became friendly with two other geometers, Claude Mylon (1618–1660) and Gilles Roberval (1602–1675). He learned of the Pascal–Fermat correspondence and attempted unsuccessfully to contact Pascal, who was then in retreat at Port-Royal. Fermat was several days' journey away in Toulouse. Through Mylon and Roberval, Huygens became aware of the mathematical problems solved by Pascal and Fermat but was apparently unable to obtain much information about their methods.

When he returned to Holland in late 1655, Huygens mounted his own attack on problems related to games of chance. By April 1656 he had produced a small treatise called *De Ratiociniis in Ludo Aleae* (*On Reasoning in Games of Chance*). This work presented his solution to the problem of points and several other gambling-related problems. Huygens submitted this work to van Schooten, who responded in short order that the tract should be published. In fact, he offered to append it to a textbook that he was writing. Huygens would of course receive full credit for this work.

Meanwhile, Huygens was seeking validation of his methods in other quarters as well. On April 18, 1656 he wrote to Roberval, sending him one of the most difficult problems he had solved and asking for Roberval's solution to compare it with his own. When he had received no reply after some time, he wrote to Mylon, posing the same problem and some additional ones. Mylon's responses were partly wrong and not very helpful. At some point, the problem Huygens had posed to Roberval and Mylon must have made its way to Toulouse, because on June 22, Carcavi sent back Fermat's correct answer. True to form, Fermat had not revealed his method of solution.

Huygens must have been relieved to learn that Fermat's answer matched his own, though frustrated that Fermat had not explained how he had arrived at this answer. Fermat also included several problems of his own for Huygens to attempt. These the young man was able to solve in a single afternoon, whereupon he sent back his answers on July 6 to Carcavi, for transmission to Mylon, Pascal, and Fermat. Anxiously awaiting confirmation of his success, he wrote to Roberval on July 27, asking why he had received no reply. Finally, in October he heard back from Carcavi, who related that Huygens had indeed used the same approach as Pascal. Carcavi also forwarded on the "gambler's ruin" problem that Pascal had sent to Fermat, along with Fermat's solution.

Meanwhile, the printing of van Schooten's textbook was proceeding at a snail's pace. At last, it was completed in August 1657 and Huygens's little treatise quickly became a great success. For the next 50 years, it remained the primary source and standard for learning about the "calculus of chance." Huygens himself had little time to spare for the subject, and returned to it only sporadically, but the book was widely circulated throughout Europe. It was also incorporated with commentary in works of several others and was translated into English twice, in 1692 and 1714. In a real sense, Huygens and van Schooten kept alive the developments of 1654. Had Huygens not been passing through Paris, and had van Schooten not encouraged and published his work, who knows whether the Pascal–Fermat breakthroughs would eventually have surfaced, and if so, when?

Reasoning in Games of Chance

It is clear from his foreword to the treatise that Huygens suspected he might be onto something big: "I would like to believe that in considering these matters closely, the reader will soon understand that I do not treat here a simple game of chance but that I have thrown out the elements of a new theory, both deep and interesting."[23] He hastened to pay his respects to Pascal and Fermat and to justify his effort on a matter that might be deemed frivolous:

> It should be said, also, that for some time some of the best mathematicians of France have occupied themselves with this kind of calculus so that no one should attribute to me the honor of the first invention. This does not belong to me. But these savants, although they put each other to the test by proposing to each other many questions difficult to solve, have hidden their methods. I have had therefore to examine and to go deeply for myself into this matter by beginning with the elements, and it is impossible for this reason to affirm that I have even started from the same principle.

To say the French mathematicians had "hidden their methods" may have been a bit strong, but in Fermat's case quite understandable.

The treatise proper begins with a set of 14 "propositions" that Huygens intends to prove. The first proposition establishes the idea of the mathematical expectation; it is an explicit version of Pascal's guiding principle. It simply states: "To have equal chances of getting a and b is worth $(a + b)/2$." His justification is essentially identical to Pascal's, but stated somewhat differently. Suppose I hold in one hand three coins and in the

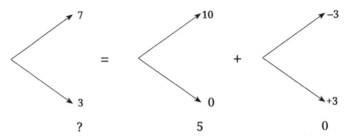

FIGURE 3.1   Illustration of the Huygens rationale for the mathematical expectation. The value of a gamble with possible outcomes 7 and 3 equaled the sum of two bets whose values were known based on previously established principles.

other seven coins, both amounts hidden from you. You can choose either hand and receive its contents. Huygens proved that the value of this gamble must be five coins.

He began by reasoning that a person who had five coins could exchange this amount for an equal chance of losing the five or winning an additional five. If he won, he would have 10 and if he lost, none. However, suppose that in addition to the original bet, the person could also make a side bet of three coins that he would lose the first bet. In that case, he would end up with either seven coins (= 10 − 3) or three coins (= 0 + 3). The situation is illustrated in Figure 3.1. Since this "hedging" bet clearly has an expected value of zero, it adds nothing to the expectation of five from the original wager. So, the total effect of both wagers must be worth five coins. Therefore, the expectation of the original wager must be the sum of the two fair bets, which equals five coins. Q.E.D.

Note that Huygens's proposition is today considered the *definition* of a mathematical expectation in this simple situation of two equal chances; we simply take the average of the two possible outcomes. More generally, if there are multiple possible outcomes and various values associated with each, the expectation is a weighted average of the different outcome values, the weights being what we now call probabilities. This, in essence, is Huygens's definition as well. However, Huygens's discussion is couched in terms of odds and expectations. Therefore, he must offer an elaborate justification for the fundamental proposition that the mathematical average of two equally likely outcomes can be interpreted as an expectation.

Huygens goes on to generalize this key result to the situation with multiple possible outcomes, and to the case of unequal numbers of chances to obtain the different prizes. On this foundation, he then proceeds to prove each of his 14 propositions. Finally, he proposes five additional problems that require extensions of the methods he has demonstrated. These "challenge" problems are presented without proof, although the solutions are provided in an appendix. He states candidly his reasons for setting forth the challenge problems similar to those posed by the French mathematicians.

> You will find at the end of this treatise that I have proposed some questions of the same kind without indicating the method of proof. This is in the first place because I think it would cost me too much work to expand succinctly the reasoning leading to the answer, and in the second place because it seems useful to me to leave something for my readers to think about (if I have any readers) and this will serve them both as an exercise and as a way of passing the time.

The five unsolved problems at the end proved a great stimulus for various alternative solutions and extensions by other leading mathematicians, intrigued by the challenge. I should mention that three of these problems were among the ones that Fermat had sent Huygens the previous year. In this way, Fermat indirectly played an important role in spreading the ideas that he and Pascal had pioneered.

In one sense, Huygens (with the help of van Schooten) was merely the conduit for transmitting these new ideas. However, his explicit formulation and generalization of the concept of mathematical expectation was a major advance. Most important, this expectation is *additive*. Consider a set of several events, of which only one will occur. The additive property means that the expectation of obtaining at least one of these events is equal to the sum of their individual expectations. This property is the critical element that facilitated the solution of many complicated mathematical problems. Indeed, this additive property is one of the axioms that define mathematical probability.[24]

Pascal and Fermat were the first to perceive how a complex problem, like the problem of points, could be resolved into several simpler problems. This insight led to ways of calculating a total expectation by adding up component parts. By formalizing the mathematical expectation as his core principle, Huygens completed this important step. However, he did not take the further step of abstracting a notion of mathematical *probability*. This may seem rather strange to us, for whom expectation seems less natural than probability, but this reaction depends on hindsight.

For Huygens, the goal was to calculate an expectation (fair share) and the implied odds associated with this expectation. His treatise contains no discussion of the *fraction* of favorable chances among all chances or the *fraction* of the total stakes that the expectation represents. With Huygens we remain firmly within the narrow realm of fair division of stakes in gambling situations. Despite his suggestion of "a new theory, both deep and interesting," there is no evidence of any idea of probability as a measure of certainty, or of an observed frequency as a way to estimate probability. Indeed, it would be another century before our modern notion of probability had fully solidified.

CHAPTER 4

HARDLY TOUCHED UPON

In the 1680s, leading mathematicians were preoccupied mainly with the new infinitesimal calculus originated by Isaac Newton and Gottfried Leibniz. The mathematics of chance was at the periphery of attention, and Huygens's little treatise was just about all that existed on the subject. After its publication in 1657, it rode the coattails of van Schooten's popular textbook all over Europe, and became a standard in its own right. Over the course of the next 50 years, it was virtually unique as a reference on the calculus of chance. During this period, there was little advancement of Huygens's ideas, with one notable exception. Jacob Bernoulli was the only person to progress substantially beyond his French and Dutch predecessors in developing the mathematics of chance.

Regrettably, Bernoulli chose not to publicize his work, and was eventually overtaken by illness and death. So his technical and philosophical achievements were not revealed until much later. Pierre Raymond de Montmort (1678–1719), learned of Jacob Benoulli's efforts from several eulogies given after his death in 1705. Based on this limited information, Montmort successfully undertook to extend Huygens's results.[1] His groundbreaking *Essay D'Analyse sur les Jeux de Hazard* (Analytic Essay on Games of Chance) was published in 1708. In an "advertisement" for the

Willful Ignorance: The Mismeasure of Uncertainty, First Edition. Herbert I. Weisberg.
© 2014 John Wiley & Sons, Inc. Published 2014 by John Wiley & Sons, Inc.

second edition in 1713, just as Bernoulli's work was finally destined to see the light of day, Montmort explained that the mathematics of chance was "a matter hardly touched upon, and entirely forgotten for 60 years."

Montmort went on to recount a brief history of the scattered developments since 1654, noting presciently that these would have "some relation to the History of Mathematics, of which the calculus of probabilities & of chances is going perhaps to become a considerable part." It is interesting that Montmort refers here to the "calculus of probabilities & of chances," although it is not clear exactly in what sense Montmort was using the word probability. His mathematical development referred to the traditional concepts of odds, chances, and expectations. On the other hand, he was aware that Jacob Bernoulli had devised some sort of "calculus" for dealing with epistemic probabilities, although he knew nothing of the details.

It is common lore that modern probability and statistical thinking burst upon the scene almost fully formed in the wake of the Pascal–Fermat correspondence. According to this view, the time was ripe for a version of mathematical probability that had a dual aspect.[2] One aspect was epistemic, reflecting the sense of a degree of belief. The other aspect related to empirical frequencies, as manifested in games of chance and certain statistical regularities in nature and society. This new probability, so the tale is told, then quickly assumed its rightful place as the dominant logic of uncertainty.

This rendition may seem plausible in hindsight, but fails to square with the known facts. The merging of qualitative probability with the combinatorial mathematics in games of chance to form mathematical probability required another century to complete. If modern mathematical probability had truly emerged around 1660, where is the evidence for its existence? The remainder of this chapter will survey what actually transpired in the decades following the Pascal–Fermat correspondence. The historical record may, of course, be incomplete, but Montmort's account in 1713 suggests that he was probably aware of just about everything that contributed to the mainstream of mathematical and philosophical thinking. If so, he was right to imply that the implications of the breakthroughs in 1654 had been essentially ignored.

Why did mathematical probability not quickly develop at this juncture? This often-asked question assumes there are strong reasons to expect that it *should* have. However, if we look closely at the existing situation, we find that the invention of modern probability was still far from preordained. Although, some of the pieces were available, the necessary and sufficient conditions to assemble them into probability were not in place.

There are three main ideas that have been subsumed in what we generally regard today under the heading of probability. First, probability is assumed to obey certain *mathematical rules* that are illustrated in their purest form by games of chance. Second, *statistical regularities* observed in natural and social phenomena are regarded as examples of probability in action. Third, probability reflects in some sense a *degree of belief* or measure of certainty. As we will see, these three tributaries of modern probability were flowing along various separate paths during the last half of the seventeenth century. They had barely begun to coalesce to form the coherent theory of probability that we recognize today. By reviewing comprehensively what actually happened during this period, we can understand better why mathematical probability was not yet ready to appear on the scene.

THE MATHEMATICS OF CHANCE

With respect to combinatorial mathematics, Pascal's *Treatise on the Arithmetical Triangle* was the premier exposition. It was published in 1665, 3 years after Pascal's death, but was not widely distributed, in part because it was written in French and was not translated into Latin. Furthermore, Pascal's treatise was really an exercise in theoretical mathematics, and only tangentially related to chance phenomena in a gambling context. So, Pascal's ideas about the mathematics of chance lived on mainly through Huygens's treatise.

Huygens himself displayed little interest in the mathematics of chance after 1657. His vast correspondence, which was preserved and eventually published, contains very little on the subject. There is some correspondence with his friend Johan Hudde (1628–1704), the political leader of Amsterdam in 1665. Huygens also received a letter sent by the French mathematician, Bernard Frenicle de Bessey (1605–1675) in 1665, and a handful of letters about various card games in 1679 and 1688. This meager record suggests that Huygens had for the most part moved on from his early interest in games of chance.

Juan Caramuel

The next point at which Huygens's influence is known to have surfaced was in a 1670 publication, *Mathesis Biceps*, by a Catholic Bishop with the unlikely moniker of Juan Caramuel Lobkowitz.[3] Caramuel (1606–1682) was born in Madrid to an engineer from Luxembourg and an aristocratic mother from Bohemia. I think of him as a cross between Gerolamo Cardano and Gottfried Leibniz. He authored over 100 books on a great variety of subjects, and achieved fluency in over 20 languages. He became a controversial figure because of his outspoken defense of sometimes unpopular views, and experienced many personal highs and lows. He was greatly admired by some for his heroism and integrity, and loathed by others, including Blaise Pascal, for his liberal religious views.

Rather like Cardano, the indefatigable Caramuel was audacious to the point of recklessness. While living in Prague in 1648, Caramuel organized and led a battalion of clergy to help defend the city from an attack by the Swedes. For his efforts, he was decorated by the Holy Roman Emperor. Besides his organizational skill, Caramuel's expertise in military architecture proved especially useful. In 1655, at great personal peril, he ministered to many victims of a plague outbreak and supervised the arrangements for numerous burials. In 1663, after having support for his controversial publications withdrawn by his patron, the Pope, Caramuel set up a printing press of his own. He even produced a treatise on the art of printing to describe the innovative methods he had devised. Given his penchant for risky enterprises, it is remarkable that Caramuel managed to attain the ripe age of 76.

Caramuel's *Mathesis Biceps* covered many mathematical topics, including number theory, mathematical puzzles (which since the age of 10 he had loved to compose and solve), and games of chance. His treatment of the latter consisted primarily of a reprinting of Huygens's *De Ratiociniis in Ludo Aleae* along with some minor elaboration. Caramuel, like others at the time, saw no connection between the mathematics of chance and the traditional concept of probability as a measure of probity or prove-ability.

Joseph Sauveur

The next work related to the mathematics of games of chance was an article in the *Journal des Sçavans* in 1679 by French mathematician Joseph

Sauveur (1653–1716), who later became famous for pioneering the science of acoustics.[4] This journal was the first academic publication in Europe, initiated in 1665. In 1678, Sauveur was asked by the Marquis de Dangeau to calculate the advantage to the "banker" in a very popular card game of the day known as Bassette. It seems that Bassette was all the rage at that time in the capitals of Europe, and had become the source of some heated disputes occasioned by the wild swings of fortune involved.

Sauveur's analysis generated several formulas but did not include the methods he had used to obtain these. Presumably, his work was influenced by Christiaan Huygens, who was residing in Paris in 1679 and had written about card games that year, as mentioned previously. An introduction to the article in the *Journal des Sçavans* mentions that:

> There is place to believe that he is not being deceived in the computation of the tables which he gives, because the first three correspond to three of those rules that Mr. Huygens has taken the pain to calculate, & of which he has given the foundation as well as some others which regard the games of chance, in the Treatise which he has published formerly on these matters.

Apparently, Sauveur's analysis caused quite a stir, and he was even invited by Louis XIV to present his theory to the French court.

Jacob Bernoulli

Six years later, the *Journal des Sçavans* carried its next item pertaining to the games of chance.[5] In the issue of August 26, 1685, Jacob Bernoulli presented a pair of challenge problems. At this point Bernoulli was not yet famous, and had held the position of lecturer in experimental physics for just 2 years at the University of Basel. He was introduced in the journal as "M. Bernoulli, mathematician of the city of Basel." For each of the following two games, Bernoulli asked for the ratio of expectations for the two players.

> A and B play with a die on the condition that the one who throws the first 1 will have won. A throws once, then B once, after which A throws two times in a row, then B two times in a row, then A three times in a row, then B three times. Or, alternately, A throws once, then B throws twice, in a row, then A three times in a row, then B four times in a row, etc., until one of them wins.

These problems are easy enough to formulate, but devilishly hard to solve, especially with the limited mathematical tools available at that time. The fact that Jacob presumably knew the answer in 1685 testifies to his superior knowledge of the mathematics of games, even at this early stage of his investigations. Indeed, for 5 years no one else responded to his challenge! Bernoulli himself finally published the solutions in 1690.

At various points between 1685 and 1692, Bernoulli gave hints of his many discoveries in his lectures.[6] In September 1685, he published a list of theses to be defended at the University of Basel. In such an exercise, a scholar would defend a set of propositions and address the criticisms and questions posed by a respondent. This form of disputation was a traditional way to advance one's candidacy for professorships that might fall open or to showcase the accomplishments of a student, who would serve as the respondent. In the September 1685 event, his precocious brother (and student) Johann, who had turned 18 in July, was the respondent. The theses included several that related to the mathematics of games of chance.

From Bernoulli's *Meditationes*, his private journal, we know that by 1689 he had moved far beyond Huygens. What remains unclear is the extent to which he shared his knowledge with other mathematicians. Before 1690, Jacob had undoubtedly related some of his discoveries to his brother Johann, who had become a close collaborator. However, by the early 1690s this filial relationship had begun to sour, as competitive jealousies flared. Jacob was not ready to reveal all the knowledge he had privately derived, although some bits and pieces must have filtered out through his lectures.

Thomas Strode

In addition to the few contributions to the mathematics of chance I have catalogued so far, there were several works related to combinatorics. However, with the exception of Jacob Bernoulli's private research, recorded in his *Meditations*, these advanced little beyond what was already known by Cardano and Galileo. Only Pascal's *Treatise on the Arithmetical Triangle* reflected a substantially higher level of development than previous work on combinatorial theory.

A minor exception was a treatise published in England by Thomas Strode in 1678.[7] Strode (1626–1699) managed to solve the problem of calculating the number of ways in which any specified total score could be achieved when rolling any given number of dice. For example, in how many ways could a total of 14 points be obtained when rolling three dice? However, rather than restricting consideration to actual six-faced dice, he generalized to deal with hypothetical dice that could have any number of sides.

Two Scottish Refugees: John Arbuthnot and David Gregory

The last significant contribution to the literature on the mathematics of gambling prior to Montmort's first edition in 1708 is the most intriguing.[8] It was written anonymously, and is usually attributed to John Arbuthnot (1667–1735), born in Aberdeen, Scotland. Around 1691, Arbuthnot emigrated from Scotland to London in order to escape a difficult religious and political climate, and to complete his education. Arbuthnot would eventually achieve celebrity as both a medical doctor and a political satirist. In the former capacity, he would become the personal physician of Queen Anne from 1705 until she died in 1713. In the latter role, he would befriend Jonathan Swift, Alexander Pope, and other literati, and he would create the immortal character John Bull, personification of the English nation.

Upon his arrival in London, Arbuthnot began teaching mathematics to the gentry as a means of supporting himself. He had received training in mathematics while at the University of Aberdeen, most likely under the direction of David Gregory (1659–1708). Gregory, 8 years older than Arbuthnot, was already well established as a mathematician, and was an early exponent of Newtonian ideas. He had assumed a professorship at Edinburgh at the age of 24. Originally intending a medical career, Gregory had learned mathematics by studying the voluminous papers left by his uncle James Gregory, a famous mathematician, who had died in 1675 at the age of 37. Like Arbuthnot and many others at the time, Gregory had also fled to London in 1691 because of the upheavals in Scotland. There, he managed to land a professorship at Oxford, with Isaac Newton's help.

By this time, Gregory and his good friend Archibald Pitcairne (1652–1713), an eminent physician, were at the center of a circle of brilliant young intellectuals. This group seems to have remained close-knit for a long time, and several members achieved fame in various fields, especially in science, mathematics, and medicine. It is quite possible that Gregory helped Arbuthnot to become established as a mathematics tutor in 1691, and then to be accepted at Oxford for medical training in 1694. It is also plausible that Gregory may have encouraged Arbuthnot to undertake the translation of Huygens's famous treatise into English.

At any rate, an anonymous author, presumed by most modern scholars to be John Arbuthnot, published in 1692 a translation of Huygens's treatise as: *Of the Laws of Chance*.[9] Whether or not he performed the translation, it is virtually certain that Arbuthnot composed the Preface, which shows signs of the spicy wit that would later contribute to his fame:

> It is thought as necessary to write a Preface before a Book, as it is judg'd civil, when you invite a Friend to Dinner, to proffer him a Glass of Hock before-hand for a Whet: And this being maim'd enough for want of a Dedication, I am resolv'd it shall not want an Epistle to the Reader too. I shall not take upon me to determine, whether it is lawful to play at Dice or not, leaving that to be disputed betwixt the Fanatick Parsons and the Sharpers; I am sure it is lawful to deal with playing at Dice as with other Epidemic Distempers; and I am confident that the writing a Book about it, will contribute as little towards its Encouragement, as Fluxing and Precipitates do to Whoring.

Arbuthnot took pains to assure readers that the work was not meant to promote gambling:

> A great part of this Discourse is a Translation from Mons. Hugen's Treatise, De ratiociniis in ludo Aleae, one, who in his Improvements of Philosophy, has but one Superior, and I think few or no Equals. The whole I undertook for my own Divertisement, next to the Satisfaction of some Friends, who would now and then be wrangling about the Proportions of Hazards in some Cases that are here decided. All it requir'd was a few spare Hours, and but little Work for the Brain; my Design in publishing it, was to make it of more general Use, and perhaps persuade a raw Squire, by it, to keep his Money in his Pocket; and if, upon this account, I should incur the Clamours of the Sharpers, I do not much regard it, since they are a sort of People the World is not bound to provide for.

The fact that this work is primarily a translation of Huygens's treatise is clearly acknowledged. Huygens's stature at the time, as second only to

Isaac Newton in the realm of natural philosophy, is intended as a great compliment, but is obviously qualified by the homage accorded to the preeminent Newton.

What seems odd, and perhaps disingenuous, is the rather breezy assertion that very little effort was required for this project. Translating Huygens's entire work from Latin to English would have been far from trivial, and must have taken some time to accomplish. Add to this the solutions of problems related to some games that were not included in the original Huygens treatise. Finally, it would have been necessary to arrange for publication and to find enough money to pay for the printing costs.

How, then, did a young immigrant fresh from Scotland, with very limited resources, manage to accomplish all this within a year of his arrival in London? Indeed, how had he even managed to come by a copy of the Huygens treatise? It was not likely to be for sale at Arbuthnot's neighborhood bookstore. My own suspicion is that he had substantial help in acquiring the necessary resources, performing the labor of translation, and extending Huygens's work. Who might have been in a position to assist him?

An obvious candidate is David Gregory, Arbuthnot's mentor and former teacher. Gregory had spent time in Holland between 1679 and 1681. He had formed a relationship with Huygens at that time, and had subsequently remained in correspondence with him. The praise for Huygens, ranking him one notch below the incomparable Newton, seems rather presumptuous for a 24-year-old unknown mathematics tutor. However, it is consistent with Gregory's position as an admirer of the older (but now fading) Huygens, while an early acolyte of Newton, the brightest star in the mathematical firmament.

Further evidence of Gregory's possible role in the Huygens translation is found in a file included among his papers at Oxford. This file, believed to have been written in 1694, contains a manuscript in Arbuthnot's handwriting that develops some extensions and practical applications of the material in Huygens's treatise. Attached to this document is a single-page abstract in Gregory's handwriting pertaining to the articles in the journal *Acta Eruditorum* in which first Jacob Bernoulli and later Leibniz offer their solutions of Bernoulli's challenge problems of 1685. So, it appears that by the 1690s Gregory was well aware of the latest developments pertaining to the mathematics of gambling. Moreover, Gregory was a world-class mathematician and an active participant in the latest developments pertaining to the infinitesimal calculus, including the contributions of Jacob Bernoulli and his brother Johann Bernoulli (1667–1748).

Arbuthnot, on the other hand, would not seem capable of producing the high-level mathematics contained in the 1694 manuscript without assistance:

> Arbuthnot was barely competent as a mathematician. Todhunter notes an incorrect solution to a problem, some problems that are not well-stated, and an approximate solution that is not very proximate. This view is not assuaged after reading the 1710 paper; the probability calculations appearing there are very elementary. The manuscript shows Arbuthnot in a much more positive mathematical light ...
>
> What appears in the manuscript is probably the upper bound on Arbuthnot's mathematical capabilities.... Curiously, the general results he obtained in this manuscript did not appear in later editions of his book.[10]

These later editions were published in 1714 and 1738, after David Gregory's death in 1708. Perhaps the explanation for his failure to include the results lies in the absence of Gregory's inspiration and assistance.

Finally, there is even some physical evidence that ties Gregory and Arbuthnot closely in producing the document.

> Because of the raggedness of the edges of the paper of the Gregory abstract, it is impossible to tell if the final page of the Arbuthnot manuscript and the Gregory abstract are from the same foolscap sheet. They were, however, placed together in the Gregory papers with the abstract following the manuscript. The other contents of the manuscript collection in the same box are written on various sizes of paper with very few, if any, of foolscap size. Finally, there exists no covering letter, or at least no letter has survived, from Arbuthnot to Gregory, or vice versa, about the manuscript. The simplest explanation for the abstract and manuscript being written on paper from the same maker, for the placement of the papers together in the manuscript collection, and for the lack of correspondence about the manuscript is that the manuscript and abstract were written in fairly close proximity, both in location and time.[11]

Indeed, the document in Arbuthnot's hand may have resulted from a joint collaboration, most likely under Gregory's direction.

Isaac Newton

To his contemporaries, Isaac Newton was more phenomenon than mortal man, and his personal idiosyncrasies were tolerated because of the awe in which he was held.[12] Along with Gottfried Leibniz, he is credited with the invention of the infinitesimal calculus and is generally hailed as the father of modern physics. His achievements are even more remarkable when we consider that Newton grew up in the most humble of circumstances and was virtually self-taught.

Newton was a loner as a youth, and remained solitary and antisocial throughout his long life, with few friends and no lovers. In splendid isolation, Newton undertook extensive research, which encompassed not only mathematics and science, but also alchemy and religion. He tended to be secretive and obsessive in his pursuits, resulting in considerable friction with his contemporaries. Most famous, of course, was his bitter dispute with Gottfried Leibniz over the origins of the infinitesimal calculus. In this, as in other disputes over scientific theory and priority, Newton could be selfish and vindictive.

John Maynard Keynes described the eerie borderland between genius and madness that Newton inhabited:

> He regarded the universe as a cryptogram ... By pure thought, by concentration of mind, the riddle, he believed, would be revealed to the initiate. He did read the riddle of the heavens. And he believed that by the same powers of his introspective imagination he would read the riddle of the Godhead, the riddle of past and future events divinely fore-ordained, the riddle of the elements and their constitution from an undifferentiated first matter, the riddle of health and of immortality. All would be revealed to him if only he could persevere to the end, uninterrupted, by himself, no one coming into the room, reading, copying, testing- all by himself, no interruption for God's sake, no disclosure, no discordant breakings in or criticism, with fear and shrinking as he assailed these half-ordained, half-forbidden things, creeping back into the bosom of the Godhead as into his mother's womb.[13]

This was not a man who made it easy on his friends and colleagues. Although a professor at Cambridge, he did not teach courses, and he had neither the time nor inclination to publicize his revolutionary ideas, which had to be wheedled out of him. Nonetheless, he attained such fame that in 1705 he was knighted by Queen Anne, the first mere man of science ever to receive such an honor.

From early in his career, Newton maintained a journal in which he jotted down extensive notes pertaining to his various projects. Between 1664 and 1666, he studied the Huygens treatise and made detailed annotations. It was during this same period that he made the initial breakthroughs that would lead to the differential and integral calculus, which he called respectively the "method of fluxions" and "method of fluents." To us, it may seem odd that the laws of chance failed to engage his creative energies. However, for Newton it was probably far from obvious how this subject would pertain to the weightier scientific and philosophical concerns that absorbed him. I believe this is further evidence of just how remote our notion of mathematical probability still was from even the most farsighted thinkers of the time.

EMPIRICAL FREQUENCIES

The mistaken belief that modern probability emerged full-blown around 1660 rests partly on an extraordinary coincidence. In 1662, the very year in which the Port-Royal *Logic* appeared in France, another publication of similar originality and significance was published. Whereas the *Logic* is often cited in connection with the emergence of probability, the *Observations on the Bills of Mortality* is considered the progenitor of statistics. Strange as it may seem, though, there was absolutely no connection between the ideas expressed in these two great works. The *Logic* made no reference to anything we would describe as statistical, and the *Observations* lacked any notion of a calculus of chance, let alone probability.

If mathematical probability, with its close connection to statistical frequencies, was indeed in the air, then why was the first true statistical exposition devoid of any reference to it? To answer this question, we must remember that measuring an empirical frequency would depend on having some relevant *data*. In 1662, data in our modern sense did not exist. For us, data are items of factual information that are viewed together as constituent elements of some aggregate. As such, each individual "datum" that is observed or measured is regarded as part of a collection of similar data. Prior to this time, there literally were no data in this sense.

There were, of course, written records that had been maintained for various legal, commercial, or administrative purposes to document certain types of significant events or commercial transactions. However, no one appeared to regard these records as useful in the aggregate. So it was a revelation when John Graunt (1620–1674) reported the results of an ingenious project he had decided to undertake. Graunt had, in effect, *invented* the idea of data. He organized and submitted to numerical analysis a set of musty documents that had been accumulating for several decades.

The cornucopia of valuable information he drew from them was startling. However, while his effort planted the seeds for a future science of statistics, it would take over a century (and the availability of vastly more data) before these ideas could take root. Graunt perceived that these records could meaningfully describe important population dynamics. In effect, he conceived of what we now call *demographics*, the statistical analysis of human populations. Graunt's methodology consisted of assembling the records into summary tables and applying a healthy dose of logic and common sense.

John Graunt

Who was this visionary? Was he an eminent natural philosopher or some privileged aristocrat? On the contrary, John Graunt was a London cloth merchant, or "draper."[14] At the age of 20, Graunt was apprenticed to his father in the London drapers' trade, and over the next 20 years managed to wax quite wealthy. Samuel Pepys recorded in his famous diary that Graunt was reputed to possess one of the finest collections of artwork in the city.[15] Well known and highly regarded, he held various civic offices in London. He also possessed considerable musical talent, and rose through the ranks of the "trained band" of the London Militias, reaching the rank of captain by around 1660.

For some unknown reason (as he tells us), Graunt became interested in the London *Bills of Mortality*, initiated during the plague year of 1592.[16] Since 1603, the *Bills* had been regularly maintained for each parish in the City of London and the surrounding areas. These documents listed the names of all those who had died during the previous week, along with the apparent cause of death. Together with this roster of the grim reaper's victims, a listing of all christenings during the week was also published.

Graunt, having been born and bred in London, was aware of these weekly notices. Like everyone else, he had paid them little mind, until he experienced an unlikely epiphany. It occurred to him that they represented a hitherto untapped resource:

> Now, I thought that the Wisdom of our City had certainly designed the laudable practice of takeing, and distributing these Accompts, for other, and greater uses

then those above-mentioned, or at least, that some other uses might be made of them ... the which, when I had reduced into Tables (the Copies whereof are here inserted) so as to have a view of the whole together, I did then begin, finding some *Truths*, and not commonly believed Opinions, to arise from my Meditations upon these neglected *Papers*.

Graunt's project was naively ambitious and completely original. The very idea of organizing such information into a tabular format was a great innovation.[17] Tabular arrangements of facts or ideas had been around almost as long as the printing press. In accounting, numerical tables had been employed. But no one, as far as we know, had previously thought to compile the frequencies of various types of events into meaningful categories and to array these "so as to have a view of the whole together." If ever a man was ahead of his time, that man was John Graunt.

As a draper, perhaps Graunt had become adept at making the most of the limited material at his disposal. If so, this ability stood him in good stead as he measured, cut, and stitched the raw facts to reveal the fabric of seventeenth-century reality. The crude information contained in the registers of christenings and deaths did not even provide the ages of the deceased, which were not to be added until 1728. Moreover, his mathematical tools consisted of the "shop Arithmetique" he had acquired in learning his trade. Drawing upon these humble resources, Graunt fashioned a remarkable chronicle that advanced human understanding significantly.

Graunt discovered empirical knowledge where previously had existed only ill-informed speculation. Graunt was well aware that his estimates were crude approximations. However, taken as a whole, his reasoning was plausible enough to debunk the wild misconceptions that prevailed at the time. He was willing to take some necessary leaps of faith that allowed derivation of ballpark figures, where almost total ignorance and superstition had previously reigned. For example, he estimated the population of London to be less than 400,000, not the millions generally presumed.

The potential importance of Graunt's *Observations* was immediately appreciated. On February 5, 1662, Graunt presented 50 copies of his report at a meeting of the Royal Society of London, which had been established 15 months earlier. It is likely that his entrée to the Royal Society was provided by his friend William Petty (1623–1687), who had been elected as one of its charter members. Just 3 weeks after his report was circulated,

Graunt himself was admitted, despite being a mere merchant. It is noted in the records that "in his election it was so far from being a prejudice that he was a shopkeeper of London, that His Majesty gave this particular charge to His Society, that if they found any more such tradesmen, they should be sure to admit them all, without any more ado." Unfortunately, it seems that Graunt was one of a kind.

Graunt's *Observations* went through five additions, the last published posthumously in 1676. The later editions, starting with two in 1665, incorporated some additional sources of data that he obtained, including the results of a partially successful census that he had organized. Word of Graunt's accomplishment spread rapidly throughout Europe, and led to the organization of systems to generate bills of mortality in other cities. Unfortunately, Graunt ran into hard times a few years later, precipitated by the Great Fire of 1666 that ravaged London. His problems were exacerbated by his conversion to Catholicism, which alienated many, and led to unfounded aspersions being cast on his work and character. He died in poverty in 1674. For some decades after, Graunt's reputation was sullied by these tragic circumstances, to the extent that some of his originality became unfairly credited to his more famous friend, William Petty.

One aspect of Graunt's work that was of particularly wide interest was the speculative "life-table" he cleverly derived. This table was included in a review of the *Observations* in 1666 published in the *Journal Des Sçavans*.[18] The life-table was incorrectly believed by many to be based on actual mortality data (i.e., records that included the age at the time of death). While not the only such life-table that was produced around this time, it became a kind of standard, despite being cobbled together from the very limited information available, which did not in fact include the age of the deceased.

Table 4.1 displays the contents of Graunt's life-table. Graunt's derivation of this table began by noting that of every 100 births, about 36 died before the age of 6. Even this "fact" was an indirect inference, based on the numbers succumbing to various diseases that mainly victimized infants and young children. Next, he imagined that only one in a hundred reached the age of 76. For each decade between 6 and 76, he seems to have assumed that approximately 5/8 would survive for a 10-year period and 3/8 would die. The implied mortality rates paint a rather grim picture of life in the seventeenth century. It is impossible to verify that Graunt's

TABLE 4.1   John Graunt's "Life-Table"

Age Attained	Frequency
Born	100
Age 6	64
Age 16	40
Age 26	25
Age 36	16
Age 46	10
Age 56	6
Age 66	3
Age 76	1

table is even roughly accurate, but his figures apparently did not surprise his contemporaries.

William Petty

William Petty, mentioned previously, was one of those profoundly influenced by Graunt's research.[19] Born in London into a family of clothiers, Petty had shipped out as a cabin boy in the Royal Navy at the age of 13 and eventually tried his hand at several occupations. From these humble origins, he had managed via a series of Horatio Alger-like adventures to achieve great wealth and celebrity. Petty must have been exceptionally charming, for he managed to wangle a series of plum appointments. In 1646, he traveled to Paris to study anatomy. There he came into contact with Descartes, Pascal, Fermat, and other luminaries. He also became acquainted with the famous philosopher Thomas Hobbes (1588–1679), and served as his research assistant.

Returning to England, he obtained in 1647 a degree in medicine and in 1650 became Professor of Anatomy at Oxford University. In the following year, he was also appointed as Professor of Music at Gresham College, with substantial help from John Graunt. While all this might seem accomplishment enough for most young men, for Petty it was merely prologue.

In 1652, Petty abandoned academia to assume the post of physician-in-chief of Oliver Cromwell's occupying army in Ireland. This position he parlayed into a vehicle for enormous personal enrichment, mainly by directing to the completion of the Down Survey of Ireland, intended to facilitate the granting of land tracts to reward members of Cromwell's army. Petty received 30,000 acres of Irish land when the Down Survey was completed in 1656. After Cromwell's defeat, Petty was among those who reestablished good relations with the restored monarchy. He was appointed as a founding member of the Royal Society in 1660, and in 1661 was knighted by Charles II.

Throughout most of his life, Petty remained an active participant in the affairs of the Royal Society, even while living mostly in Ireland. Ultimately, he became one of the largest landowners in Ireland. In 1682, he helped to form the Dublin Society, patterned after the Royal Society. In his scholarly pursuits, Petty specialized in studying the history of trades and technology (naval architecture was a particular specialty). His "political arithmetic" involved the use of statistical information to support various theories. It is often considered a precursor of the field of *political economy* that developed throughout the eighteenth century, concerned primarily with the economic activities of countries.

Petty, like his friend Graunt, was a pioneer in appreciating how numerical data could be used. However, his personality and approach were quite different from his friend's. Graunt is widely admired even today for his careful, objective, and thoughtful reasoning, and for the transparency of his assumptions. Petty, on the other hand, was a high roller who was not above coaxing the facts to support his ambitious ends. In essence, while Graunt can be said to have invented the science of data analysis, Petty may have pioneered the political art of "inventing the data."

Petty's political arithmetic, which was based in part on numerical data, was criticized for treating people as a commodity to be exploited. In fact, Petty's writing became the model upon which John Arbuthnot's friend Jonathan Swift (1667–1745) based his famous satirical essay "A Modest Proposal," published in 1729.[20] In earnest tones, Swift's fictional essayist offers a well-reasoned proposal, supported by creative statistical evidence and dubious authority, in the manner of Petty. The horrific idea that the Irish ought to export their excess children to England as a source of food is intended to highlight the abysmal social and economic situation of Ireland and to parody Petty-esque proposals:

> A child will make two dishes at an entertainment for friends; and when the family dines alone, the fore or hind quarter will make a reasonable dish, and seasoned with a little pepper or salt will be very good boiled on the fourth day, especially in winter.

Swift discusses the many economic benefits that would accrue to Ireland, which could improve its balance of trade, while providing a commodity that would not compete with anything produced by England.

Graunt and Petty are both justifiably deemed to be founders of statistical disciplines. However, it is noteworthy that neither of these men utilized any sophisticated mathematics or related their statistics in any way to games of chance. The kind of basic enumerations and simple summaries they employed provided the pattern for many "political economists" and other policy analysts in the following century.

Three Dutch Masters: Huygens, Hudde, and De Witt

The excitement that greeted Graunt's data and analysis underlines how narrow was the existing worldview of even the most educated. Virtually nothing quantitative was known about the most basic facts of human populations. Graunt's life-table, in particular, aroused much interest, because it provided actual evidence about a question of vital importance to everyone: How long can a person reasonably expect to live? The idea that mortality might follow some universal law that could potentially be discovered was new.

One of those who became very interested in Graunt's table was Ludwig Huygens, whom we last encountered in 1655 in Paris during his youthful travels with brother Christiaan. By 1669, Ludwig had become a prominent politician and diplomat in the Netherlands, and Christiaan the foremost scientist of Europe. In a letter to Christiaan that year, Ludwig mentioned that he had used Graunt's life-table to calculate the expected years of life remaining to a person at any particular age. In fact, he projected that his brother, who was then 40, could expect to survive for another 16 years.

Christiaan was familiar with Graunt's *Observations*, having been sent a copy by Sir Robert Moray (1608–1673), first president of the Royal Society, on March 16, 1662. Thanking Moray for this gift,[21] he wrote back on June 9, 1662:

> The discourse of Graunt is very worthy of consideration and pleases me greatly, he argues well and cleanly and I admire how he is prudent in drawing all those consequences out of those simple observations, which don't seem to have served

for anything until him. In this country now people do not do it at all, although it would be wished that one had this curiosity and the thing is easy enough, principally in the city of Amsterdam, which is entirely divided into quarters, and in each there are some prefects who know the number of the persons and all that which happens there.

Perhaps surprisingly, there is no evidence of any effort on his part to advocate for such a program. Moreover, Huygens apparently saw no important connection between Graunt's inferences based on compilations of data and the mathematics of games of chance. However, stimulated by his brother's letter, Huygens thought more about the life-table and its possible uses.

In his initial response to his brother, Christiaan pointed out that Graunt's table is only approximate. To be exact "it would be necessary to have a table which indicates from year to year how many die of the 100 persons that one supposes." Nonetheless, Christiaan went on to develop a theory that is grounded in an analogy between individual life spans and outcomes in a game of pure chance. So, he became the first of many to view human mortality as a process that could be viewed as analogous to a game of chance. This was to become the main practical application of the calculus of chance for nearly a century.

Specifically, Huygens regarded the life-table figures as if they were generated by a lottery with 100 tickets, each of which was marked with a number corresponding to a particular life span. He set the proportions of these "prizes" in the lottery to correspond approximately with the data in Graunt's table. For example, since 36 per 100 were expected to die before age 6, Huygens assumed that 36 of the 100 tickets would have the number 3 (half-way between 0 and 6). For this hypothetical lottery, Huygens could apply the rules he had developed in his famous treatise 12 years earlier.

Here we have the first known example of an analogy between empirical data about a complex causal process, like mortality, and a lottery. As we will see in Chapter 5, this idea was central to the breakthroughs achieved by Jacob Bernoulli about 20 years later. Based on this analogy, Christiaan Huygens confirmed Ludwig's computation of the life expectation at any age, which corresponded to the mathematical expectation for the lottery. He went on to calculate as well the *median* years of remaining life, that is, the number of years that were equally likely to be exceeded or not.

He astutely observed that both measures could be useful, but for different purposes:

> There are thus two different concepts: the expectation or the value of the future age of the person, and the age at which he has an equal chance to survive or not. The first is for the calculation of life annuities, and the other for wagering.

Life annuities at this time played an important role in public financing. Suppose that a local or national government needed to raise funds for a major construction project or military operation and direct taxation was not feasible. One way to "borrow" money was to sell life-annuities. The purchaser would receive an annual or semiannual payment of a fixed amount for life. The price paid for the annuity was driven primarily by supply and demand (and perhaps an implicit rate of interest), but was generally not related to the individual's age or health status.

Given the high (and unknown) mortality rates prevailing at all ages, this failure to account for the annuitant's age is not as bizarre as it may seem. Huygens's insight that the individual's mathematical "expectation of the value of the future age" should be the theoretical basis for pricing of an annuity was quite remarkable. It represents perhaps the first explicit linkage between real-world data and the mathematical concepts developed in connection with the games of chance. Likening the distribution of ages at death in a human population to the mixture of tickets in a lottery was a major conceptual leap. In fact, it entailed what I have called the principle of willful ignorance. By ignoring the potentially relevant differences among individuals and treating the population as a group of indistinguishable objects (like lottery tickets), general statements about life expectancy became possible.

Huygens went on to discuss multiple-life annuities, which were sometimes sold, usually involving two lives. In this case, the payments would continue for as long as one of the annuitants remained alive. Of course, the cost of such a joint annuity would be higher than that for a single annuity. Huygens specifically considered the hypothetical case of a man of age 56 who marries a woman aged 16. He asks how long the two can expect to live together, the expected length of the longer life, and the expected length for the one who dies first. These problems appear to be presented as mathematical curiosities, rather than as practical advice for reforming the arbitrary pricing policies for annuities that were common at that time.

However, soon there were two serious attempts to put such ideas into practice. Not surprisingly, both of these involved friends of Christiaan Huygens.

In 1671, the military and political situation confronting the Dutch Republic was dire, as war with France loomed. It was imperative to raise funds to outfit and support the army. The political leader of the Dutch Republic at this time, with the odd title of Grand Pensioner of Holland, was Johan de Witt (1625–1672).[22] de Witt received degrees in both law and mathematics. In fact, he was another of the wunderkinds under the tutelage of Frans van Schooten, along with Johan Hudde (1628–1704) and Christiaan Huygens. In 1649, de Witt had written a book on analytic geometry that was subsequently published as part of a van Schooten textbook. This work was esteemed by Isaac Newton, and Huygens regarded de Witt as a mathematical genius. However, de Witt's political talents and family connections had by 1653 propelled him to the pinnacle of power in the Dutch Republic, whose leadership he would hold for nearly two decades.

In 1671, the issuance of life annuities seemed a viable option for raising the funds needed by the Dutch government. However, de Witt believed that annuities were being sold too cheaply. The going rate for a single-life annuity was "14 years' purchase." This meant that to receive 1 florin per year for life, an annuitant would pay 14 florins. At a zero interest rate, this price would imply a life expectancy of 14 years. Taking account of the time value of money (the effective interest rate) things would become more complicated. What we now call the "net present value" of the annuity can be calculated by discounting the flow of future payments in accordance with an assumed rate of interest.

De Witt had corresponded with Johan Hudde regarding the pricing of annuities as early as September 1670. It seems likely that Hudde, at least, was aware of the correspondence between the brothers Huygens on the subject. Hudde was the political leader of the city of Amsterdam, which had often used annuities as a financing technique, and had been conducting his own research on this subject. Like de Witt and Huygens, Hudde believed that prices for life annuities ought to be based on their expected value, which ought to take into account the annuitant's age.

De Witt formally presented his proposal for increasing the price of annuities, along with his method and calculations, in a pamphlet, *The*

Value of Life Annuities Compared to Redemption Bonds, which was presented to the legislative body of the Dutch Republic (The Estates General) and was later published. de Witt's report was the first to explain how to combine an assumed rate of interest with a life-table to compute the fair value of an annuity. His approach was mathematically correct given his assumptions, and drew directly on the methodology of Huygens's treatise.

For the interest rate, he assumed 4% per annum. For the life-table, he made some rough (and in his view conservative) assumptions about mortality rates at different ages. After Herculean calculations, he obtained the result that a fair price for a life annuity on a young child would be almost exactly 16 florins. Moreover, he argued that in view of several circumstances potentially favorable to the annuitant, this would actually be a bargain. (Of course, the risk of a default by the government was not mentioned.)

De Witt seems to have been somewhat insecure about the accuracy of his assumptions related to mortality. In a supplement to his main report, he provided some data he had obtained from the registers of Holland and West Friedland. For approximately 1000 annuitants, he knew their age at purchase and age at death. For each annuitant he calculated the present value of actual payments that had been made, and then averaged these for several age-classes of individuals. To his delight, the results revealed that in all classes the actual value exceeded his conservative estimate of 16 florins.

De Witt also solicited and obtained from Hudde a formal certification of his methods and calculations. Hudde, meanwhile, had been gathering data from the records of a set of annuities that had been issued in Amsterdam between 1586 and 1590 on 1495 lives. These he had compiled into a table that was organized according to the age of the annuitant at purchase, and listed the ages at death for each age category. Being well aware of the exigencies under which de Witt was operating, Hudde sent this table of mortality data to de Witt immediately upon completion, the day after de Witt's report was submitted to the Estates General. (Three weeks later he also sent a copy to Christiaan Huygens). In subsequent correspondence with Hudde, de Witt noted that his hypothetical assumptions for the death rates were somewhat higher than the actual rates derived from his own and Hudde's data. Thus, a typical annuitant might expect to live longer (and therefore receive a greater amount of money) than de Witt had assumed.

The work on life annuities by Huygens, Hudde, and de Witt embodied important aspects of what would eventually become the modern statistical framework. For probably the first time, the empirical data pertaining to a set of real-world events (deaths of annuitants) were analyzed as if they were the outcomes from a game of chance. To justify these analyses, an explicit analogy was drawn between the events and the outcomes of a chance mechanism. If one accepted the analogy, then Huygens's mathematical expectation would provide the fair value of the annuity.

De Witt went even further by explaining how in calculating a mathematical expectation, the absolute number of "chances" for a particular outcome was not important. Rather the *relative* proportion of chances to the total number of chances was the key: "It plainly results from the foregoing proposition, that in a strict sense it is not the number of chances of each value which we must consider, in the application of the aforesaid rules, but solely their reciprocal proportion." de Witt understood that, unlike the situation in a game of chance, there is no possibility of obtaining the actual number of "chances" that a person will die at any given age. However, he believed that plausible estimates of the *relative* chances of death for an individual at any age could be made. From these, he constructed what we would call a *probability distribution*. This is a remarkable accomplishment on de Witt's part and suggests that he was close to formulating the modern notion of probability as a proportion (fraction) of both total chances and of certainty.

Moreover, de Witt (along with Huygens and Hudde) apparently regarded the historical record of mortality for past annuitants as providing relevant data to estimate the future relative mortality rates at different ages. Thus, the data could provide a means of assessing whether the theoretical "model" that de Witt had proposed appeared reasonable. In many respects, it seems that this extraordinary triumvirate was well positioned to formulate the synthesis of ideas that would eventually become the modern view of probability and statistics. On the other hand, their collaboration was firmly rooted in an attempt to solve a particular pressing problem, not to propose a general theoretical approach for dealing with uncertainty.

It is possible that de Witt would have continued to pursue these matters, in collaboration with Hudde and Huygens, and perhaps created our theory of mathematical probability. We will never know, as fate intervened. On August 8, 1672, de Witt was forced to resign his office after France and England invaded Holland. Twelve days later, a tragic and grisly sequence of events ensued; Johan de Witt and his brother Cornelis were lynched by a mob organized by their political opponents. Their corpses were mutilated, and their body parts were put on display. The details of these events were dramatically portrayed in the opening chapters of a famous historical novel, *The Black Tulip*, written by Alexandre Dumas (1802–1870) in 1850.[23]

De Witt's proposal for pricing annuities based on the expected duration of future life was never implemented by the Dutch government. In Amsterdam, Hudde's recommendations did lead to age-related pricing of annuities that were issued in 1672 and 1674. However, the prices were much lower than those that de Witt's calculations suggested. For example, in 1672, the cost of a life-annuity on a child was only 10 years' purchase. It seems likely that in the uncertain political climate of that time, the risk of default may have played a role in driving down the price that could be realistically demanded by the city. Subsequent to this brief outburst of relative rationality in pricing behavior, annuities continued to be sold in Amsterdam, as elsewhere, without any relation to age or health condition.

Jacob Bernoulli

As early as 1685, Bernoulli had come to believe that the mathematics of games of chance could be applied to many practical problems. He had conceived a sophisticated theoretical rationale for inferring the expectation of a certain event with "moral certainty" based on observed frequencies of occurrence. However, he had not yet fully developed his ideas about when such an inference would be appropriate and reliable as a guide to practical actions. By 1689, he had privately elaborated these ideas in a mature form, but was not yet prepared to share them broadly. Possible reasons for this reluctance will be discussed in Chapter 5.

One set of applications that was clearly in Jacob's sights pertained to certain legal issues related to inheritance and other matters that depended on life expectancies.[24] These were mentioned in several of his academic disputations at the University of Basel. For example, in 1686 he discussed a hypothetical marriage contract with different consequences if one or the other of the fathers of the couple died before the wife, or vice versa. The expectation of the inheritance for the husband under the terms of the contract would depend on the odds that the wife would outlive both of the fathers. Bernoulli asserted that it might seem impossible to make such a calculation, but that the bills of mortality from London or Paris would provide a basis for obtaining an approximate solution.

In an article published in the *Journal des Sçavans* in 1686, Bernoulli did in fact offer a solution to a simpler version of this problem.[25] He stated (without proof) that the odds were 101:59 that a 16-year old would outlive a 56-year-old person. This result was based on the "data" contained in Graunt's life-table, available in the review that had been published in this journal in 1666. Writing in 1685 in his private journal, he mentioned several types of problems for which data about observed frequencies might be useful. He stated that such information would allow one to conjecture about such diverse questions as how many births and deaths would occur in a given city each year, after how many years a contagious epidemic will recur, the average barometric pressure, and the trustworthiness of a witness.

Edmond Halley

Edmond Halley (1656–1742) is of course most famous today for the eponymous comet that arrives on schedule every 76 years.[26] In 1705, Halley predicted that this comet would appear next in 1758. It did, although Halley did not live to witness the event. In his time, however, Halley was a major figure who made many important contributions to several scientific disciplines, especially astronomy and mathematics.

Halley was the son of a wealthy soap manufacturer, who was able to provide young Edmond with a first-rate education. In 1673, Halley entered Oxford University and pursued the interest in astronomy he had already developed, becoming a student of John Flamsteed (1646–1719), the first Astronomer Royal. In November 1676, the multitalented Halley was recruited for a scientific mission to chart the stars visible in the southern hemisphere, so off he went to the island of St. Helena to set up a telescope and make observations. When he returned to England 2 years later, he registered 341 newly discovered stars. This greatly pleased King Charles II, who had supported the expedition, and the king arranged for Halley to receive his Master of Arts (M.A.) degree from Oxford.

Shortly afterward, Halley was elected as a member of the Royal Society. Just 6 months later, the intrepid 22-year old was sent by the Royal Society on a diplomatic mission to Danzig to help settle a touchy dispute between two famous scientists, Robert Hooke (1635–1703) and Johannes Hevelius (1611–1687) regarding techniques of astronomical observation. After successfully accomplishing this delicate task, he traveled to Paris, where in 1680 he spent time with the famous astronomer Giovanni Cassini (1625–1712), who was then director of the Paris Observatory. While there, he may have met Christiaan Huygens, who was working there at the time.

Returning home in 1682, Halley married and settled down to continue his researches in astronomy and related areas of mathematics. These pursuits led him to become aware of the remarkable discoveries of Isaac Newton, which were not yet widely known. In 1684, Halley traveled down to Cambridge to seek guidance from the inscrutable Newton. During the course of their discussions, Halley realized the full importance of Newton's revolutionary findings and offered to assist with and even pay for their publication. Halley was the driving force behind the appearance in 1687 of probably the most influential scientific work ever printed, Newton's *Principia Mathematica*:

> He paid all the expenses, he corrected the proofs, he laid aside his own work in order to press forward to the utmost the printing. All his letters show the most intense devotion to the work.[27]

During the next 55 years, Halley would go on to a varied and distinguished career, which included a 2-year stint as deputy comptroller of the Royal Mint (under Newton), followed in 1698 by command of a warship, the Paramore. The purpose of this naval commission was to conduct an investigation of terrestrial magnetism over a wide area of the globe. In addition to his research on astronomy and geophysics, he contributed significantly to archeology, and translated several important ancient mathematical treatises from Latin, Greek, and even Arabic sources.

In 1704, Halley became the Savilian Professor of Geometry at Oxford, after the death of John Wallis (1616–1703), and in 1720, he succeeded

Flamsteed as Astronomer Royal. Unfortunately, Halley's liberal religious views and close association with Newton had over the years caused a rift with his old mentor. Indeed, in 1691 Halley had been rejected for the Savilian Professorship of Astronomy, which went to David Gregory, in part because of Flamsteed's opposition. When Halley was appointed as Astronomer Royal, Flamsteed's widow was so infuriated that she sold off all of her late husband's instruments at the Royal Observatory to prevent Halley from getting his hands on them!

Halley and Gregory, on the other hand, maintained amicable relations, despite their rivalry for the Oxford Astronomy Chair in 1691. They became allies in staunchly supporting Newton's position during the famous priority disputes with Leibniz over discovery of the calculus. From 1704 until Gregory's death in 1708, the pair also collaborated on a translation from Greek into Latin of a famous mathematical text from antiquity, the *Conics* of Apollonius.

Halley seems to have been an exceptionally able individual who was willing to pitch in wherever he perceived that something important needed doing. It was in this spirit that he undertook a task that would make him a founder of actuarial science. In 1689, the Royal Society was seeking data that might allow improvements on the demographic research of Graunt and Petty. Through Gottfried Leibniz, the Society had learned of a remarkable source of data being maintained by Caspar Neumann (1648–1715), a priest in Breslau (in Silesia, now part of Germany).

Neumann had been meticulously maintaining a registry of all births and deaths in Breslau that included the age and sex of the deceased. He had written up a few observations on mortality and sent these to Leibniz, along with a table that contained the data upon which these were based. Richard Waller (1660–1715), Secretary of the Royal Society, wrote to Neumann in 1689 to request a copy of Neumann's records, and received them in 1692. Halley was deputized to analyze the Breslau data and prepare a report on his findings. In 1693, Halley presented his results, which were then published the following year in the *Philosophical Transactions* of the Royal Society.[28]

Halley's paper opens by discussing the main limitations that had been acknowledged by Graunt and Petty in their studies of London and Dublin, respectively. First, the total populations of these metropolises were unknown. Second, the ages of the deceased were not recorded in the Bills of Mortality on which Graunt and Petty had relied. Third, there was no information about patterns of migration. The total population of Breslau was likewise unknown, but Neumann had captured the age and sex of each decedent. Furthermore, owing to Breslau's isolated location, the amount of migration was believed to be minimal. Thus, the data were far superior to any previous resource for calculating a true life-table.

Halley's analysis began by deriving a mortality rate at each attained age from 1 to 100. The result of his analysis was the first true life-table for the city of Breslau. From Halley's table, he estimated that the total population of Breslau was 34,000, which had not previously been known. Halley knew that his table was a major improvement on Graunt's, which he characterized as "an imaginary valuation." Table 4.2 shows a comparison of the Halley's mortality rates with those Graunt had generated. Halley's results appeared to demonstrate that rates of mortality after childhood were much lower than Graunt had obtained, though still appalling by modern standards.

Halley then went on to develop seven different uses for this remarkable table.

First, he determined the proportion of men in the population between the ages of 16 and 56, and therefore deemed capable of performing military service, and the proportion of women between 16 and 45, and thus presumably capable of bearing children. Second, he explained how to calculate the *odds* that a person would survive from a given age to another

TABLE 4.2   **Edmond Halley's Life Expectancies Compared with John Gaunt's**

Age Attained	Graunt (London)	Halley (Breslau)
Born	100	100
Age 6	64	55
Age 16	40	48
Age 26	25	43
Age 36	16	37
Age 46	10	30
Age 56	6	22
Age 66	3	14
Age 76	1	6
Age 84	0	2

specified age. He gave as an example that the odds in favor of a person of age 25 living for at least one more year were 80 to 1. This he termed a measure of *vitality*, the inverse of mortality. Third, he defined the median years of remaining life for a person of a given age, which is simply the future age at which half the individuals of this age will still be living, since it will then be "an even lay" that the individual would reach this age. For example, he observed that a man of age 30 had an even chance of surviving for another 27 or 28 years.

Fourth, Halley proposed that the price of a term insurance policy should be regulated in accordance with the actual odds of survival. Fifth, Halley derived a method for calculating the value of a life annuity at any age and interest rate. He illustrated his calculations by deriving and presenting a table of these values for life-annuities on individuals of various ages, at an assumed 6% interest rate. He remarked that at the standard price of only 7 years' purchase, an annuity was a real bargain. His sixth and seventh uses were extensions of the logic for annuity valuation to the cases of annuities on two or three lives.

Halley's paper was remarkable for its sophistication and is hailed as a seminal contribution to actuarial science, although this topic was a sideline to which Halley never again returned.[29] His definition of the median length of remaining life was, as far as we know, preceded only in Huygens's correspondence with his brother in 1669. Relating survival odds to insurance seems an original idea, as does his method of analysis for annuity prices, which appears superior to the methods derived by de Witt and Hudde (of which he was presumably unaware).

Halley had an intuitive feeling for random variability, as he observed that the irregularities in the counts of deaths at different ages can be "attributed to Chance" and "would rectify themselves, were the numbers of Years much more considerable." Finally, he considered whether the data from Breslau were likely to generalize to other cities, inferred that they offered a valid standard for London, and advocated collection of similar data in other locales.

Like the Dutch efforts to rationalize the pricing of annuities based on statistical analysis, Halley's innovative proposals fell on deaf ears. It would be several decades more before men of business would perceive practical advantage in these mathematical calculations. Moreover, the systematic collection of data upon which actuarial calculations could be solidly made was also far off. Indeed, Halley's table based on the little city of Breslau would remain a standard of reference until well into the next century.

While in some ways strikingly modern, Halley's study in 1693 was grounded in a traditional framework that did not include the notion of probability in the modern sense. Throughout his exposition, Halley utilizes the standard language of chances and odds. He does not mention the word probability, and does not explicitly refer to games of chance. Though recognizing that data for more years would somehow reduce the chance fluctuations in the counts, he offers no theory as to *why* this should be so, or *how many* years would be adequate. Finally, like de Witt, Halley appears on the verge of defining probability as a ratio of favorable to total chances, but fails to take this step.

Halley's methodology for obtaining the fair price of an annuity at a given age (e.g., 30 years) hinges on the ratio of chances of surviving to some future age (e.g., 60 years) relative to the chances of surviving to the current age. We would view these quantities as estimates of *conditional probabilities.* For example, the expected stream of income for a woman of age 30 would depend on her probabilities of reaching age 31, 32, 33, and so on given that she had already survived to age 30. Like de Witt, Halley developed the ratios in his formula as a means of solving a particular practical problem. He could not foresee that this fraction of chances would one day become the basis for a general theory of probability.

A QUANTUM OF CERTAINTY

The third aspect of our modern conception of probability is its epistemic connotation. Probability is a numerical measure of certainty, whether framed as a subjective degree of belief or as an objective frequency of occurrence. However, in the seventeenth century, as I discussed in the last chapter, this concept did not exist. Rather the idea of probability was associated with the degree of certainty about a proposition. A proposition was more or less probable (prove-able) depending on the arguments that supported it. However, there was no attempt to quantify the weight of these arguments or to place the probability on a scale between zero and one.

Of course, empirical frequencies could sometimes shed light on how much probability to attribute to a particular event. Such evidence could be enlisted as an argument for or against the existence of the event. However, no one imagined that a precise numerical ratio of happenings to nonhappenings in a specified situation could actually be computed. Where would the data for such a calculation have been found? Rather, a general sense of the magnitude of this ratio was the best to which even the wisest and most experienced could aspire.

Here is how John of Salisbury (1120–1180) wrote in 1159 about the relation between frequency and probability:

> Something that is always or usually so, either is or seems, probable, even though it could possibly be otherwise. And its probability is increased in proportion as it is more easily and surely known by one who has judgment. There are things whose probability is so lucidly apparent that they come to be considered necessary; whereas there are others that are so unfamiliar to us that we would be reluctant to include them in a list of probabilities.[30]

He seemed to be saying that "one who has judgment" pertaining to some matter knows "more easily and surely" the extent to which something "is always or usually so." We must remember that John of Salisbury lived in a world filled with many opinions but precious few facts.

It is hard to imagine life in a world devoid of systematically collected data. However, before the last 300 years, the extent to which things could be categorized and counted was incredibly limited. It took the genius of John Graunt to imagine the possibility of assembling data in our modern sense about even the most fundamental of human events: births and deaths. Prior to that, the odds of a particular occurrence could only be guessed by those few experts with some relevant experience and judgment.

As late as the seventeenth century, the connection between probability as a degree of belief and the principles that determined odds or expectations in gambling remained tenuous. Relating decisions under uncertainty as analogous to wagers based on rolls of dice or draws in a lottery was a figure of speech, not a literal statement. Julius Caesar's famous pronouncement on crossing the Rubicon that *alea iacta est* (the die is cast) was presumably meant to convey the idea that "fortune" would determine the outcome of his momentous act of rebellion.

Shakespeare's use of the odds of "ten to one" merely indicated something was unlikely, not that it would happen precisely 10/11 of the time. The philosopher Thomas Hobbes referred to odds of twenty to one as a way to express the idea that frequent occurrence provides strong support for believing something will happen, but not full proof: "If the signs hit twenty times for one missing, a man may lay a wager of twenty to one on the event: but may not conclude it for a truth."[31] Such allusions to betting odds were meant as general indications, and thus expressed as round numbers. No one would think of estimating the odds of rain by nightfall at 5:2 or 7:3.

Outside the artificial realm of gambling, the estimation of probabilities mathematically by somehow linking the "play of chance" in life with a precise numerical measure was almost inconceivable. To make such a connection would require an act of genius. Perhaps the two most likely candidates for such an assignment, besides Isaac Newton, were Christiaan Huygens and Gottfried Leibniz.

Why not Huygens or Leibniz?

Huygens traveled and corresponded widely and was eventually in contact with most of the scientific movers and shakers of his time. In 1672, while in Paris, he met the 26-year-old Gottfried Leibniz, already well on his way to becoming a one-man nerve center for the intelligentsia of Europe. He took Leibniz under his wing, introducing him to the work of other leading mathematicians, including René Descartes and Nicolas Malebranche (1638–1715). In 1673, Huygens again met with Leibniz and suggested an extensive reading list for him.

Leibniz was to become famous for his encyclopedic knowledge related to a variety of subjects, including law, philosophy, mathematics, history, politics, and literature.[32] His quixotic ambition was to assemble, organize, and codify virtually all facets of human knowledge. In this quest, he was eventually to engage in regular correspondence with hundreds of leading scientists and other intellectuals. His base of operations was the position as librarian and advisor to the Duke of Hanover, which he assumed at age 30 in 1676 and held for the remaining 40 years of his life. Beginning around 1676, Leibniz also developed his version of the infinitesimal calculus.

In 1666, at the age of 19, Leibniz had written an essay on the "combinatorial arts," which included some fairly rudimentary combinatorial analysis in the context of an early attempt to unify all forms of knowledge.[33] At the time, Leibniz was not yet aware of Huygens's treatise. Throughout his career, Leibniz at several points referred to the potential of combinatorial methods and also to various concepts of probability as a "degree of possibility." However, he invested little effort in these topics and his knowledge of the mathematics of chance was not very deep. In his correspondence, Leibniz often expressed a desire that someone take up the task of fruitfully linking combinatorics with uncertainty. He did not realize until the last decade of his life that Jacob Bernoulli had in fact done so.

We might surmise that, while mentoring the young Leibniz, Huygens did not emphasize the calculus of games of chance as a particularly important area of study. As mentioned previously, Huygens was devoted almost exclusively to scientific and mathematical pursuits; perhaps he lacked the temperament for abstract philosophical contemplation. Moreover, his scientific interests generally did not encompass political and social issues. So, thinking deeply about the potential applications and limitations of his calculus of chance to human affairs would not have come naturally to him. Leibniz, on the other hand, possessed philosophical depth and interest in spades, but seemed unable to find the time to make probability a high enough priority.

What about Probabilism?

I mentioned that the philosopher/priest/mathematician Juan Caramuel incorporated Huygens's treatise in his 1670 mathematical masterwork *Mathesis Biceps*. Caramuel was interested in the calculus of chance and in the philosophical idea of probability. Indeed, earlier in his career he was a leading spokesman for the philosophy of "probabilism," which had emerged in the late sixteenth century. Ironically, this background may have worked against any inclination to find common ground between chance and probability.

Bartolomé de Medina (1527–1581), a Spanish Dominican theologian, is considered the originator of probabilism. The basic idea was that when there was uncertainty about the wisdom or propriety of a course of action, it was permissible to rely on what was merely probable, as opposed to certain.[34] Certainty could be derived only from scripture (as interpreted by the Catholic Church) or by logical deduction. Probable reasoning, on the other hand, could be supported by sound inductive arguments or by the opinions of established authorities.

Probabilism was motivated by a desire to loosen religious strictures in order to deal with apparent ambiguities or certain unavoidable practical realities. However, there was much debate about the extent to which such liberties could be taken. For example, was it acceptable to adopt a probable position even if there was arguably a *more* probable one? Writing in 1577, de Medina first lays out several apparently cogent arguments that support the common view, which held that:

> When the doubt is not equal on either side, and there are more urgent reasons for one side than the other, that part is to be preferred that is confirmed by more arguments; for the excess of reason makes that part preponderate.

However, he disagrees that what is confirmed by more arguments must necessarily dictate morality:

> These arguments certainly seem very good, but it seems to me that if an opinion is probable it is licit to follow it, though the opposite be more probable. For, a probable opinion in speculative matters is one that we can follow without danger of error and deception; therefore a probable opinion in practical matters is one that we can follow without danger of sin.

To our modern way of thinking, this position makes no sense. James Franklin explains what de Medina had in mind:

> This is completely impossible on a usual understanding of *probable*, since the opposite of a proposition is more probable than it, then the proposition itself is not probable but improbable. But this is only so if *probability* is taken to mean, as it should, probable on one's total evidence, that is after all consideration of reasons both for and against.[35]

However, this assumes (as we do) that "one's total evidence" can be woven into a coherent picture. The evidence for and against may be contradictory, so that such an integration is impossible. Moreover, in de Medina's time, the dividing line between "evidence" and "argument" was far more ambiguous than today. For example, the testimony of a learned expert was one of the main sources of evidence.

As I explained in Chapter 3, probability connoted something more like an amount of justification for believing something, or its prove-ability. An argument in support of a proposition would address the ambiguity of the circumstances plus the doubt about which course of action was warranted. As Keynes explained, unless the bodies of evidence adduced in support of a proposition and opposing it are identical, there is no single dimension along which the probabilities for and against can be arrayed numerically. In the face of the extreme ambiguity of the moral issues being debated, uniformity of opinion regarding the relevant evidence was rare.

Caramuel's extremely liberal views earned him the sobriquet "prince of laxists." Caramuel's ideas were in direct opposition to Jansenism, of which Pascal's friend Arnaud at Port-Royal was a leading figure.[36] The Jansenists, so-named from the originator of the movement, Cornelius Jansen (1585–1638), opposed probabilism. Their theology was very complex, but generally emphasized the importance of unwavering faith over human rationality. Caramuel was a strong advocate of reasoning about probabilities. Pascal after adopting Jansenism took up the cudgel against Caramuel in his *Provincial Letters* of 1656.

Because of its religious and philosophical overtones, probability might have been too loaded a term for either Caramuel or Pascal to associate with the calculus of chance. Indeed, in his writing Pascal lampooned the abuses to which "probable" arguments had been put in sanctioning highly questionable behavior based on flimsy rationalizations. So, it is perhaps surprising that the Port-Royal *Logic*, on which he advised, offers the first hint of a connection between probability and chance.

At the tail end of a very long exposition, a few modern-*seeming* concepts have been tucked in.[37] For example, many have interpreted Pascal's Wager as an early exercise in probabilistic utility theory. What we find in the *Logic* is perhaps the *germ* of an idea that games of chance have something important to teach us about making rational decisions under uncertainty. However, it is highly doubtful that anything like our concept of mathematical probability had begun to replace traditional probability here. Indeed, the only person before 1700 to think *seriously* about games of chance as a model for uncertainty was just 7 years old when the Port-Royal *Logic* appeared in 1662.

Bernoulli's Meditations

Sometime in the mid-1680s Jacob Bernoulli conceived a revolutionary notion.[38] He believed that games of chance could serve as a useful model for dealing with many situations involving decisions in the face of uncertainty. In his *Meditationes*, he expressed his nascent thoughts about the relationships between the mathematics of gambling, the potential to make inferences from observations of event frequencies and the idea of probability as a numerical measure of uncertainty. His extensive elaboration of these ideas would not appear until 1713, 8 years after his death. However, by 1689 nearly all of his *Ars Conjectandi* (*The Art of Conjecturing*) had already been completed.

What was known to his contemporaries is not clear. A few students may have been privy to some aspects of his thinking. In his public disputations involving his brother Johann and others, Jacob alluded to the potential importance of combinatorial mathematics for a variety of practical problems and provided many specific examples of potential applications. Moreover, in his inaugural lecture upon becoming dean of philosophy at the University of Basel in 1692, he asserted that "the use and necessity of the art of combinations is universal: without it neither the wisdom of the philosopher, nor the exactness of the historian, nor the dexterity of the physician, nor the prudence of the politician could be established." Bernoulli was the first to attempt a systematic formulation of the connection between probability and the combinatorial mathematics that governs games of chance.[39]

Certainly, Johann Bernoulli must have had some inkling of Jacob's insights, since the brothers had worked closely together until their alienation in the early 1690s. In 1692, Jacob apparently wrote to Johann, who was then in Paris teaching the infinitesimal calculus to the Marquis de l'Hôpital (1661–1704), about his work on the *Ars Conjectandi*. In particular, he may have boasted about his Golden Theorem, though probably without providing details of the proof. To an inquiry from Leibniz in 1697 regarding Sauveur's article in 1679 on Bassette, mentioned earlier in this chapter, Johann responded:

> Until now I did not know that he (Sauveur) wrote something mathematical on the game of Bassette. I would like to see it, because my brother already a long time ago endeavored to write a book entitled *Ars Conjectandi*, in which would be

provided not only a mathematical treatment of all kinds of games, but also means of reducing to calculations other probabilities in every area of life. I do not know, however, whether the book is still unfinished or not, only that while he once judged that to consult anything of mine was not to be spurned, now, agitated by his usual rivalry, he scarcely ever fails to attack.[40]

So, it seems that during the 1690s word of Jacob's achievements may have begun to leak out. However, the specifics of his approach remained a mystery.

Across the Channel

On the Continent during the 1690s, there was only a hint of the conceptual and mathematical breakthroughs that Bernoulli had made. However, in England we know of three publications that express ideas about probability that appear at least parallel to, if not influenced by, those expressed by Jacob Bernoulli. Were these simply the natural flowering of an idea whose time had come, or perhaps inspired somehow by Bernoulli's work? This remains a mystery that has yet to be solved.

One clue lies in the Preface to the first of the three publications, the 1692 translation of Huygens's famous treatise I mentioned earlier.[41] In the Preface by John Arbuthnot, the word "probability" is mentioned no fewer than five times. This is curious because nowhere in Huygens's treatise does the word probability appear. Moreover, Arbuthnot never actually refers to probability as a fraction of favorable to total cases, either here or in any later writing. So, I believe he was using probability in its traditional sense. However, he might have become aware in some way of Jacob's general idea that epistemic probability and games of chance could somehow be linked.

Remarkably, Arbuthnot's Preface suggests that the "Calculation of the Quantity of Probability might be improved to a very useful and pleasant Speculation, and applied to a great many Events which are accidental, besides those of Games." Except for Jacob Bernoulli, no one else in 1692 had so clearly enunciated such an idea, as far as we know. The Preface continues:

> … these Cases would be infinitely more confus'd, as depending on Chances which the most part of Men are ignorant of; and as I have hinted already, all the Politicks in the World are nothing else but a kind of Analysis of the Quantity of Probability

in casual Events, and a good Politician signifies no more, but one who is dexterous at such Calculations; only the Principles which are made use of in the solution of such Problems, can't be studied in a Closet, but acquir'd by the Observation of Mankind. There is likewise a Calculation of the Quantity of Probability founded on Experience, to be made use of in Wagers about any thing; for Example, it is odds, if a Woman is with Child, but it shall be a Boy; and if you would know the just odds, you must consider the Proportion in the Bills what the Males bear to the Females.

Both the ideas and their expression here sound quite Bernoullian. For example, compare Jacob's pronouncement in his inaugural lecture about combinatorics as critical to "the dexterity of the physician" and "the prudence of the politician" with Arbuthnot's remark that "a good Politician signifies no more, but one who is dexterous at such calculations." In another paragraph reconciling human perception of chance with divinely ordained necessity, Arbuthnot states that:

It is impossible for a Dye, with such a determin'd force and direction, not to fall on such a determin'd side, only I don't know the force and direction which makes it fall on such a determin'd side, and therefore I call that Chance, which is nothing but want of Art.

This seems like an abbreviated paraphrasing of Bernoulli's a passage in the *Ars Conjectandi*:

It is most certain, given the position, velocity, and distance of a die from the gaming table at the moment when it leaves the hand of the thrower, that the die cannot fall other than the way it actually does fall ... Yet it is customary to count the fall of the die ... as contingent. The only reason for this is that those things which ... are given in nature, are not yet sufficiently known to us.[42]

Hmmm! Arbuthnot's later writing about chance did not display a similar degree of originality, philosophical sophistication, or usage of the term probability. So, how was young Arbuthnot inspired to propound these ideas? As I suggested earlier, David Gregory may have been the connecting link.

The two other English contributions to quantitative probability concerned the credibility of testimony. Both of these were published in 1699, and both have been attributed to mathematically literate English clergymen. One of these mathematical theologians was John Craig (1663–1731), who was born in Dumfries, Scotland. Craig was trained in mathematics at Edinburgh in 1684–1685 under the tutelage of David

Gregory. In 1685, he traveled to Cambridge and there became inspired by Newton, resulting in a short mathematical treatise, which subsequently embroiled him in a long-running dispute with Johann Bernoulli.[43]

By the mid-1690s, Craig had obtained an M.A. in theology, moved back to England and embarked on a career in the Church of England. However, he also remained active as a mathematician, pursuing research related to the new infinitesimal calculus and tutoring private students to supplement his income. Craig was one of the earliest to recognize the significance of Newton's scientific and mathematical achievements, and was an early disciple. He maintained an active correspondence with David Gregory and other "Newtonian" mathematicians. Craig's mathematical contributions were recognized by his contemporaries, and he was elected in 1711 to the Royal Society.

Around 1696 Craig authored a tract, eventually published in 1699, that combined his religious and mathematical interests.[44] This he rather grandiosely dubbed Mathematical Principles of Christian Theology. Obviously influenced by Newton's *Philosophiae Naturalis Principia Mathematica* (Mathematical Principles of Natural Philosphy), this work was intended to defend Christian faith against certain heretical beliefs. Like many others at the time, he took Newton's brilliant exposition of God's governing *physical* laws as a model for how truth in many other domains of knowledge could be revealed.

Craig disputed the popular misconception that the Second Coming was close at hand. He had found evidence in the Gospels that suggested the return would happen at a time when faith had dissipated completely. To estimate when that loss of belief would happen, he developed an elaborate mathematical analysis of the rate at which the credibility of historical testimony would erode over time. His discussion began with a definition of probability as "the appearance of agreement or disagreement of two ideas as through arguments whose conclusion is not fixed, or at least is not perceived to be so."

This rather obscure formulation was perhaps inspired by the famed philosopher John Locke (1632–1704), who discussed probability in *An Essay Concerning Human Understanding*, published in 1690:

> Therefore, as God has set some things in broad daylight; as he has given us some certain knowledge, though limited to a few things in comparison ... so, in the greatest part of our concernments, he has afforded us only the twilight, as I may so say, of probability; suitable, I presume, to that state of mediocrity and

probationership he has been pleased to place us in here ... Men often stay not war-
ily to examine the agreement or disagreement of two ideas which they are desirous
or concerned to know; but ... lightly cast their eyes on, or wholly pass by the
proofs.[45]

For Locke and Craig, judgments of probability entailed a necessarily
imperfect weighing of evidence to decide whether to infer that one idea
implied another idea. Like the staunch Newtonian he was, Craig explicitly attempted to derive a general mathematical law to describe the mental "forces" at work and the "velocity" of changing opinions over time.
Craig's notion of probability was quantitative, but cannot be translated
into a degree of certainty in the modern sense. Rather, it was an attempt
to reduce the old-style probability to a mathematical logic:

> The key, we must realize, is that Craig's 'probability' was not our probability. He
> was writing at a time ... before probability came to be nearly universally taken
> to be a measure of uncertainty on a scale of zero to one, where, in the case of
> independent events, combination was by multiplication.[46]

Craig concluded that belief in the historical veracity of the Biblical
accounts would not evaporate until the year 3150. Craig's attempted
application of Newtonian mathematical analysis may seem peculiar, but
his methodology should not be dismissed too lightly. Craig drew an analogy between the dynamics of belief and the physical dynamics that governed the universe. Had it taken root, this idea might have resulted in
an alternative version of mathematical probability. What is important to
understand is that defining probability as a fraction of chances had not
yet been established.

The third English publication on probability in the 1690s is in some
ways the most extraordinary and enigmatic.[47] It appeared as an anonymous paper in the *Philosophical Transactions* of the Royal Society in
1699 entitled "A Calculation of the Credibility of Human Testimony."
Since that time, its authorship has been debated. Most scholars currently
attribute the work to the Reverend George Hooper (1640–1727), a well-
known clergyman who later became Bishop of Bath and Wells. Hooper
was known as a brilliant student with diverse academic interests, including mathematics, graduating from Oxford in 1660 and obtaining graduate
degrees there in 1673 and 1674. He published many essays, including in

1689 a commentary on the reliability of historical evidence based on oral and written transmission.

This essay published by Hooper in 1689 did not contain a mathematical treatment of the subject. Ten years later, however, the paper in the *Philosophical Transactions* revisited this topic, but with a far more sophisticated mathematical slant. Indeed, it appears to be the work of a mathematical maestro; if truly written by Hooper, then this unusually tardy mathematical debut at age 59 may represent some kind of world record. Karl Pearson, nearly a century ago, attributed the work to Edmond Halley, in part because of the advanced probabilistic treatment: "The man who wrote this paper knew how to measure probability and what is meant by odds.[48] He also knew something of insurance work." Indeed, the author was also conversant with the use of algebraic notation, the concept of present value of a future payment, and the use of logarithms.

In this paper, the author draws another kind of analogy. He likens the degradation of credibility associated with a historical event to the present value of a future asset. As an example, he assumes that with each transmission of a report about the event, our confidence in the report's veracity would decrease by 6%. He observes that "the Proportion of Certainty after Twelve such Transmissions will be but as a Half, and it will grow by that Time an equal Lay, whether the Report be true or not."

The choice of 6% is interesting because it would have allowed the author to piggyback on a table in Halley's 1693 paper on the Breslau data. Halley provided a table showing the present value at 6% interest as a function of the number of years until payment. Halley's table indicated that an amount owed would be worth precisely 0.497 of its current value if paid 12 years later. Halley's discussion of the difficulties in performing such calculations shows that logarithms were still cutting-edge technology at that time. It seems unlikely that Reverend Hooper would be proficient in their use.

Perhaps even more astounding than the level of technical virtuosity is the surprisingly modern probabilistic reasoning. Although the paper refers to "credibility" rather than probability, this credibility of testimony obeys the basic axioms of modern mathematical probability. It *seems* that this paper must be using our probability, but the conceptual underpinnings are quite different. The conceptual model involves financial computations (present value) rather than games of chance. In a sense, the mathematical formulation of modern probability has been foreshadowed, although the conceptual foundation appears to be different.

Could Hooper really have been author of this impressive work? Since his voluminous writings include nothing even remotely comparable, this seems unlikely. Moreover, he was not even a member of the Royal Society, so how did this paper come to be published in the *Philosophical Transactions*? It seems likely that a member of the Royal Society must have been involved in some way, possibly even as the true anonymous author.

In 1699, there were only three Fellows of the Royal Society who appear to be plausible candidates.[49] One of these was Edmond Halley, Karl Pearson's nominee. However, Halley between 1698 and 1700 was far from England, sailing the high seas on his expedition to map patterns of magnetic forces. The second was Abraham De Moivre, who would later become the dominant figure in extending the mathematics of gambling. However, there is clear evidence that de Moivre's interest in probability was not sparked until he encountered Montmort's *Essay* a decade later. There remains one qualified candidate, David Gregory.

Could Gregory have played a role in either or both of the papers attributed to Craig and Hooper? If so, what might have been his motivation for analyzing the transmission of testimony? Gregory, like Isaac Newton, is known to have harbored doubts about some orthodox tenets of Anglican Christian beliefs. Newton, Gregory, and their friends held that the original scriptures were true and reliable, but that some errors or distortions had been introduced over the centuries since Biblical times.[50] In particular, they privately rejected the doctrine of the Trinity, believing that various passages appearing to support Trinitarianism were a result of "faulty copies, imperfect translations, and purposeful tampering by Trinitarian scribes."

Perhaps Gregory became interested in the credibility of historical testimony as a result of such heterodox views.[51] Indeed, in a book written in 1696 by a theologian named Stephen Nye, the following appears:

> Mr. Gregory of Oxford says in his preface to some critical notes on the scriptures that he published, there is no author, saith this learned critick, that has suffered so much by the hand of time, as the Bible has.

John Friesen, the historian reporting this quote mentions that he has been unable to locate a work of this description, which, he says, may have been published anonymously or circulated privately among a circle of friends. Perhaps these "critical notes" would, if they ever come to light, reveal what role if any David Gregory might have played in the evolution of "probability" in the 1690s.

CHAPTER 5

A MATHEMATICIAN OF BASEL

It is a frigid morning in early December of 1687 in Basel, Switzerland.[1] A few snowflakes are visible through the small window in the dining room of the Bernoulli house. Jacob stokes the fire before settling down to a light breakfast. Judith, his wife of 3 years, nurses their first child, Nicholas, born just a few months ago. As usual, Jacob is lost in thought; there is much on his mind these days.

It is less than a year since he finally garnered the prize he had coveted for so long, the professorship in mathematics at Basel University. Quite an accomplishment, he muses, for a self-taught mathematician with degrees in theology and philosophy. He has no regrets about refusing to enter his father's lucrative trade in medicinal herbs or perhaps becoming a respectable clergyman. Jacob has insisted on following his true calling, mathematics. He has already become one of the leaders in the new infinitesimal calculus devised by Gottfried Leibniz and has published several articles related to it.

His father, after whom young Nicholas was named, cannot understand the value of abstruse mathematics, and Jacob's unconventional career choice has led to much dissension. The vigorous new grandson bearing his name has certainly helped to mollify his father somewhat and ease

Willful Ignorance: The Mismeasure of Uncertainty, First Edition. Herbert I. Weisberg.
© 2014 John Wiley & Sons, Inc. Published 2014 by John Wiley & Sons, Inc.

the tension between the two strong-willed men. Jacob feels more than ever that his mission is to demonstrate the practical value as well as the beauty of mathematical analysis. This sense of destiny is reflected in his chosen motto: *Invito patre sidero verso* (Despite my father I turn toward the stars). Once he had meant the stars literally, but now he has turned from astronomy to the realm of abstract ideas. He has even dared to believe that mathematics can lead to solutions for many important practical problems.

"Doctor Leibniz is most assuredly a brilliant geometer," he tells Judith, "but I find the presentation of his new calculus lacking in rigorous proof and often very difficult to follow. Sometimes I wonder if the printer has made an error in reproducing his words." Surprisingly, she responds with a suggestion: "Why don't you stop complaining and just write to the great man and ask him?" Jacob, who has already been contemplating such a course, resolves to do so as soon as his lecturing responsibilities will allow. In addition to initiating a discussion related to the infinitesimal calculus, he plans eventually to raise another issue with Leibniz, but not just yet.

For the past 3 years, Jacob has been fascinated by the calculus of games of chance. He has made much progress in understanding and extending the ideas in Huygens's treatise, which he first came upon while visiting Holland 6 years ago during his period of youthful travel and study. Already, he believes, he has surpassed Huygens and the few others he knows of who have written on these matters. Indeed, the challenge problem he posed 2 years ago in the *Journal des Sçavans* (Journal of the Savants) has yet to be solved by any of its distinguished readers. But Jacob's interest in the subject goes far beyond mere gambling problems. He perceives combinatorial mathematics as the key to an "art of conjecturing" about many things that are uncertain, extending to the spheres of legal, social, and economic affairs. He suspects that Leibniz, whose interests and contacts are so broad, would be more capable than anyone of offering wise counsel about this subject.

Returning from his brief reverie, Jacob sighs and turns his attention to present concerns. He has an appointment to meet with his younger brother Johann in 1 hour. Teaching Johann, now 20, has been a mixed blessing. On the one hand, Jacob enjoys their collaboration in penetrating the mysteries of the new Leibnizian calculus. On the other hand, introducing Johann to mathematics has put him even further in his father's bad graces, as Johann is supposedly destined for a medical career.

Moreover, his precocious sibling's attitude has begun to cause some friction of late; Johann seems to relish any opportunity to display his mathematical talent, whether in private conversation or in public disputations. This can often be at the expense of others less quick and clever, and at times even of Jacob himself. "Perhaps he will mellow with age," thinks Jacob.

PUBLICATION AT LAST

During the 18 years that Jacob occupied the Chair of Mathematics at Basel, his record of accomplishment elevated him to the first rank of European mathematicians. He and his younger brother Johann became the primary exponents and developers of Leibniz's calculus and were responsible for many refinements and fundamental advances. When Jacob finally succumbed to tuberculosis in 1705, at the age of only 50, several written eulogies attested to the high esteem in which he was held. In addition to his extensive research on the infinitesimal calculus, these encomiums alluded to his unfinished masterpiece, *Ars Conjectandi* (The Art of Conjecturing).

Based mainly on information provided by Jacob's student and colleague Jacob Hermann (1678–1733), a lengthy eulogy was written by Bernard le Bovier Fontanelle (1657–1757) and delivered before a general assembly of the French Royal Academy of Sciences on November 14, 1705.[2] Referring to the *Ars Conjectandi*, Fontanelle stated:

> He achieved a great work De Arte Conjectandi, & although nothing of it has appeared, we are able to give an idea of it on the testimony of M. Herman ... Some great Mathematicians, & principally Messers Pascal & Huygens, have already proposed or resolved some Problems on this matter, but they have done only to touch it lightly, & Mr. Bernoulli embraced it in a greater extent, & studied it thoroughly much further. He carried it even to Moral & Political things, & it is there that the Work must have more new, & more surprise.

So, the broad outlines of Bernoulli's work were known, but the specifics remained obscure.

As the potential importance of his advances became more widely circulated after his death, interest grew in having the *Ars Conjectandi* completed, if possible, and published. Leibniz, among others, urged Jacob's widow to allow the publication, possibly edited by Johann. However, by then the internecine rivalry between Jacob and his brother had become so acrimonious that his wife Judith and son Nicholas (by that time a promising young painter) refused to allow Johann access to the manuscript. Only Jacob Hermann was trusted to help organize his master's papers but wrangling over the conditions of publication persisted for several years.

Eventually, the responsibility for overseeing the publication devolved upon another Nicholas Bernoulli (1687–1759), a nephew of both Jacob and Johann (the son of their brother Nicholas, a well-respected portrait painter), who had studied mathematics under Jacob. Keeping the Bernoullis all straight, especially the Nicholases, is no easy matter. This particular Nicholas was born in 1687, graduated from the University of Basel in 1704, and subsequently completed a doctoral degree in law and mathematics in 1709. His thesis drew heavily upon the unpublished work of his uncle, to which he had access while a student of Jacob's. Nicholas agreed to supervise the publication.[3]

Ironically, by the time *Ars Conjectandi* finally appeared in 1713, its impact was muted by several other developments that had been inspired by its anticipation. These include Pierre de Montmort's *Essay D'Analyse* in 1708, Nicholas Bernoulli's doctoral thesis in 1709, and Abraham de Moivre's *De Mensura Sortis* (On the Measurement of Chances) in 1711. Nonetheless, Bernoulli's unfinished opus was immediately recognized as a masterpiece and became highly influential. To maintain your temporal bearings, it might be helpful to refer to the Timeline once again.

THE ART OF CONJECTURING

The *Ars Conjectandi* was a 239-page book that consisted of four separate sections, or Parts, each a gem in its own right.[4] The title was chosen to highlight Jacob's purpose of extending the subject treated in the *Ars Cogitandi* (Port-Royal *Logic*) of Arnaud and Nicole. While the Logic dealt with rationality in general, Bernoulli aspired to treat the art of thinking about uncertain matters. Since pure logical deduction could not adequately deal with the challenges posed by such problems, he would propose a parallel art of conjecture.

The first three Parts comprised a summary and extension of what had gone before, which was then capped by Bernoulli's bold vision of the art

Landmarks of Probability

1600		
	1654	Pascal & Fermat
	1657	Huygens
1700		
	1713	**Bernoulli**
	1718	De Moivre
	1764	Bayes & Price
	1774	Laplace
1800		
	1837	Poisson
	1838	De Morgan
	1843	Mill
	1843	Cournot
	1849	Ellis
	1854	Boole
	1866	Venn
	1892	Peirce
1900		
	1921	Keynes
	1921	Knight
	1922	Fisher
	1926	Ramsey
	1926	Neyman & Pearson
	1928	Von Mises
	1937	De Finetti
	1949	Reichenbach
	1954	Savage
	1959	Popper

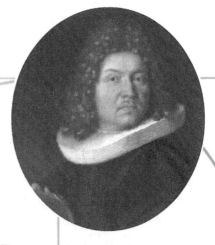

JACOBI BERNOULLI,
Profeff. Bafil. & utriúfque Societ. Reg. Scientiar.
Gall. & Pruff. Sodal.
MATHEMATICI CELEBERRIMI,

ARS CONJECTANDI,

OPUS POSTHUMUM.

Accedit

TRACTATUS
DE SERIEBUS INFINITIS,

Et Epistola Gallicè scripta

DE LUDO PILÆ
RETICULARIS.

BASILEÆ,

Jacob Bernoulli

of conjecturing in the unfinished Part Four. From Bernoulli's perspective, the first three Parts, while interesting and important, served mainly as a prelude to the revolutionary conceptual and mathematical breakthrough in Part Four: "The Use and Application of the Preceding Doctrine in Civil, Moral, and Economic Matters."

Part One: The Annotated Huygens

The first section of the *Ars Conjectandi* consisted of a reprinting of Huygens's treatise in its entirety, along with extensive explanatory notes. These notes, much longer than the Huygens text itself, served two purposes. First, they provided a helpful elaboration of the rather cryptic discussion contained in Huygens's original presentation. Jacob's clear and detailed exposition offers us a hint of why he was regarded so highly as a mentor and lecturer. Second, the notes extended and generalized the mathematical analysis in many ways.

Bernoulli begins by explaining the fundamental concept of mathematical expectation, by which "account is taken of the extent to which our hope of getting the best is tempered and diminished by fear of getting something worse." The expected value is "something intermediate between the best we hope for and the worst we fear." Recall that Huygens's original definition (his first Proposition) appealed to a rather complicated scenario of "hedging" bets to justify the mathematical expectation on general principles of fairness. Bernoulli justifies the concept more straightforwardly, illustrating by reference to Huygens's example of 7 coins (or a coins in general) hidden in one hand and 3 coins (or b) in the other.

If I will receive the contents of whichever hand I choose, and you will receive what is in the other hand, what is my expectation?

> In this case both of us together will acquire without fail and therefore ought to expect what is hidden in both hands, namely 10 coins or $a + b$. But it must be conceded that each of us has an equal right to what we expect. Therefore it follows that the total expectation should be divided into two equal parts, and to each of us should be attributed half of the total expectation, that is 5 coins or $(a + b)/2$.[5]

So, in this simple case, my expectation is simply my fair share of the total expectation.

Bernoulli goes on to deal with the various problems considered by Huygens, including the five challenge problems. In many cases he generalizes the problem and often adds helpful commentary. For example, in discussing the famous problem of points first solved by Pascal and Fermat, he points out how our intuitions can lead us astray. He mentions the fallacy that the ratio of the expectations for the players in a discontinued match ought to reflect simply their ratio of games needed to win. For example, if I lack 3 games and you lack only 2, a naïve division would award 2/5 of the pot to me and 3/5 to you.

> So this should warn us to be cautious in our judgments and to avoid the habit of immediately drawing conclusions from any proportion we find in things, something that very frequently happens, even with those who seem to know a very great deal.[6]

He also condemns the idea that experiencing good fortune is some kind of habit that confers on someone a right to expect it to continue.

In one of his most remarkable comments, Jacob essentially states the modern definition of probability without actually using the term:

> We can use the letter *a*, as the author [Huygens] does, to denote monetary stakes that can be divided among the players in proportion to their expectations. But as we shall show more fully in the last part of the book, it can also be used more generally to denote anything that, even if it is inherently undivided, can be *conceived* as divisible with regard to the number of cases in which it can be gained or lost, happen or fail to happen. Things that can be divided *in this conceptual way* include any reward, triumph, or victory, the status or condition of a person or thing, any public office, any work undertaken, life or death and so on (emphasis added).[7]

In this passage, the connection between an expectation and a specific gambling context is cleanly severed. Jacob is stating that for virtually any imaginable thing, we can *conceive of* the expectation that it will happen.

Expectation is not necessarily a monetary value, but rather a measure of how much confidence we have (or ought to have) that the event will come to pass. Jacob is well aware that his remark about the "number of cases" is not to be taken literally. He tells us that things like reward and triumph "can be divided in this conceptual way." This is an essential point that has been much misunderstood. Bernoulli's notion of cases is intended to be interpreted metaphorically, not literally.

For Jacob, the concept of expectation relates not only to fairness, as for Huygens, but has explicitly taken on an *epistemic* connotation as well. Expectation expresses something about our *knowledge* or *belief* regarding whether or not the event is apt to occur. Probability for us can be interpreted as the expectation of something *in the abstract*, stripped of an associated outcome value. But this was far from the case when Jacob wrote in the 1680s. Jacob highlights the strangeness of this new idea by the example of a prince who decrees that two condemned criminals can play a fair game to decide which of the two will be pardoned. Since the expectation for each would then be 1/2 of life, each man could in a sense be considered half dead and half alive.

Jacob derives solutions to many other gambling problems and suggests how his approach can be extended to other problems. One result he obtains is of particular value and is especially important for the application he has in mind in Part Four. He considers the general problem in which a gamester attempts to obtain a particular result within a given number of trials. For example, he may need to roll a 6 at least once in four rolls of a standard die. Pascal and Fermat had already solved this problem in 1654, but Bernoulli went on to consider the player's expectation if he must roll *exactly* two 6s within four rolls. In fact, he solved the general problem of this type for *any* number r of "successes" in any number n of total "trials," and with any number b of chances for success on each trial and c chances for failure.[8]

Part Two: Permutations and Combinations

The second section of the *Ars Conjectandi* provides a thorough analysis of the ways in which various things can be arranged and combined. A *permutation* is a shuffling, or re-ordering, of a given set of objects or elements. For example, the letters a, b, and c can be ordered in six possible ways: *abc, acb, bac, bca, cab, cba*. For any number n of distinct objects (letters, numbers, words, people, etc.) there is a simple formula that can be used to calculate the number of possible arrangements. This formula is simply the product $n(n-1)(n-2) \ldots 1$. For example, the number of permutations of four objects is 24 ($= 4 \times 3 \times 2 \times 1$). Mathematicians express such a product as $n!$ (n-factorial).

There are also many possible complications that can be introduced. For example, some of the elements may appear more than once, or various restrictions may be placed on the positions that can be occupied by some of the elements. We can also consider arrangements of a subset of the total set. For example, the number of ordered pairs that can be formed from n objects is $n(n-1)$. Thus, twelve pairs can be composed using four letters: *ab, ac, ad, ba, bc, bd, ca, cb, cd, da, db, dc.*

Calculating the number of permutations of things under different specified conditions is part of the subject of combinatorial mathematics, or *combinatorics.* An even more important branch of the subject pertains to the number of combinations. A *combination* is a selection of a certain number of elements from a larger total set. For a combination, as opposed to a permutation, the order of selection does not matter. For example, there are six ways of choosing two out of four elements. It is no coincidence that six is half of twelve. In the list of twelve permutations above, each combination appears twice. That is, there are two permutations of each pair of two elements.[9]

Combinatorics plays a central role in the analysis of gambling. Some obvious examples are games of cards, in which the numbers of selections (e.g., poker hands) leading to particular outcomes (e.g., full house, flush) determine the chances of winning. However, the theory of combinations enters in more subtle ways into games involving dice, coins, or other "random" mechanisms. Of particular importance is the formula for the number of combinations of r things taken out of n total. This formula played a central role in the derivation of Jacob's Golden Theorem in Part Four.

The modern derivation of this formula is quite simple and familiar to many high school students. But in Bernoulli's time this formula was not widely known or at all obvious. Rather, the number of combinations for various values of n and r would typically be obtained from a table similar to Table 5.1. Note that this table can be extended indefinitely by following a simple rule. To find the number that corresponds to any n and r, simply add the number immediately above to the number above and one column to the left.

Table 5.1 is actually one version of what has come to be known as Pascal's Arithmetical Triangle, although it was known long before Pascal's famous *Treatise on the Arithmetical Triangle.* This method of calculation works perfectly but is too cumbersome for the analysis of complex

TABLE 5.1   Pascal's Arithmetical Triangle

1	1	1	1	1	1	1	1	1	1
1	2	3	4	5	6	7	8	9	
1	3	6	10	15	21	28	36		
1	4	10	20	35	56	84			
1	5	15	35	70	126				
1	6	21	56	126					
1	7	28	84						
1	8	36							
1	9								
1									

problems, such as the problem of points. Blaise Pascal, had written his *Treatise* shortly before his correspondence with Pierre Fermat.[10] This little monograph summarized and expanded upon the esoteric knowledge that had grown over the centuries regarding these marvelous numbers.

One of the important formulas derived by Pascal provided a convenient way to calculate the number of combinations for any values of n and r. Unfortunately, Jacob was unaware of Pascal's book, which had been published only in French and not widely circulated. This is strange, since the *Ars Conjectandi* does mention the famous correspondence between Pascal and Fermat, which Jacob knew about from Fermat's collected works, published in 1679.[11] However, while Pascal alludes to his unpublished treatise in the letters sent to Fermat, there is no detail about the book's contents, and it was not published until 1665. Since Fermat died in 1665, he would not have possessed a copy.

At any rate, Bernoulli has to start essentially from scratch, independently deriving much of the same material.[12] He also derives several combinatorial results that are completely new, or are improved versions of what had gone before. In his Introduction to Part Two, Jacob highlights the importance and the difficulty of accounting for *all* the complex ways that various parts can be assembled to produce natural phenomena and human actions.[13] In a famous passage originally read in his 1692 inaugural oration, he motivates the study of combinatorics by emphasizing its potential value as a mental discipline.

> … there is no error into which even the most prudent and circumspect more frequently fall than the error that logicians commonly call the *insufficient enumeration of the parts*. This is so true that I dare say this is almost the only source from which

spring the countless and most serious errors that we daily commit in our thinking, whether about things to be understood or things to be done. As a result, the Art called Combinatorics should be judged, as it merits, most useful, because it remedies this defect of our minds and teaches us how to enumerate all possible ways in which several things can be combined, transposed, or joined with each other, so that we may be sure that we have omitted nothing that can contribute to our purpose.[14]

This is a remarkably strong statement, which we may be tempted to dismiss as mere hyperbole. But Jacob Bernoulli was a man who did not use words loosely. I believe he meant that errors in judgment occur primarily because we are *ignorant* regarding certain relevant aspects of a given situation, pertaining either to the existence of an unrecognized factor or to the way in which different factors interact with each other. Combinatorics, he asserts, can sensitize us to the critical importance of considering all relevant information. Furthermore, as he goes on to elaborate in Part Four, it may in some cases undergird a calculus of probability.

As a prime example of how the insufficient enumeration of cases can trip us up, Bernoulli, discusses the so-called "Proteus verses," a term coined over a century earlier by a philosopher of great pretension and ambition aptly named Julius Caesar Scaliger (1484–1558).[15] Part of Scaliger's renown rested on his devastating 900-page critique of a widely read work by our old friend Gerolamo Cardano. While this caused Cardano some consternation, he managed, in a comedy of errors, to exact retribution when Scaliger mistakenly came to believe a report that Cardano had died shortly after receiving this screed. Upon learning of this, Cardano deliberately stalled in correcting this misunderstanding, motivating the guilt-ridden Scaliger to retract some of his accusations.

A Proteus verse was a Latin verse that conformed to a certain very particular poetical form but could be permuted in many ways that would still maintain the same metrical rhythm (though the meaning might be nonsensical).[16] One of the most famous of these was a hexameter by a Jesuit priest, Bernard Bauhuis (1575–1616):

Tot tibi sunt dotes, Virgo, quot sidera coelo

This translates as "You have as many virtues, Virgin, as there are stars in the heavens." The challenge that had occupied several eminent mathematicians over the course of a century was to calculate the exact number of different permutations of the words that would still satisfy the complex metrical rules. In all, there are 40,320 possible permutations of the eight words, so an attempt to list them all and evaluate each one would have been impractical.

A variety of different answers had been proposed, including 2196 by the French mathematician Jean Prestet (1648–1690), which he later amended to 3276, and 3096 by John Wallis (1616–1703). Bernoulli attempted to set the record straight. However, his correct answer to this problem continued to be disputed right into modern times. It was not finally settled until the advent of electronic computers. Remarkably, Jacob's answer of 3312 is the only correct solution by hand calculation that is known! Moreover, it turns out that he had developed and meticulously applied a sophisticated technique that would much later be known to computer scientists as the "backtracking algorithm."[17]

Finally, Jacob suggests that combinatorics is important not only in artificial problems, such as counting verses, but potentially in many endeavors of practical importance:

> Although, indeed, this is a mathematical matter insofar as it ends in calculation, nevertheless if one looks to its use and necessity, it is absolutely universal and so well established that neither the wisdom of the philosopher nor the exactitude of the historian, neither the dexterity of the physician nor the prudence of the statesman can stand without it. As an argument for this, let it suffice that the work of all of these kinds of individuals depends upon *conjectures*, and every conjecture involves weighing complexions or combinations of causes.[18]

Bernoulli seems to be saying that sound judgment, the art of conjecture, boils down to accurate comprehension and appropriate weighing of all the types and quantities of evidence that are available. This problem, he believes, is fundamentally a matter of combinatorial mathematics, although the nature of the causal factors involved or their interconnections may be unknown to us.

Part Three: Games of Chance

The third section of the *Ars Conjectandi* provides a thorough analysis of the ways in which the theory of permutations and combinations can be applied to solve many problems related to various games of chance. His introduction to this long section of the book is succinct, and has the tone of someone dutifully satisfying an onerous but necessary obligation.

> Having completed in the preceding Part of this work the doctrine of permutations and combinations, methodical order demands that we explain in this Part its fullest use in determining the expectations of players in various ways of drawing lots and games of chance. The general foundation of this investigation consists in taking all the combinations or permutations of which the subject matter is capable as so many equipossible cases and in diligently considering how many of these cases are favorable to or opposed to this or that player. After this, the rest is solved by the doctrine of Part I.[19]

This contrasts sharply with his almost lyrical introduction to the "art of combinatorics" in Part Two.

It is apparent that Jacob has little enthusiasm for the art of gambling *per se*. However, he soldiers on through 70 pages of densely worded text, dealing in great detail with arcane aspects of many popular games that involved cards or dice. He devotes 10 pages to a card game called *Trijacques* (Three Jacks) and 9 pages to *Bassette*. He describes the results obtained by Joseph Sauveur in 1679 related to the expectations for the players in various situations. He then diplomatically points out some errors committed by Sauveur:

> If anyone has compared the Tables of Dr. Sauveur with ours, he will understand that the former, in some places, and especially in the last, require some emendations. Concerning what is added there to the observations containing the proportion of the increase and decrease of the advantage to the banker as the number of cards is increased or decreased, it would gain nothing to say anything, since from the inspection of the Tables they are manifest to anyone.[20]

Part Four: Civil, Moral, and Economic Matters

Part Four was entitled "The Use and Application of the Preceding Doctrine in Civil, Moral, and Economic Matters." It consisted of 20 pages, divided into five chapters. Although it is a brilliant and original exposition, Jacob apparently looked upon it as somehow incomplete, or perhaps even defective. He pondered the implications of his theory off and on for

20 years, and remained unsatisfied, but was unwilling to publish—exactly why, remains a mystery.

Chapter 1: Some Preliminaries   The full title of Chapter 1 was "Some preliminaries on the certainty, probability, necessity, and contingency of things."[21] As a trained philosopher and theologian, Bernoulli was sensitive to the potential quagmire of attempting to reconcile concepts like certainty, probability, and contingency with religious faith. So, he acknowledges that God is the primary cause of all that exists, but sets such potential distractions aside: "Others may dispute how this certainty of future occurrences may coexist with the contingency and freedom of secondary causes; we do not wish to deal with matters extraneous to our goal."

He then proceeds to make clear that he is writing about *epistemic* probability, something that exists in our minds:

> Seen in relation to us, the certainty of things is not the same for all things, but varies in many ways, increasing or decreasing. Those things concerning the existence or future occurrence of which we can have no doubt ... enjoy the highest, and absolute, certainty. All other things receive a less perfect measure of certainty in our minds, greater or less in proportion as there are more or fewer probabilities that persuade us that the thing is, will be, or was.

This measure of certainty about something (proposition, event, conjecture) is an aspect of our mental state, which may or may not correspond with external reality. Moreover, its strength is in proportion to the reasons that persuade us. Jacob then offers his novel definition of probability as a numerical measure of belief whose value can range between 0 and 1:

> *Probability*, indeed, is degree of certainty, and differs from the latter as a part differs from the whole. Truly, if complete and absolute certainty, which we represent by the letter a or by 1, is supposed, for the sake of argument, to be composed of five parts, or probabilities, of which three argue for the existence or future existence of some outcome and the others argue against it, then that outcome will be said to have $3a/5$ or $3/5$ of certainty.

It is tempting to interpret Bernoulli's concept of probability as identical to our familiar mathematical probability, but there is an important difference. To grasp his meaning, imagine that our certainty can be represented by the height of the liquid in a cylindrical glass, or tube. A full glass would equate to complete certainty about some event (or statement). Each relevant argument would increase the height of the liquid to the degree that it tends to prove the existence of the event (or truth of the statement). The height at any moment as a fraction of the glass's total height is the probability in favor of the event (or statement).

According to *our* concept of probability, the liquid's height would of course represent our degree of certainty that the event will happen (or statement is true), and the empty space above it our certainty that the event will *not* occur (or statement is false). But that is not how Bernoulli, or anyone in his time, saw things. In effect, Bernoulli imagined that there were two separate glasses that could potentially be filled: one glass for evidence that supported the *existence* of the event (or truth of the statement), and another glass for evidence that supported the *non-existence* (or falsity). Each glass could potentially be filled to any extent, based on the arguments supporting the corresponding hypothesis. There was not *necessarily* any relationship assumed between the arguments on both sides. From this perspective, there were two competing, but not fully complementary, measures of the two competing absolute probabilities to be considered.

Bernoulli was attempting to quantify the type of thinking about probability that would have been familiar to Pascal and Caramuel. He regarded Huygens's calculus of chance as providing a potential means toward this end. However, he did not have our brand of probability in mind. His version of probability was implicitly more ambitious, in the sense of addressing uncertainty quite generally, including its aspects related to what I have termed ambiguity as well as to doubt. Like Bartolomé de Medina, the father of probabilism, Bernoulli assumed that the evidentiary bases pro and con were not necessarily identical. So uncertainty could not be placed on a single continuum.

Bernoulli states that something "is *possible* if it has even a very small part of certainty, *impossible* if it has none or infinitely little." Something "is *morally certain* if its probability comes so close to complete certainty that the difference cannot be perceived." He offers 999/1000 as an example of a possible criterion for moral certainty but indicates that the context must be taken into account in setting such a standard. "By contrast, something is *morally impossible* if it has only as much certainty as the amount by which moral certainty falls short of complete certainty."

By defining impossibility as having no certainty or an infinitely small part of certainty, Bernoulli was not suggesting *physical impossibility.* Rather, he meant that our arguments would be incapable of inducing even a smidgen of confidence that the event did exist. However, this would not necessarily also mean that the event had been proved *not* to exist. *Our* version of probability implicitly assumes that we are always deciding *between* existence and non-existence. Bernoulli's assumed that we are building an argument about *whether* the event exists.

Chapter 2: On Knowledge and Conjecture   Jacob defined probability as a personal "degree of certainty" regarding any proposition or event.[22] This degree of certainty was likened to the fraction of probabilities that "argue for" the event out of all such probabilities that can be brought to bear. So, he viewed the "probability" as both the fraction of certainty in total and also the sum of supporting component "probabilities" that together sum to this total. This unfamiliar formulation required amplification, as he well appreciated. So, he provided an extensive discussion of what he meant by "arguments" and how a probability can be fashioned from them.

The discussion begins with a sweeping statement that indicates the ambitious scope of his project:

> We are said to *know* or *understand* those things that are certain and beyond doubt, but only to *conjecture* or have *opinions* about all other things. To conjecture about something is to measure its probability. Therefore, we define the *art of conjecture*, or *stochastics*, as the art of measuring the probabilities of things as exactly as possible, to the end that, in our judgments and actions, we may always choose or follow that which has been found to be better, more satisfactory, safer, or more carefully considered. On this alone turns all the wisdom of the philosopher and all the practical judgment of the statesman.

Jacob explains that by weight he means the "probative force" of the argument. He further mentions the traditional distinction between *internal* and *external* (intrinsic and extrinsic) arguments. Internal arguments are based on what we might call logic and hard evidence. External arguments are based on "human authority and testimony."

Bernoulli's conception seems to be that the probability is determined by the total weight of the various relevant supporting arguments. Thus, at least conceptually, the probability (probative force) associated with each argument is a component of the total probability. However, he does not yet indicate how various probabilities lent by the individual arguments can be combined to produce a total degree of certainty. In terms of my metaphor of filling a glass, how exactly do several arguments combine to increase the height of the liquid?

Before undertaking that task, however, Jacob offers "some general rules, or axioms, which simple reason commonly suggests to a person of sound mind, and which the more prudent constantly observe in civil life." He offers with brief explanations nine general axioms of prudence, to which, he indicates, other maxims applicable in various specific circumstances could easily be added.

1. There is no place for conjectures in matters in which one may reach complete certainty.
2. It is not sufficient to weigh one or another argument. Instead we must bring together all arguments that we can come to know and that seem in any way to work toward a proof of the thing.
3. We should pay attention not only to those arguments that serve to prove a thing, but also to those that can be adduced for the contrary, so that when both groups have been properly weighed it may be established which arguments preponderate.
4. Remote and universal arguments are sufficient for making judgments about universals, but when we make conjectures about individuals, we also need, if they are at all available, arguments that are closer and more particular to those individuals.
5. In matters that are uncertain and open to doubt, we should suspend our actions until we learn more. But if the occasion for action brooks no delay, then between two actions we should always choose the one that seems more appropriate, safer, more carefully considered, or more probable, even if neither action is such in a positive sense.
6. What may help in some case and can harm in none is to be preferred to that which in no case can help or harm.

7. We should not judge the value of human actions by their results, since sometimes the most foolish actions enjoy the best success, while the most prudent actions have the worst results.

8. In our judgments we should be careful not to attribute more weight to things than they have. Nor should we consider something that is more probable than its alternatives to be absolutely certain, or force it on others.

9. Because, however, it is rarely possible to obtain certainty that is complete in every respect, necessity and use ordain that what is only morally certain be taken as absolutely certain.

These maxims are not formulas, but guidelines. They represent a summary and distillation of the principles that are followed intuitively by a wise philosopher or prudent statesman.

Chapter 3: Various Kinds of Arguments

Jacob makes an important distinction that seems paradoxical from our perspective, but was quite sensible in his conceptual framework.[23] Some arguments, he points out, support one side of an argument only, while others can support both sides, usually to different degrees. The former can bolster our certainty about something, but have no effect on our certainty regarding the contrary. Bernoulli referred to such a one-sided argument as a *pure argument.* "Pure arguments prove a thing in some cases in such a way that they prove nothing positively in other cases."

As an example, Jacob discusses the demeanor of a defendant accused of murder. Suppose, he says, that upon questioning about the crime, the accused turns pale and appears guilty. Such evidence might add some amount of probative liquid to the guilt-glass but would not affect the innocence-glass. Conversely, evidence of the defendant's good character might increase the level in the latter but not the former. Note that in this framework, unlike ours, there would be no way that additional evidence could ever *decrease* the level in either glass. The function of evidence is to build a case on one side or the other. These two separate opposing cases are then compared. This process is somewhat analogous to the way evidence and arguments are evaluated in a modern-day court of law.

In contrast to a pure argument, a mixed argument might provide some evidence for both sides. "*Mixed* arguments prove a thing in some cases in such a way that they prove the contrary in the other cases." A mixed argument can be imagined as an amount of liquid that will be contributed to both glasses. However a different proportion of the total amount can go into each of the glasses. So, part of the mixed argument's "probative force" or "weight" goes to one side of the issue and the remainder to the other. Bernoulli's notion of a mixed argument is essentially the same as our modern conception of how evidence operates to swing the balance of belief in one direction or the other.

Perhaps, most typically, mixed arguments refer to the kind of evidence that is sometimes indicative of the event and sometimes of its contrary. Bernoulli describes a hypothetical case in which a murderer was wearing a black cloak, and the accused man wore such a cloak, but so did three others in the same vicinity. Suppose this argument is deemed to be worth four "units" of certainty. One unit would be added to the hypothesis that the suspect is guilty but three units of certainty to the hypothesis that he is innocent. Note, however, that in Bernoulli's system, this argument might comprise only part of the evidence needed to achieve certainty. So, it would need to be combined in some way with any other relevant arguments until a sufficient volume of "probative force" had accumulated.

For this purpose, Jacob developed a rather elaborate system for weighing and combining the various individual arguments to arrive at an overall probability in favor of the event (or statement). Similarly, the arguments relevant to the contrary must be weighed and combined in like manner. Then, the two composite arguments would be compared:

> Now if, besides the arguments that tend to prove a thing, other pure arguments for the contrary arise, then both categories of arguments must be weighed separately according to the preceding rules so as to establish the ratio that holds between the probability of the thing and the probability of the contrary. Here it should be noted that, if the arguments adduced on each side are strong enough, it may happen that the absolute probability of each side significantly exceeds half of certainty, that is, that both of the contraries are rendered probable, though relatively speaking one is less probable than the other. Thus it can happen that one thing has 2/3 of certainty, while its contrary has 3/4; in this way both contraries will be probable, yet the first less probable than its contrary, in the ratio 2/3 to 3/4, or 8 to 9.

Our version of probability implicitly assumes that there is a *single body of evidence* upon which all the probabilities are predicated. Jacob's version does not impose this restriction, except in the context of games of chance.

A game of chance can, in principle, always be resolved into a known number of possible cases, all equally likely to happen. A player's probability of winning depends only on the number of cases that are favorable relative to the number that are unfavorable. Each case (chance) represents a single unit of argument that points either in favor of or against a win. In effect, there is only a single well-defined mixed argument that is fully specified by the equipment and rules of the game. Furthermore, this argument is definitive, because one of the cases must occur. Therefore, the total number of arguments (cases) always adds up to certainty. That is, the amount of metaphorical liquid in the two glasses must add to certainty. As a result, Bernoulli's probability of winning and probability of losing are complementary events that add up to 1 (certainty), just as our probabilities would.

Except in games of chance, however, Jacob's theory can have some surprising consequences. Most notably, he proposed a rule for combining the evidence based on pure arguments with the evidence based on mixed arguments. To illustrate the dilemma, suppose that as a result of the pure arguments, we obtain a probability of 3/4 for guilt. What would happen if we were to add a mixed argument that implied a certainty of innocence? According to Bernoulli's rules, the probability of guilt would remain 3/4, even though the event is "impossible" according to the mixed argument!

Some later analysts have seized on this "paradox" to suggest a flaw in Jacob's reasoning, but he was much too careful and thoughtful to make such an elementary error.[24] (Recall his solution of the exacting problem of the Proteus verses). To him, the consequences were undoubtedly well understood and made perfect sense. Adding an argument that provides *no justification* for believing in guilt would indeed simply *add nothing* to the justification resulting from the pure arguments. (The guilt-glass would remain 3/4 full.)

It would not nullify this justification. However, this mixed argument *would* imply complete certainty for innocence. Thus, we would have a situation in which P (Guilt) $= 3/4$, but P (Innocence) $= 1$. The apparent contradiction arises for us because we assume that both probabilities must be based on the same body of evidence.

Although there was no logical error in Bernoulli's reasoning, he was somewhat diffident regarding his rules for combining arguments. He recognized in particular the mental tension inherent in believing that something and its contrary could *both* enjoy an "absolute probability" greater than half of certainty. Such a situation, he suggests, might require us to reconsider our assumptions:

> I cannot conceal here that I foresee many problems in particular applications of these rules that could cause frequent delusions unless one proceeds cautiously in discerning arguments. For sometimes arguments can seem distinct that in fact are one and the same. Or, vice versa, those that are distinct can seem to be one. Sometimes what is posited in one argument plainly overturns a contrary argument.

Here he seems to be struggling with the conundrum of how to quantify our uncertainty in the face of the ambiguity of the evidence. As an example, he discusses a problem that had been discussed in the Port-Royal *Logic*. The problem involves a hypothetical dispute pertaining to whether a certain written contract was fraudulently predated. On the one hand, there is a strong presumption that the notary who witnessed the contract and attested to its validity was honest. Bernoulli assigns a probability of 49/50 to the proposition that the contract is authentic based on this argument alone. On the other hand, an argument alleging fraud could be based on the notary's "very bad reputation," which renders the inference of fraud virtually certain.

> We should not, however, ... conclude from this that the probability of authenticity and the probability of fraud are in a ratio of 49/50 to 999/1000, that is, that they are in a ratio close to equality. For when I posit that the fidelity of the notary is in dispute, by this very fact I posit that he is not to be included with the case of the 49 honest notaries who abhor fraud, but that he himself is himself the 50th who does not take his oath to heart and conducts himself faithlessly in office. This is what completely obviates or destroys the force of the argument that might otherwise have proved the authenticity of the document.

Bernoulli astutely recognizes that the arguments pro and con can be based on different assumptions that may be impossible to reconcile. He counsels us to consider carefully whether one side of the evidence is really obviated by the other.

This is sound advice, but I suspect he remained uneasy about the possibility of other difficulties "that could cause frequent delusions" in various specific situations. For example, an argument in favor of something (e.g., fraud) might be based on an assumption that merely *decreased* our confidence in the contrary (e.g., authenticity) without fully destroying its probative force. Can we devise general principles for dealing with such complex considerations? More than three centuries later, we can say little that is definitive regarding how we actually *do*, or how ideally we *should*, weigh the merits of such apparently conflicting evidence.

Chapter 4: On a Double Method of Finding the Number of Cases

Jacob now comes to his most exciting discovery, for which the earlier chapters have paved the way.[25] He has previously explained how combinatorics can remedy the "defect of our minds" that can result in the "insufficient enumeration of cases." In Part Two he has noted that the art of combinatorics "teaches us how to enumerate all possible ways in which several things can be combined, transposed, or joined with each other, so that we may be sure that we have omitted nothing that can contribute to our purpose."

In Chapters 1–3 of Part Four he has shown that the probability for anything can be considered a problem in combinatorics. Just as in a game of chance, it is necessary to count accurately the numbers of "cases" in which something specified can occur and not occur. However, the rules for calculating the probability (conjecturing) based on several arguments are more complex than those governing games of chance and also may require subjective judgment to apply appropriately.

> It was shown in the preceding chapter how, from the number of cases in which arguments for things can exist or not exist, indicate or not indicate, or also indicate the contrary, and from the forces of proving proportionate to them, the probabilities of things can be reduced to calculation and evaluated. From this it resulted that the only thing needed for correctly forming conjectures on any matter is to determine the numbers of these cases accurately and then to determine how much more easily some can happen than others.

Bernoulli recognized that his calculus of argumentation had to account not only for how many cases existed, but also for "how much more easily some can happen than others." In many situations, this assessment would obviously pose great difficulties, but these could be circumvented *conceptually* by assuming that a more likely case was equivalent to several equally likely cases, just as in a game of chance.

I assume that all cases are equally possible, or can happen with equal ease. Otherwise a correction must be made. For any case that happens more easily than the others as many more cases must be counted as it happens more easily. For example, in place of a case three times as easy I count three cases each of which may appear as easily as the rest.

In this way, he reduced the art of conjecturing to an implicit counting of equally likely cases (chances), analogous to the indistinguishable tickets or tokens drawn from an urn in a hypothetical lottery. Once again, we must remember that this presumed resolution into equally possible cases is metaphysical; it does not imply that we can actually count the cases, except in games of chance.

So, at this point it seems as if Bernoulli is about to offer a method for calculating the probabilities in civic and economic matters. But immediately upon seeming to promise this in the beginning of Chapter 4, he seems to pull the rug out from under us:

> But here we come to a halt, for this can hardly ever be done. Indeed, it can hardly be done anywhere except in games of chance. The originators of these games took pains to make them equitable by arranging that the numbers of cases resulting in profit or loss be definite and known and that all the cases happen equally easily. But this by no means takes place with most other effects that depend on the operation of nature or on human will.

In other words, real life *would* be like a game of chance, and potentially subject to combinatorial analysis, but we can hardly ever ascertain the true numbers of underlying equally likely cases and the rules of the game.

Bernoulli elaborates this critical point by discussing three examples of matters upon which we might wish to conjecture: the age at which a particular person will perish, the weather at some given date, and the victor in a game that depends on skill. For example, with regard to predictions of mortality he argues:

> But what mortal, I ask, may determine, for example, the number of diseases, as if they were just as many cases, which may invade at any age the innumerable parts of the human body and which imply our death? And who can determine how much more easily one disease may kill than another – the plague compared to dropsy, dropsy compared to fever? Who, then, can form conjectures on the future state of life and death on this basis?

Who indeed? So it seems that we are at an impasse if we wish to apply his calculus to arrive at a degree of certainty in such cases. But wait! There may be a way around this dilemma:

> Nevertheless, another way is open to us by which we may obtain what is sought. What cannot be ascertained a priori, may at least be found out a posteriori from the results many times observed in *similar situations*, since it should be presumed that something can happen or not happen in the future in as many cases as it was observed to happen or not to happen in *similar circumstances* in the past. If, for example, there once existed 300 people of the *same age and body type* as Titius now has, and you observed that two hundred of them died before the end of a decade, while the rest lived longer, you could safely enough conclude that there are twice as many cases in which Titius also may die within a decade as there are cases in which he may live beyond a decade (emphasis added).

Jacob has here implicitly introduced two critical conditions that can sometimes allow us to learn the ratio of underlying cases. The first necessary condition is that the relevant aspects of reality must remain essentially stable. For example, the potential causes of mortality and their relative frequencies must be assumed to change very slowly if at all. Second, the situation whose outcome is uncertain must be considered not in its individuality, but rather as a member of some class of similar past instances. For example, Titius must be regarded not as a distinct person but as a man of given age and body type. These two conditions treat the event of interest as essentially analogous to the outcome of a drawing from a lottery.

Bernoulli is not saying that individual characteristics are irrelevant to a prediction of Titius's prospects for longevity. Remember his axiom that "when we make conjectures about individuals, we also need, if they are at all available, arguments that are closer and more particular to those individuals." But when such specific arguments are *not* available, it is safe enough to rely on the evidence provided by a substantial body of experience for the *class* of men who are generally similar to Titius. This substitution of *quantitative* information for a relevant reference class in place of the unattainable *qualitative* detail for the individual is the essence of what I have termed willful ignorance. Ironically, by treating Titius as a faceless member of a large reference class, we can extract valuable information about his expectation for future survival.

Jacob's core insight was that individual details can be willfully *ignored* as long as the basic relevant conditions of the world remain stable. The situation is similar to that prevailing when dice are rolled or a token selected from an urn. Which particular token is drawn would be determined by the laws of physics and thus, theoretically subject to calculation. As a practical matter, though, such a calculation must always exceed human capabilities. Similarly, predicting individual mortality is impossible, but observing outcomes for a large number of "draws" from the urn of nature can reveal the expectation for a class of individuals whose personal characteristics are ignored.

Bernoulli asserts that fundamentally "this empirical way of determining the number of cases by experiments is neither new nor uncommon." He alludes to the *Ars Cogitandi* as having previously endorsed this empirical approach and mentions that "everyone does the same thing in daily practice." Moreover, he notes that "even the most foolish person, alone and with no previous instruction, (which is truly astonishing), has discovered that the more observations of this sort are made, the less danger there will be of error." However, the reason *why* this should be so, he believes, is connected to the art of conjecturing, and in particular to combinatorics.

Furthermore, through mathematical analysis it is possible to answer a critical question that has never before been posed, let alone answered.

> Something else remains to think about, which perhaps no one else has considered up to this point. It remains, namely, to ask whether, as the number of observations increases, so the probability increases of obtaining the true ratio between the numbers of cases in which some event can happen and not happen, such that this probability may eventually exceed any given degree of certainty. Or whether, instead, the probability has an asymptote, so to speak; whether, that is, there is some degree of certainty that may never be exceeded no matter how far the number of observations is multiplied, so that, for example, we may never be certain that we have discovered the true ratio of cases with more than half or two-thirds or three-fourths parts of certainty.

Note that Bernoulli refers to "the true ratio between the numbers of cases in which some event can happen and not happen," which in a game of chance would be the odds in favor of the event. For example, his canonical example is an urn that contains 3000 white tokens and 2000 black ones. The hidden ratio to be discovered in the experimental way is in this case a ratio of 3:2.

An event in the real world (e.g., surviving for a decade, rain tomorrow, making a point in a tennis match) can be regarded *as if* it were the outcome of a metaphorical lottery. The prize in this metaphorical lottery is *certainty* that the event will occur. Observing the outcomes from many "similar" situations is therefore conceptually and mathematically equivalent to observing the outcomes of drawings from such a lottery.

> And indeed, if in place of the urn we substitute, for example, the air or a human body, which contain within themselves the germ [*fomitem*] of various changes in the weather or diseases just as the urn contains tokens, we will be able in just the same way to determine by observation how much more easily in these subjects this or that event may happen.[26]

The number of events observed in a given number of homogeneous real-life situations (e.g., men of the same age and body type as Titius) is governed by the same mathematical rules as the lottery. In fact, if we observe enough such situations, Bernoulli asserts, the hidden proportions of the cases can be ascertained (within very narrow limits) and with moral certainty. (This assumes, of course, that we have no relevant arguments available *other* than the observed outcomes. If other arguments *are* available, they must presumably be combined with this empirical evidence according to the second and fourth of his axioms of prudence in Chapter 3 of Part Four).

According to Bernoulli, an event of interest such as succumbing to disease had some unknown expectation of occurring. However, he was certainly not implying that each known disease was equally likely to occur, which would be absurd. Rather, he claimed that there existed some unknown propensity for each disease to cause death to happen within a decade. Some of these diseases were associated with more chances than others, but that does not really matter. "For any case that happens more easily than the others as many more cases must be counted as it happens more easily." But this counting is conceptual, metaphysical. It suffices for us to act *as if* such cases are in some sense real and that their relative proportions remain fixed.

From this perspective, the proportion of events (e.g., survival for 10 years, rain tomorrow) among a given number of indistinguishable total trials follows the same *mathematical laws* as the number of white tokens drawn from an urn. So, the critical question becomes how many such draws must be observed in order to be "morally certain" that the ratio of favorable to unfavorable trials will closely approximate the true unknown ratio. If such moral certainty about the hidden ratio could be achieved, the resulting fraction of favorable chances out of the total chances would be the expectation of certainty or equivalently the amount of probability.

Bernoulli poses the question of whether it is possible to achieve such moral certainty. He refers to a hypothetical experiment in which independent trials are performed. Each trial consists of selecting a token randomly (and with replacement after each trial) from an urn that contains 3000 white and 2000 black tokens:

> It is asked whether you can do this so many times that it becomes ten, a hundred, a thousand times more probable (that is, that in the end it becomes morally certain) that the number of times in which you have chosen a white and in which you have chosen a black will have to each other the same ratio of three to two that the numbers of tokens or of cases secretly enjoy than some other ratio. Unless, indeed, this happens, I confess it will be all over with our effort to investigate the numbers of cases by experiments. But if it does happen and if in the end moral certainty is acquired in this way (how this will happen I will show in the following chapter), we will have found the numbers of cases a posteriori almost as certainly as if they were known to us a priori. This, surely, in the practice of civil life ... more than suffices for directing our conjectures in any contingent matter no less scientifically than in games of chance.

This statement seems to imply that the *exact* ratio of favorable to unfavorable cases can be discovered with moral certainty. While rhetorically impressive, it promises slightly more than Bernoulli can actually deliver. So, he hastens to qualify this claim:

> Rather, the ratio should be defined within some range, that is, contained within two limits, which can be made as narrow as anyone might want. Indeed, if, in the example of the tokens just discussed, we take two ratios, say 301/200 and 299/200, or 3001/2000 and 2999/2000, etc., of which one is just larger and the other just smaller than the ratio of three to two, it may be shown that the ratio found by many repeated experiments will fall within these limits around the ratio of three to two rather than outside.

Chapter 5: Solution of the Preceding Problem

In this final (and presumably unfinished) chapter, Jacob presented an elegant and rigorous mathematical proof of the result promised in Chapter 4. He demonstrated that, indeed, the probability (expectation of certainty) can be made arbitrarily close to 1 by performing a large enough number of trials. Later mathematicians would come to describe this result as the "weak law of large numbers." While acknowledging its originality, these followers were in a position to compare it to several "stronger" versions that were later derived. These improvements were stronger in the sense of requiring fewer trials to achieve a specified level of probability.

To demonstrate how his Golden Theorem could be applied, Jacob considered a hypothetical situation analogous to the lottery described above. He assumed that, as in this lottery, there were three "fertile" cases in which a certain event would occur for every two "sterile" cases. He found that it would require 25,550 trials to be 1000 times more likely that the proportion of fertile observations would lie between 29/50 and 31/50. This was a dauntingly large number to contemplate, and must have given him pause. Indeed, as statistician Arthur Dempster has suggested, it might well explain his hesitancy to publish.[27]

Bernoulli must have known it would be possible to reduce somewhat the required number of observations by further mathematical analysis. A mathematician would say that 25,550 was *sufficient*, but might not be *necessary*. So, he was aware that a substantially smaller number might suffice, although he lacked the tools to find the exact number. As it turns out, it would take slightly over 6000 trials to observe a fraction of events between 29/50 and 31/50 with a probability 0.999. This would be substantially better, but still hardly practical.

To lower the required number of trials much more would necessitate either widening the acceptable range of uncertainty around the true values (say to between 28/50 and 32/50) or settling for a probability that would not constitute moral certainty (say 0.99). Neither of these options would have appealed to Jacob, because he was wedded to the notion that the observed ratio of cases could simply be *substituted* for the unknown ratios. Anything less than a very small range and a very high probability would not (in his mind) have allowed such a substitution. Perhaps like Moses, having come so far, he lacked the physical and emotional stamina to push on into the uncharted territory where potential solutions to this conundrum might be found and left this task to his successors.

A TRAGIC ENDING

In a letter to Leibniz dated October 3, 1703, Jacob pleads ill-health and "natural laziness" as the reasons why he has not completed his magnum opus.[28] Here he is responding to a letter in which Leibniz had inquired about Jacob's "theory of the estimation of probabilities," about which he had been hearing rumors. Suspicious that his brother Johann was the source of this information, Jacob asks Leibniz how he has learned of the work: "I would very much like to know, dear sir, from whom you have it that a theory of estimating probabilities has been cultivated by me."

It is clear that there were few, if any, in whom Jacob had confided extensively on matters of probability. Perhaps his brother was the only one who knew any details about his Golden Theorem, which had been mentioned in a letter sent to Johann in 1692, when the two were still on somewhat civil terms.

> Nevertheless, I have completed most of the book, but there is lacking the most important part, in which I teach how the principles of the art of conjecturing are applied to civil, moral, and economic matters ... having solved finally a very singular problem, of very great difficulty and utility. I sent this solution already twelve years ago to my brother, even if he, having been asked about the same subject by the Marquis de l'Hôpital, may have hid the truth, playing down my work in his own interest.

Jacob's serious health problems and the burden of many weighty responsibilities were certainly real. However, this seems disingenuous; although he tells Leibniz that the work is incomplete because he has been "most reluctant to get to writing," we know that he had penned over 200 pages of carefully reasoned analysis. The problem was apparently not one of execution, but rather of a psychological block that had induced 20 years of paralysis.

What might have been the critical element that Jacob felt was lacking before his theory could be shared with the world? He never really says. Indeed, he may never have been consciously aware of what was holding him back. Perhaps he was simply unhappy about the impractical data requirements and too exhausted to carry on. Or, possibly he feared that he might be accused of trafficking in forbidden knowledge. This was a major concern at the time, as the propriety of "natural philosophy" was still doubted in some quarters.[29]

All of these reasons have some plausibility, but in addition, he may also have suffered from doubts about his basic assumptions. In his mathematics he could have full confidence, but its applicability to real-world matters had yet to be demonstrated. Were matters in fact so constituted as to justify his analogy between events in the world and the tokens in an urn? Were classes of similar situations really like sets of independent draws from an urn of nature?

In several letters between 1703 and 1705, Jacob paraded his main ideas before the one person whose opinion he probably valued above all others, Gottfried Leibniz. What has survived of this correspondence offers the best evidence of where he may have felt most vulnerable. First let us consider some issues that did not seem to trouble him. In the version of the treatise that was ultimately published, he responded to "a few objections that learned men have raised." He then replies to three points that Leibniz had mentioned to him in their correspondence[30]:

1. They object first that the ratio of tokens is different from the ratio of diseases or changes in the air: the former have a determinate number, the latter an indeterminate and varying one.

2. Second, they object that the number of tokens is finite, but the number of diseases etc., infinite.

3. Third, they add that the number of diseases does not always remain the same, but new diseases spring up daily.

To the first objection, Jacob replies that "both are posited to be equally uncertain and indeterminate with respect to our knowledge." The hidden contingencies involved must be the result of *some* underlying causal process that is fully determined, but the causal rules are unknown to us. This causal process, however it might generate observable outcomes, has a dual aspect. It is fully determined by God but perceived by us as contingent (random).

For both ratios (in the hypothetical urn and in the wider world), "that either is indeterminate in itself can no more be conceived by us than it can be conceived that the same thing at the same time is both created and not created by the Author of nature." Whether Titius dies within a decade or it rains on a given day are events that are fully determined. However, we cannot begin to approach exact knowledge of these outcomes, which must remain a divine prerogative. Nonetheless, we can obtain partial knowledge by observing the results in many similar situations.

To the second objection, Jacob states first that the numbers of cases are likely to be "astonishingly large" but not truly infinite. However, "even if it were actually infinite, it is known that there can be a determinate ratio even between two infinities, a ratio that can be expressed by finite numbers, either exactly or at least as closely as anyone might want." Jacob's metaphor of the urn is not meant to be taken literally but as a way of conceptualizing the enormous variety of different contingencies that exist in nature. Nature is far more complex than any actual urn filled with tokens, but it is essentially *like* an urn (from our perspective), regardless of how many contingencies may exist. When we observe the outcome of some situation, it is *as if* we are drawing from a huge urn with a possibly unlimited number of tokens.

The third issue raised by Leibniz concerned the assumption of a stable world that implicitly underlies Jacob's urn model. "Third, they add that the number of diseases does not always remain the same, but that new diseases spring up daily." Jacob's response indicates his awareness that this objection could indeed have some force. However, he is concerned primarily with processes like mortality and the weather that remain stable for long periods.

> We cannot deny that the number of diseases multiply with the passage of time, and anyone who wanted to draw an inference from today's observations to the antediluvian times of the Patriarchs would surely stray very far from the truth. But from this it only follows that new observations should be made in the meanwhile, just as with the tokens, if their numbers in the urn were assumed to change.

Bernoulli seemed to have all the answers but was missing one important piece of the puzzle. Could his theory be substantiated by testing its implications with actual empirical data? To test this supposition he would need actual data, such as the real durations of life for a large group of individuals of a specified age. But in the 1600s, compilations of such data were exceedingly rare. Recall that Graunt's *Observations*, published in 1662, created a sensation, despite its severe limitations. In 1686, Jacob had applied Graunt's "life-table" to reckon that the odds were 101:59 that a wife of age 16 would outlive her husband aged 56. However, Graunt's table was a very crude approximation, based on the London Bills of Mortality, which did not even include the age of death for each individual. To verify his calculated odds, for example, Bernoulli needed data on the actual ages at which death occurred for a large sample. Even better would be data on *pairs* of individuals who had been followed from a given date until their deaths.

In the letter to Leibniz written on October 3, 1703, Jacob explains what he has in mind:

> I began to inquire whether what is hidden from us by chance a priori can at least be known by us a posteriori from an occurrence observed many times in similar cases, i.e., from an experiment performed on many pairs of young and old men. For had I observed it to have happened that a young man outlived his respective old man in one thousand cases, for example, and to have happened otherwise only five hundred times, I could safely enough conclude that it is twice as probable that a young man outlives an old man as it is that the latter outlives the former.

At the end of this letter, he mentions de Witt's treatise on annuities, which he believes may contain the kind of source data he needs: "Perhaps he has something doing here; whatever it is, I would very much wish to obtain his source from somewhere." In the ensuing correspondence with Leibniz, Jacob mentions his interest in de Witt's report and underlying data no fewer than five times!

Leibniz indicates that he believes the de Witt pamphlet lies somewhere among his voluminous stacks of letters and books. His repeated pledges to unearth it are well-meaning, but reflect no sense of urgency. He fails to grasp why Jacob is so desperate to obtain this little treatise.

> The dissertation of Pensioner Witt, or rather the printed paper concerning annuities on a life, reasonably brief, certainly exists among my books, but since I wished to send it to you, I have not yet found it. I shall nevertheless surrender the work when found, where in the first place it will be permitted to be brought to light being hidden somewhere at home. It contains nothing besides, which can be very new to you.

In his final petition, just a few months before his death, Jacob responds: "I beg again you remember to pass to me the treatise of Mr. de Witt, if ever meanwhile it will have fallen into your hands; for no matter what it contains, they are not able to not be to me completely new things."

Leibniz may have believed that Bernoulli was seeking some mathematical or philosophical insight from de Witt's writing. Jacob had not made clear enough his reasons for wanting de Witt's *sources*, that is, the underlying *data*. Had he done so, Leibniz might have connected the dots between this request and the Breslau data of Caspar Neumann that he had helped Halley to obtain in 1692. That data would undoubtedly have been helpful to Jacob, although de Witt's perhaps even more so, since it contained actual outcomes for pairs of annuitants.

Leibniz may also have been somewhat skeptical of Jacob's claims regarding the broader application of mathematics in the social and political spheres, especially in legal matters: "The estimation of probabilities is extremely useful, although in several political and legal situations there is not much need for fine calculation as there is for the accurate recapitulation of all the circumstances."

Although these two intellectual giants tragically miscommunicated, their interchange of ideas highlights the inherent tension that underlies all practical applications of probability. On the one hand, our deliberations should ideally depend on "accurate recapitulation of all the circumstances." On the other, we must be *willing to overlook* some of these individual circumstances, so "what is hidden from us by chance a priori can at least be known by us a posteriori from an occurrence observed many times in similar cases." How are we to reconcile these two contradictory mandates? We have been wrestling with this conundrum ever since.

CHAPTER 6

A DEFECT OF CHARACTER

Before 1700, probability had a somewhat nebulous connotation, referring to a qualitative degree of certainty based on evidence, argument, and authority. In this broad sense, probability described the partial knowledge humans could obtain, in contrast with God's perfect understanding. In John Locke's famous phrase, probability expressed a kind of twilight knowledge suitable "to that state of mediocrity and probationership he has been pleased to place us in here."[1] For us, because of our limited capacities, the world can appear confusing and uncertain.

Jacob Bernoulli was the first great thinker to attempt a *quantitative* formulation of this uncertainty. This quantification depended on drawing an analogy between our uncertainty in the moral, political, and economic spheres on the one hand and the randomness in games of chance on the other. In many practical situations, the outcomes are completely unpredictable except to the extent that previous experience provides some rough indication of their propensity to occur. *In effect*, therefore, life can be regarded as *just like* a lottery in which there exists an unknown proportion of winning tickets. In these situations, the probability of a particular outcome could be conceived of as the proportion of "fertile" or "favorable" chances in this lottery of life.

Willful Ignorance: The Mismeasure of Uncertainty, First Edition. Herbert I. Weisberg.
© 2014 John Wiley & Sons, Inc. Published 2014 by John Wiley & Sons, Inc.

This formal equivalence provided a way to calculate the hidden ratio of chances. However, Jacob never took the further step of *identifying* the fraction of fertile cases with the probability. In Bernoulli's framework, the probability depended on all the relevant arguments that could be brought to bear. Only when we are ignorant of any specific arguments pertaining to the case of interest (as we often are) would Bernoulli regard the fraction of cases as the appropriate measure of probability. As I have explained, the link between epistemic probability and observed frequencies for Bernoulli was dependent on his notion of a mixed argument.

Bernoulli's law of large numbers is often interpreted today as demonstrating that by increasing the sample size we can estimate an underlying *probability* of a favorable outcome (on any single trial) within arbitrarily narrow bounds. However, this interpretation anachronistically attributes to the word "probability," a connotation that was unknown to writers in the late seventeenth and early eighteenth centuries. For them, probability was essentially psychological, while the ratio of chances pertained to the objective nature of things.

During the course of the eighteenth century, a remarkable transformation occurred. An entirely new meaning of probability, less ambiguous but more circumscribed, was forged and gradually gained currency as its potential utility became manifest. This new probability *merged* two intellectual streams: an epistemic interpretation of probability as a degree of certainty and a mathematical interpretation as a *fraction* of total chances. This hybrid is often called classical probability by historians of science.

Classical probability had deep roots in traditional qualitative probability, with one important difference. Probability was reduced in scope by implicitly assuming that all probability statements about a particular event referred to a common totality of evidence. Thus, the probability of an event A and its contrary $\sim A$ (not-A) must add to 1, representing certainty. The amount of evidentiary liquid in the metaphorical two glasses must always total certainty (a full glass). As a result, Bernoulli's broader algebra of combining arguments, and his distinction between pure and mixed arguments, got lost. The ambiguity that Jacob's system attempted to encompass was no longer recognized; all types of evidence became implicitly treated like mixed arguments.

This new mathematical probability had the great advantage of being expressed on a single numerical scale. At one end of the spectrum was impossibility and at the other end, certainty. Probability represented a *relative* degree of certainty, especially suitable for placing bets. Jacob Bernoulli's complex algebra for combining various arguments was eventually relegated to the scrap heap of science, a relic of a vanishing way of thinking. Along with it went the awkward possibility that the probabilities derived from the arguments for and against a proposition might not add to 1.

By around 1750, mathematical probability was becoming established. By the turn of the following century, it had sloughed off its explicit dependence on earlier concepts and attained a kind of freestanding status. The underlying "chances" had receded into the background, and "odds" had been largely supplanted by the more convenient fractional form for expressing uncertainty. This probability came to seem more tangible and intuitively meaningful; it could be manipulated in useful ways both algebraically and linguistically. It became an essential element of scientific discourse and even everyday life, but unlike its ancestral namesake, this modern version of probability was governed by the increasingly sophisticated mathematics of chance.

The driving forces for this amazing transformation were in part technical and in part pragmatic. On the one hand, the emphasis on probability as a *fraction* began to yield enormous technical dividends, facilitating the mathematical development of the theory of probability. On the other hand, this new sense of probability found application in a number of different areas. Probability began to seem a natural tool for describing and analyzing problems related to astronomy, demography, medicine, insurance, and political economy. These were subjects for which relevant data on outcomes (e.g., births, marriages, deaths) were just starting to be amassed. As Jacob Bernoulli had anticipated, the outcomes could be regarded as if they had arisen from a lottery.

The pivotal step in this transformation was the mathematical *definition* of probability as the fraction of favorable chances out of the total chances. Associating the word "probability" exclusively with this fraction, rather than with the odds, expectation, or any other mathematical expression, had subtle and momentous unforeseen consequences. As Jacob Bernoulli averred, "probability is indeed a degree of certainty, and differs from the latter as a part differs from the whole." But in place of Jacob's tortuous logic needed to link epistemic probability and empirical observations, there was now a direct and "obvious" connection. Probability was now by definition *both* the proportion of chances *and* the proportion of certainty. Within this new framework the applicability of mathematical probability to practical problems came to be regarded as self-evident.

The primary architects of this reengineering of probability were two geniuses whose careers spanned over a century. Both were born in France, Abraham de Moivre in 1667 and Pierre-Simon Laplace in 1749, but their lives could hardly have been more different. De Moivre experienced a great deal of hardship, struggle, and frustration, while Laplace rocketed to the pinnacle of preeminence, influence, and privilege. This chapter will focus on the first half of the transformation, from about 1700 to 1750, during which de Moivre was the dominant figure. The next chapter will deal with the consolidation and perfection of mathematical probability during the subsequent half-century.

MAN WITHOUT A COUNTRY

Had life been easier for Abraham de Moivre (1667–1754), the course of probability and statistics might have been quite different.[2] De Moivre was born in the Champagne province of France, about 100 miles northeast of Paris. His father was a surgeon who, while not wealthy, managed to provide for his precocious son an excellent early education. Young Abraham proved especially adept at mathematics and devoured Prestet's text on combinatorics and Huygens's famous treatise. Unfortunately, however, the timing of his birth was not fortuitous.

While Protestants had enjoyed a fair degree of religious tolerance in predominantly Catholic France since the Edict of Nantes in 1598, that was all about to change. In October of 1685, Louis XIV revoked the Edict, with disastrous consequences for all Protestants, including the 18-year-old de Moivre. Within a short time, de Moivre found himself virtually incarcerated in the Priory of St. Martin, a residential academy devoted mainly to indoctrinating young Huguenots into the Catholic faith. When he was finally released in 1687, de Moivre fled the country and, along

Landmarks of Probability

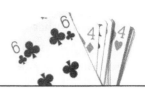

1600

1654   Pascal & Fermat
1657   Huygens

1700

1713   Bernoulli
1718   **De Moivre**

1764   Bayes & Price
1774   Laplace

1800

1837   Poisson
1838   De Morgan
1843   Mill
1843   Cournot
1849   Ellis
1854   Boole
1866   Venn

1892   Peirce

1900

1921   Keynes
1921   Knight
1922   Fisher
1926   Ramsey
1926   Neyman & Pearson
1928   Von Mises
1937   De Finetti
1949   Reichenbach
1954   Savage
1959   Popper

THE
DOCTRINE
OF
CHANCES:
O R,
A Method of Calculating the Probability
of Events in Play.

By A. De Moivre. F. R. S.

L O N D O N:
Printed by W. Pearson, for the Author. MDCCXVIII.

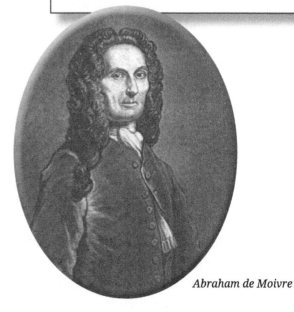

Abraham de Moivre

with his mother Anne and his younger brother Daniel, arrived in London. His father could not manage to escape and perished in France a few years later.

An Itinerant Teacher

Once settled in England, de Moivre capitalized on his mathematical training and set up shop as a tutor, cultivating contacts among the nobility and establishing an excellent reputation. In this way, he was able to support a modest but comfortable lifestyle. However, the work was arduous, often requiring him to trek all over London to meet with his well-heeled clients.

> I am obliged to work almost from morning to night; that is, teaching my pupils and walking. But since the city is very large, a considerable part of my time is employed solely in walking. That is what reduces the amount of profit I can make, and cuts into my leisure for study. Moreover one is obliged here more than anywhere else in the world to maintain a certain appearance; that is almost as essential as scientific merit. What remains to me at the end of the year is that I have indeed lived … but without having anything to spare.[3]

His base of operations when not making house calls was Slaughter's Coffee House, where he not only gave math lessons, but also offered consulting to gamblers and insurance brokers. In his day, many coffee houses served as informal centers of education and commerce.

While apparently successful as a teacher, and increasingly well-known as a leading mathematician, de Moivre was never able to obtain a position commensurate with his extraordinary abilities. Despite many close contacts with London's scientific and social elite, and a growing reputation within the international mathematical community, he failed repeatedly in attempts to garner a university appointment. Some have suggested that his foreign origins were responsible for a lack of full acceptance among the English. However, there is evidence that his personality may also have been a contributing factor.

While his relations with colleagues and clients were generally cordial, he apparently lacked close personal friendships and never married, or indeed displayed any romantic leanings. His "passions" were intellectual rather than emotional. Besides an intense, almost obsessive, absorption in solving difficult mathematical puzzles, he enjoyed classical literature and music. (His brother Daniel became a professional flautist of some note.) According to de Moivre's biographer Matthew Maty, who interviewed him near the end of the famous mathematician's long life:

> His favorite authors were Rabelais and Moliere, and he could recite them by heart. He once told one of his friends that he would rather have been Moliere than Newton. He recited scenes from *Le Misanthrope* with all the flare and wit that he recalled seeing them presented with on the day he saw the play performed in Paris 70 years earlier by Moliere's own company. It is true that misanthropy was nothing new to him. He was a stern judge of men and at times, a glance was all that was required for him to form a judgment. He was unable to conceal sufficiently his impatience with stupidity and his hatred of hypocrisy and lies.[4]

De Moivre seemed to get along well enough with others on a superficial level, but was perhaps not capable of feeling or inspiring real affection:

> On the whole, he seems to have been a friendly person, but patience and forbearance may have been thrust upon him by his humble circumstances. There is a certain defect of character somewhere, for none of his friends exerted their influence on his behalf, although it would probably have been easy for them to do so.[5]

As indicated by Maty, he could be prickly and did not suffer fools gladly. He also exhibited a tendency toward insensitivity to the feelings of others.

By the early 1700s, de Moivre was in close contact with most of the leading mathematicians both in England and on the Continent. In 1692, he had met Edmond Halley, and through Halley had become part of Newton's circle of early supporters. In 1695, Halley (ever helpful) was instrumental in having a paper of de Moivre's on the Newtonian calculus published in the *Philosophical Transactions* of the Royal Society. As a result, de Moivre was introduced to the London mathematical community, and in 1697 he was elected to the Royal Society. Around that time, he began to interact with a number of other eminent mathematicians who shared in the development of the theory of "fluxions," as Newton had called his version of the differential calculus.

In 1703, de Moivre became embroiled in a dispute over the publication of an expository text on fluxions by George Cheyne (1671–1743).[6] Cheyne was a Scottish physician who, like Gregory, Craig, and Pitcairne, had emigrated from Scotland to England. He was notorious for his personal struggles with obesity, his weight at times exceeding 400 pounds! He became an advocate of vegetarianism, for which he claimed numerous health benefits, including weight loss.

Cheyne was also a mathematician of some note and, like his mentor Archibald Pitcairne, sought to apply Newtonian methods in medicine. Unfortunately for him, his book managed to upset Newton, who encouraged de Moivre to reply. Newton was frequently involved in disputes caused by his tendency to conceal his discoveries until forced to divulge them. The controversy with Leibniz a decade later over the calculus would eventually have very serious repercussions. Newton's reaction to Cheyne's apparently well-meant effort in 1703 was a sign of things to come.

De Moivre harshly criticized Cheyne's book, defending his own claims to priority in certain matters, as well as Newton's. This public spat brought de Moivre to the attention of the leading Continental mathematicians, including Leibniz and Johann Bernoulli. Thus began a regular correspondence between de Moivre and Johann that lasted for a decade, ending presumably because the conflict between Newton and Leibniz over the origins of the calculus had become too heated. De Moivre was, by practical necessity, forced into Newton's camp; he was enlisted in 1712 into the rubber-stamp committee of the Royal Society that validated Newton's claims. Bernoulli, meanwhile, became "Leibniz's bulldog."

Turning Point

Before 1710, de Moivre's major mathematical interests and contributions had revolved around pure mathematics, especially the infinitesimal calculus. He had apparently lost interest in the problems of combinatorics and the laws of chance that had captivated him in his youth. By 1709, however, Montmort's *Essay on the Analysis of Games of Chance* had made its way across the Channel and had soon been brought to de Moivre's attention.[7] Recall that Montmort's interest had been stimulated by the eulogies to Jacob Bernoulli. Starting with a rather vague idea of what Jacob had accomplished (his *Ars Conjectandi* would not be published until 1713), Montmort independently derived many previously unpublished results.

Francis Robartes (1649–1718), who would a few years later become the third Earl of Radnor, was an amateur mathematician and patron of the sciences who had received a copy of Montmort's *Essay*. Robartes prevailed on de Moivre to attempt some problems he believed were more difficult than any of those considered by Montmort. De Moivre rose to this challenge and in the process began to think more deeply about the mathematical principles involved. The result was a short treatise presented to the Royal Society in 1711 and published the following year: *De Mensura Sortis* (*On the Measurement of Chance*). De Moivre's dedication to Robartes provides some background and perhaps exemplifies the lack of tact that tended to land de Moivre in hot water:

> Huygens was the first that I know who presented rules for the solution of this sort of problems, which a French author has very recently well illustrated with various examples; but these distinguished gentlemen do not seem to have employed that simplicity and generality which the nature of the matter demands: moreover, while they take up many unknown quantities, to represent the various conditions of gamesters, they make their calculation too complex.[8]

De Moivre sent out copies of *De Mensura Sortis* to Newton, Halley, and Montmort among others. Montmort was not pleased with the characterization of his work as a mere illustration of Huygens's methods and lacking in generality. Furthermore, when de Moivre had written *De Mensura Sortis*, he was unaware that Montmort had been in consultation with Nicholas Bernoulli, Jacob's nephew who had in 1709 written his doctoral thesis that expanded upon his uncle's pioneering work.

This collaboration between Montmort and Nicholas Bernoulli had led to advances that paralleled those presented by de Moivre, so that in some cases it became difficult to sort out who could justifiably claim priority. Montmort wrote to Nicholas that he had found little in de Moivre's opus that was really new to them. Meanwhile, Nicholas was spending time visiting in England and had met with both de Moivre and Newton. Upon returning home, toward the end of 1712, Nicholas wrote to Montmort, indicating that he believed the apparent slight was inadvert and that de Moivre was actually quite a decent fellow.

In 1713, Montmort was preparing a second edition of his *Essay* that would incorporate his correspondence with Nicholas, which contained many new discoveries. He and Nicholas worked together for 3 months at

Montmort's estate to edit the manuscript. When the revised and expanded *Essay* was published later that year, Montmort shot back at de Moivre:

> Mr. Moivre has judged well that I would have need of his Book in order to respond to the Critique that he made of mine in his Foreword. The laudable intention that he has had to elevate & to give his Work value, has carried him to debase mine & to dispute to my methods the merit of novelty. As he has believed to be able to attack me without giving me my subject to complain of him, I believe to be able to respond to him without giving to him reason to complain of me. My intention is not at all to critique his Work; beyond that it is above criticism, one would be much annoyed to diminish the merit of it: this is too removed from our character; but because it is permitted to defend oneself, & to conserve one's property, I myself am proposed to respond to him.[9]

Montmort did indeed respond, detailing his various grievances. Soon after clearing the air, however, Montmort seems to have moved on, and it seems that relations between the two mathematicians were soon patched up. By all accounts, Montmort was a very personable chap and not inclined to hold a grudge.[10]

In 1715, Montmort visited London to witness a total eclipse of the sun that had been predicted by Halley. This highly anticipated event had attracted scientists from near and far, and they were not disappointed; the eclipse occurred within 4 minutes of when Halley had prognosticated! During these festivities, de Moivre and Montmort spent some time together, apparently on good terms. Moreover, in a letter in 1716 to the British mathematician Brook Taylor (1685–1731), Montmort expressed admiration for de Moivre and wondered why de Moivre had not written back to him for some time.[11]

Meanwhile, back in London, de Moivre was undertaking his own campaign to master the mathematical analysis of games. He had apparently become determined to conquer this intellectual domain, and was hard at work on an expanded version of his 1711 paper. Such a publication could enhance his reputation and perhaps open up new avenues of professional opportunity. Interest in this subject had been stimulated not only by Montmort's *Essay*, but also by the appearance (at last) of Jacob's *Ars Conjectandi* in 1713, as well as a new 1714 translation of the Huygens treatise by William Browne (1692–1774).[12]

Sometime in 1717, the shrewd and distrustful de Moivre placed a copy of his draft manuscript into Newton's care as a kind of insurance policy against potential challenges to the work's originality. In 1718, *The Doctrine of Chances: or, A Method of Calculating the Probability of Events in Play* was published.[13] The book was certainly the most advanced and comprehensive treatment of the mathematics of chance published up to that point. Most important, it introduced explicitly the definition of probability as a fraction of chances, thus initiating mathematical probability as we know it.

Apparently determined not to repeat the faux pas that had kindled Montmort's uncharacteristic umbrage, de Moivre's took pains to explain the background of his work and its relation to previous publications. He detailed the circumstances that had led to *De Mensura Sortis* in 1711:

> I had not at that time read anything concerning this Subject, but Mr. Huygen's Book de Rationciniis in Ludo Aleae, and a little English Piece (which was properly a translation of it) done by a very ingenious Gentleman, who, tho' capable of carrying the matter a great deal farther, was contented to follow his Original; adding only to it the computation of the Advantage of the Setter in the Play called Hazard, and some few things more. As for the French Book, I had run it over but cursorily, by reason I had observed that the Author chiefly insisted on the Method of Huygens, which I was absolutely resolved to reject, as not seeming to me to be the genuine and natural way of coming at the Solution of the Problems of this kind. However, had I allowed myself a little more time to consider it, I had certainly done the Justice to its Author, to have owned that he had not only illustrated Huygen's Method by a great variety of well chosen Examples, but that he had added to it several curious things of his own Invention.[14]

It is interesting that his allusion to *Of the Laws of Chance*, usually attributed to John Arbuthnot, mentions that it was done by "a very ingenious Gentleman, who, tho' capable of carrying the matter a great deal farther, was contented to follow his Original."

I have suggested previously that, while Arbuthnot almost certainly wrote the Preface, the actual translation may have been the work of David Gregory. Arbuthnot was by all accounts a distinguished physician and a great wit, but would hardly have been deemed ingenious by de Moivre's lofty standards. On the other hand, there is evidence that de Moivre was not especially fond of Gregory.[15] So, he may have actually meant Arbuthnot. Or, the remark may indeed refer to Gregory, if we interpret it as chiding him for failing to do more despite his mathematical abilities.

In addition, de Moivre took note of the second edition of Montmort's *Essay* and included some flattering words:

> Since the printing of my Specimen, Mr. de Montmort, Author of the Analyse des jeux de Hazard, published a Second Edition of that Book, in which he has particularly given many proofs of his singular Genius, and extraordinary Capacity; which Testimony I give both to Truth, and to the Friendship with which he is pleased to Honour me.

However, once again, De Moivre was being either oblivious or disingenuous. He failed to give credit for many original discoveries by Montmort and Nicholas Bernoulli that he had incorporated in his own book.

Upon receiving a copy of the book, Montmort flew into a rage. In a letter to his collaborator Nicholas Bernoulli in June of 1719, he complained that their results had been appropriated by de Moivre without giving them due credit.[16] Undoubtedly, a major dispute would have ensued had Montmort lived longer, but a few months later he died of smallpox in Paris. Nicholas, meanwhile, had no real desire to enter this fray. So, the kingdom of chance was left wide open for de Moivre to dominate for several decades.

By the time the *Doctrine of Chances* was published, the *Ars Conjectandi* had been in print for 5 years. From a mathematical viewpoint, much of its novelty had worn off. Jacob's findings had been transmitted through his nephew Nicholas, and to a much lesser extent his brother Johann, or discovered and extended independently by de Moivre, Montmort, and Nicholas. However, Bernoulli's proposed extension to "civil, moral and economic matters" was a hot potato that was unceremoniously dropped by all.

De Moivre discharged whatever sense of responsibility he felt by appealing to Nicholas and Johann Bernoulli, neither of whom heeded the call. Lacking much interest in the philosophical questions that motivated Jacob Bernoulli to derive his Golden Theorem, de Moivre placed no special emphasis on this pioneering result. The time was not yet ripe for the widespread "statistical" applications of probability that Jacob had imagined. Only a few small shoots that would eventually blossom into what we now call statistics were beginning to sprout.

Expanding His Empire

In de Moivre's time, the main practical application of the "doctrine of chances" that had been recognized, though hardly developed, was the "actuarial" analysis of mortality data. Edmond Halley, in his paper of 1693 on the Breslau life table had suggested that insurance policies and life annuities should be based on empirical data about life expectancies. This was a radical idea and impractical at the time because there was no reliable data upon which to base the estimation of longevity. At any rate, Halley's sound advice seems to have fallen on deaf ears.

De Moivre must have encountered many insurance brokers and underwriters at Slaughter's Coffee House, where he often gave lessons to students, and elsewhere (perhaps even at Edward Lloyd's coffee house, birthplace of today's Lloyd's of London). Being familiar with Halley's paper, de Moivre realized that the mathematical principles related to chance could be applied to the pricing of annuities and various other complex risk-management arrangements that were then in vogue. In 1725, he published *Annuities upon Lives*, which was essentially a manual for underwriters.[17] This book proved very successful, and four later editions were published between 1743 and 1756. Remarkably, de Moivre relied for his data on Halley's original table from 1693, which remained the only available source.

Meanwhile, the *Doctrine of Chances* had become the definitive text on the mathematics of gambling, which it would remain throughout most of the eighteenth century. A second edition, trumpeted as "fuller, clearer and more correct than the first," was issued in 1738.[18] While it may have been fuller and clearer, it was also less magnanimous to the late Montmort; the laudatory passage mentioning "proofs of his singular Genius, and extraordinary Capacity" was expunged from this later edition.

Most noteworthy among many upgrades in this second edition was a landmark result that de Moivre had first derived in a paper in Latin circulated among a few friends in 1733. It is for the contents of this paper more than anything else that de Moivre is known to modern mathematical statisticians.[19] The main formula discovered by de Moivre has been considered a refinement of Jacob Bernoulli's law of large numbers and as the earliest version of what would much later be termed the *Central Limit Theorem* of statistics.

Suppose we conduct an "experiment" in which there are numerous "trials." For example, each trial might consist of a single draw from an urn that contains 50 white and 50 black balls, with replacement of the ball after each trial. Jacob's Golden Theorem, and his nephew Nicholas's refinement, each provided a method for finding the number of trials necessary to be assured that the observed percentage of white balls would fall within any specified distance of 50%. However, their estimates of this number were conservative, in the sense of being sufficient, but perhaps larger than actually necessary. De Moivre tackled the more difficult problem of finding a close approximation to the *exact* number required.

De Moivre began the presentation of his solution by alluding to the previous discoveries made by the two Bernoullis:

> Besides *James* and *Nicolas Bernoulli*, two great Mathematicians, I know of no body that has attempted it; in which, tho' they have shewn very great skill, and have the praise which is due to their Industry, yet some things were farther required. For what they have done is not so much an Approximation as the determining very wide limits, within which they demonstrated that the Sum of the Terms was contained.[20]

De Moivre could not resist the urge to crow a bit about this amazing achievement:

> Now the Method which they have followed has been briefly described in my *Miscellanea Analytica*, which the Reader may consult if he pleases, unless they rather chuse, which perhaps would be the best, to consult what they themselves have writ upon that Subject: for my part, *what made me apply myself to that Inquiry was not out of opinion that I should excel others, in which however I might have been forgiven*; but what I did was in compliance to the desire of a very worthy Gentleman, and good Mathematician, who encouraged me to it (emphasis added).

In this case, de Moivre's pride was justified. If Jacob's was a golden theorem, then de Moivre's was platinum.

Rather than a conservative lower *limit* for the probability that an observed ratio of chances would lie in a particular range around the true value, de Moivre was able to derive a close approximation to the *exact* probability. His approximation formula was based on what would later be called the Gaussian, or *normal*, probability distribution, graphically represented as the famous bell-shaped curve (see Figure 6.1).

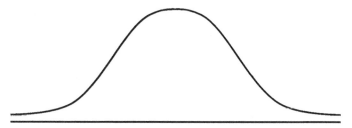

FIGURE 6.1 The normal distribution (bell-shaped curve).

Furthermore, de Moivre's formula could be used in reverse to determine for a given number of trials, the probability of obtaining a number of successes between any two values. Suppose, for example, that a fair coin is tossed 100 times and the number of heads is noted. What is the probability that the total number of heads is between 40 and 60? De Moivre's formula indicated that this probability is close to the area under a normal curve (see Figure 6.2). That area could be found using methods of integral calculus. According to de Moivre's approximation, the probability to three decimal places in this example would be 0.955, which is very close to the exact answer of 0.965.[21]

When de Moivre completed the second edition of the *Doctrine* in 1738, he was 70 years of age, but still at the top of his mathematical game. He was internationally known, having added membership in the Berlin Academy of Sciences to his Royal Society affiliation a few years earlier. Yet, he was still unable to attain the academic appointment he craved, with "age discrimination" now compounding his disadvantages. In 1739,

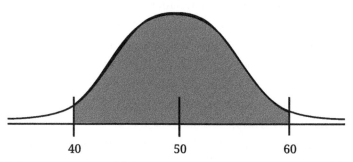

40   50   60

FIGURE 6.2 An example of de Moivre's approximation to the binomial distribution. The area under the curve approximates the probability that the number of successes in 100 trials is between 40 and 60 when the probability on each trial is 0.50.

he was put forward as a candidate for the prestigious Lucasian Chair in Mathematics, once held by Sir Isaac himself (and, until his recent retirement, occupied by Stephen Hawking). This would have been a fitting capstone for an extraordinary, if rather unorthodox, career.

De Moivre was actually admitted to Cambridge in order to receive an obligatory M.A. degree in 1739, a formality necessary in order to be appointed. However, in the end, he was rejected in favor of the competent but pedestrian John Colson (1680–1760). A historian in 1889 noted that this decision was rationalized at the time by the belief that "de Moivre was very old and almost in his dotage."[22] This commentator observed cryptically that "the appointment was admitted to be a mistake."

Dotage indeed! Even in old age, Abraham de Moivre never stopped toiling, or continuing to defend his hard-won intellectual empire. Perhaps the rigors of his existence even contributed somehow to his longevity and vigor. All that constant walking around London to meet with his far-flung students may have helped to keep him fit.

Defending His Empire

In 1743, de Moivre felt called upon to confront a challenge posed (he believed) by an upstart teacher of mathematics (and part-time weaver) by the name of Thomas Simpson (1710–1761). Simpson was self-taught and in addition to his day job as a weaver, earned his living mainly by giving lectures in various London coffee houses and publishing books and articles on mathematical topics. In 1743, he was appointed as a professor of mathematics at the Royal Military Academy at Woolwich.

Simpson was a talented mathematician, but was mainly a popularizer of mathematical ideas rather than an originator.[23] He must have been quite a flamboyant character. He wrote under several colorful pseudonyms, including Marmaduke Hodgson, Anthony Shallow, and Hurlothrumbo. His articles and responses to questions posed by readers appeared in such varied publications as *Gentleman's Magazine*, *Miscellanea Curiosa Mathematica*, and the *Ladies Diary*.

In 1740, Simpson had first intruded on de Moivre's turf by publishing a text, *On the Nature and Laws of Chance*, based largely on de Moivre's work. Simpson's avowed purpose was not to eclipse the master, but primarily to "bring down some of the most useful things already known to the level of ordinary capacities."[24] In addition to making the subject matter more accessible, he also sought to make it more affordable. In the preface he was critical of all potential competition for his book, with the lone exception of the *Doctrine of Chances*:

> There is indeed but one, that I have met with, entirely free from this Objection; and tho' it neither wants Matter nor Elegance to recommend it, yet the Price must, I am sensible, have put it out of the Power of many to purchase it; and even some; who want no Means to gratify their Desires this way, and who might not be inclinable to subscribe a Guinea for a single Book; however excellent, may not scruple the bestowing of a small Matter on one, that perhaps may serve equally well for their Purpose.

Where de Moivre had catered to the carriage trade, Simpson aimed to bring "the doctrine" to the masses. Priced at a guinea in 1742, when Simpson published his text, de Moivre's *Doctrine* would have been prohibitively expensive.

This venture met with no obvious objection from de Moivre, but 2 years later Simpson crossed the line. He presumed to publish a treatise on annuities that must have cut closer to the nub.[25] Indeed, this unwelcome competition inspired de Moivre to come out the following year with a second edition of his own *Annuities upon Lives*, which he now called *Annuities on Lives: Plainer, Fuller, and more Correct than the Former.*[26] In the preface, de Moivre attacked Simpson:

> After the pains I have taken to perfect this Second Edition, it may happen, that a certain Person, whom I need not name, out of Compassion to the Public, will publish a Second Edition of his book on the same Subject, which he will afford at a very moderate Price, not regarding whether he mutilates my Propositions, obscures what is clear, makes a Shew of any Rules, and works by mine; in short, confounds, in his usual way, everything with a crowd of useless Symbols; if this be the Case, I must forgive the indigent Author, and his disappointed Bookseller.

Simpson was indignant at this sarcastic rebuke, and responded in kind by penning an "Appendix Containing some Remarks on a Late Book on the Same Subject, with Answers to some Personal and Malignant Misrepresentations in the Preface thereof."[27] Among these remarks was the opinion that de Moivre had been guilty of "self-sufficiency, ill-nature, and inveteracy, unbecoming a gentlemen." The gauntlet had been thrown down and de Moivre's natural impulse was to pick it up, but his friends successfully counseled him to let the matter drop.

A Mixed Legacy

On November 27, 1754, Abraham de Moivre passed away at the age of 87. He had continued to be productive right to the end, and a final version of the *Doctrine of Chances*, which incorporated *Annuities on Lives* as well, was published posthumously in 1756.[28] De Moivre was a truly great mathematician, but his apparent "defect of character" may have prevented him from becoming a truly great man. In his dealings with the rich and powerful, he could be somewhat obsequious in public, but highly critical behind the scenes.

Whether constrained mainly by circumstances or by temperament, he seems to have been too insecure to take a firm stand on matters of principle. Nowhere was this quality more consequential than in the "calculus wars" over the origins of the infinitesimal calculus. De Moivre may have been especially well positioned to perform a great service to science by attempting to mediate between the British Newtonians and the Continental defenders of Leibniz.

De Moivre's intellect had won the respect of the leading mathematicians in both camps, including Isaac Newton, Gottfried Leibniz, and Johann Bernoulli. Indeed, Newton in his later years reportedly responded to mathematical questions by saying: "Ask Mr. de Moivre[29]; he knows all that better than I do." Leibniz and Johann Bernoulli for their part had attempted unsuccessfully to obtain a university post in Germany for de Moivre in 1713. But instead of trying to find some common ground between Newton and Leibniz, de Moivre apparently fell in quietly with Newton's self-serving agenda.[30] Did he really believe that Newton was completely in the right? Perhaps he felt a debt of loyalty to a man he considered a friend and benefactor. Surely he must have perceived the growing rift that would be disastrous for scientific progress, and would cut him off from his valuable contacts on the Continent.

Ironically, being somewhat isolated from mathematical developments in Europe may have motivated him to pursue his fortune in another direction. So, had matters stood otherwise, Abraham de Moivre might have been instrumental in defusing the destructive conflict between Newton and Leibniz. But, had things been otherwise, he might not have invented modern mathematical probability.

A FRACTION OF CHANCES

In 1711, de Moivre was just beginning to learn about the new calculus of chance. He had been encouraged by Robartes to look into the recent developments published by Montmort. De Moivre's initial efforts were summarized and presented to the Royal Society in *De Mensura Sortis*. This work was certainly substantial, but not earthshakingly original. He had accepted the intellectual challenge of solving several difficult mathematical problems, but did not regard these as especially worthy of major attention on his part.

Five years later, de Moivre's interest in the mathematics of gambling had been ignited, and he was rapidly extending the mathematics of chance. By then, he had been inspired by Jacob Bernoulli's *Ars Conjectandi*. Foreseeing the potential importance of combinatorial mathematics, he had perhaps begun to regard Montmort as a rival. That would explain the unusual step of "registering" his intellectual property with Isaac Newton and of curtailing his correspondence with Montmort. What epiphany had occurred around 1716 that transformed de Moivre's attitude toward the subject so profoundly?

De Mensura Sortis

When he first dealt with the mathematical analysis of chance in 1711, de Moivre adopted the time-honored epistemic and ambiguous connotation of probability. Here is how he begins *De Mensura Sortis*:

> If p is the number of chances by which a certain event may happen, and q is the number of chances by which it may fail, the happenings as much as the failings have their degree of probability; but if all the chances by which the event may happen or fail were equally easy, the probability of happening will be to the probability of failing as p to q.[31]

De Moivre assumes that there are p different possible chances for the "happening" of an event, and q chances for the "failing" of the event. In general, some chances are more likely than others to occur, with each chance having its own "degree of probability." Without any further ado, however, he immediately moves on to consider the special case of games of chance, in which all the chances are "equally easy."

Now he can get down to business:

> If A and B, two gamesters, were so to contend about events, that if p chances should happen A wins but if q chances should happen B wins, and there were a sum, *a*, placed down, the 'sors' or expectation of A will be *pa/(p + q)* and the 'sors' or expectation of B will be *qa/(p + q)*, and moreover, if A or B should sell his expectations, it is fair that they should receive *pa/(p + q)* and *qa/(p + q)* for them, respectively.

Note that de Moivre does not define the probability to be the fraction $p/(p + q)$, as we would today. Rather, like Huygens and Montmort, he refers to the *expectations* of the two players. Furthermore, the entire presentation that follows is couched in the traditional terms of odds and expectations. Chances, odds, and expectations were the accepted ways to talk about probability in the context of games of chance. However, except in Bernoulli's as yet unpublished *Ars Conjectandi*, there was no formal concept of probability as a fraction between 0 and 1 within the mathematical theory.

So, when de Moivre first turned his attention to the calculus of chance, mathematical probability did not yet exist. When de Moivre uses the word probability in his 1711 text, he seems to mean the relative number of chances, not the fraction of the total chances.

In his mathematical analyses, de Moivre invariably referred either to the odds or the expectation. However, there is one indication to suggest a dawning awareness, perhaps not even conscious, of what was to come. In several of the more complicated problems, he simplifies the mathematical expressions by letting the "sum deposited or the prize to be won" have a value of 1 instead of an amount *a*. By dispensing with the irrelevant stakes of an actual game, the expectation corresponds essentially to our probability.

De Moivre's Epiphany

By the time de Moivre published his *Doctrine of Chances* in 1718, something had definitely changed. That something, I conjecture, was

Bernoulli's *Ars Conjectandi*, which was the most likely stimulus for the breakthrough in de Moivre's thinking. Bernoulli had explained clearly how (at least in games of chance) probability could be measured as a fraction of chances. On the opening page of de Moivre's *Doctrine* we find a clear statement of modern mathematical probability:

> The Probability of an Event is greater, or less, according to the number of Chances by which it may Happen, compar'd with the number of all the Chances, by which it may either Happen or Fail. Thus, if an event has 3 Chances to Happen, and 2 to Fail; the Probability of its Happening may be estimated to be $\frac{3}{5}$, and the Chances of its Failing $\frac{2}{5}$.[32]

Perhaps the choice of the fraction 3/5 here, the same fraction used by Bernoulli in defining probability as a degree of certainty, was coincidental, but I think not.

I rather imagine that upon reading the *Ars Conjectandi*, the pieces fell into place for de Moivre. He must have grasped the centrality of the *fraction* of chances for the mathematics of chance. However, unlike Jacob Bernoulli, de Moivre was not particularly interested in the broader implications of the doctrine of chances for moral, political, and economic judgments. He was concerned with the mathematics arising out of games of chance. For him, the primary motivation for casting probability as the fraction of favorable chances out of all possible chances was *pragmatic*.

De Moivre realized, as no one before, that framing many problems in terms of this fraction, rather than the odds or expectation, could greatly facilitate the mathematical analysis. I believe that the connotation of the word probability as a "degree of certainty" was of secondary importance for him. This association certainly fit well with the mathematical concept, and reinforced its intuitive appeal, but was probably not the driving force in his thinking.

Immediately after introducing, without comment or explanation, this radically new definition of probability, De Moivre continues:

> Therefore, if the Probability of Happening and Failing are added together, the Sum will always be equal to Unity. If the probabilities of Happening and Failing are unequal, there is what are commonly call'd Odds for, or against, the Happening or Failing; which Odds are proportional to the number of chances for Happening or Failing. The expectation of obtaining any Thing is estimated by the Value of that Thing multiplied by the Probability of obtaining it.[33]

Now this is a truly remarkable quantum leap. For all practical purposes, our modern theory of mathematical probability has (finally) been conceived, although it would not truly be born for many years.

First, de Moivre states explicitly that the probability of an event and the probability of its negation must add to one. This is essentially the "additive" property at the core of mathematical probability. It is obviously true in games of chance, but was not assumed for the epistemic probability of Jacob Bernoulli and his predecessors. It is only true when the arguments supporting each of the two possibilities assume the *same* base of evidence. Interested mainly in games of chance, de Moivre was probably unconcerned (or unaware) that his definition had imposed such a restriction.

Second, he presents the idea of probability as fundamental, and the concepts of odds and expectations as derivative from it. For us, this seems the obvious way to proceed, but it represented a dramatic reversal in de Moivre's time. To de Moivre it had become clear that defining probability as a fraction of chances was a magic key to unlock the mysteries of chance.

A few paragraphs later, he mentions almost in passing another major insight, the multiplication principle for independent events:

> From what has been said, it follows, that if a Fraction expresses the Probability of an Event, and another Fraction the probability of another Event, and those two Events are independent; the Probability that both those Events will happen, will be the Product of those two Fractions.[34]

He illustrates with an example of two wagers, one with odds of 3:2 for event A and the other with odds of 7:4 for event B. What are the odds against winning both of these bets? Without turning the odds into probabilities, this would not be easy to solve. However, by transforming the odds of 3:2 into a probability of 3/5, and the odds of 7:4 into 7/11, we can apply de Moivre's nifty multiplication rule.

The resulting probability for both to occur is 21/55 ($= 3/5 \times 7/11$). In terms of odds, this becomes 34:21 against the event that both A and B will occur. In Chapter 3, I mentioned Oystein Ore's puzzlement at the much more laborious method employed by the brilliant Gerolamo Cardano 150 years earlier. Wouldn't Cardano have loved to know this trick? De Moivre then extends this approach to several independent events.

Having proceeded along this path, he was able to generalize the multiplication principle still further. He considered the case when two (or more) events are *not independent.* That is, the probability of an event may depend on whether or not some other event has occurred. He gives several examples that involve playing cards drawn from a deck *without replacement.* Suppose we are interested in the probability of drawing a heart from a well-shuffled deck of 52 cards. On the first draw, the probability is 13/52, or 1/4. If we shuffle and draw again from the remaining cards, the probability becomes 12/51. To find the probability of drawing two consecutive hearts, therefore, we must multiply the initial probability for the first draw times the *conditional probability* for the second, given the outcome of the first.

These basic laws of probability were developed in de Moivre's lengthy Introduction and then used to yield many clever solutions of various particular problems. However, while the new concept of probability was put to excellent use, it did not completely replace the more traditional odds and expectations. Rather, it functioned as a useful expedient for obtaining an intermediate expression that he could then translate back into the more familiar form of the odds. Furthermore, in algebraic expressions, de Moivre expressed a probability in the form $a/(a + b)$, where a represents the number of *chances* favoring the event and b, the number of *chances* unfavorable. The notion of chances remained the bedrock upon which the probabilities (along with odds and expectations) were firmly supported.

For the remainder of the eighteenth century, mathematical probability retained the classical definition as a fraction of chances. However, the explicit representation of chances receded more and more into the background, and the centrality of probability fractions became more prominent. In the 1738 second edition of the *Doctrine of Chances*, de Moivre explicitly recognized the technical convenience of representing a probability directly by a single symbol or letter in an equation[35]:

> Before I put an end to this Introduction, it will not be improper to shew how some operations may often be contracted by barely introducing one single Letter, instead of two or three, to denote the Probability of the happening of one Event.[36]

After illustrating this point at some length with several examples, he concludes:

> And innumerable cases of the same nature, belonging to any number of Events, may be solved without any manner of trouble to the imagination, by the mere force of a proper Notation.

Nonetheless, throughout most of the work he continued to frame problems in terms of chances, rather than directly in terms of probabilities. It was not until sometime after de Moivre's passing in 1754 that the further step of using a single symbol for a probability became more common, as probability in its fully modern sense finally came into being.

De Moivre died in 1754, one hundred years after the correspondence between Pascal and Fermat. Yet, after all that time, our modern notion of probability had just begun to gain wide acceptance. Moreover, the relevance of this new type of probability to the frequencies of certain real-world events, such as births, deaths, and astronomical observations was becoming recognized. However, mathematical probability was still associated mainly with games of chance and served primarily a technical function. It had not yet acquired the intuitive and universal character that we now attribute to probability.

CHAPTER 7

CLASSICAL PROBABILITY

In a letter written in September 1749 to Frederick the Great, the King of Prussia, the great mathematician Leonhard Euler (1707–1783) wrote:

> My researches on the hydraulic machine occupying me again for some days, I take the liberty to render account of the examination of the Italian Lottery, for which it has pleased Your Majesty to charge me so graciously. First I have determined by the calculus of probabilities, how much each player ought to pay in order that the advantage were so much equal for him as for the bank.[1]

This is one of the first clear references to the *calculus of probabilities*. Before 1750, the mathematical analysis pertaining to games of chance had almost always been known as the *doctrine of chances*. After that, this subject was more frequently termed the calculus of probabilities or sometimes the *theory of probability*.

This change in terminology reflected a major shift in thinking. From this point on we can find several writers referring to the calculus of probabilities in addition to, or in place of, the doctrine of chances. Moreover, the mathematical expositions became increasingly framed in terms of probability directly, although references to chances, odds, and expectations still occurred as well. By the 1760s, the idea of mathematical

Willful Ignorance: The Mismeasure of Uncertainty, First Edition. Herbert I. Weisberg.
© 2014 John Wiley & Sons, Inc. Published 2014 by John Wiley & Sons, Inc.

Landmarks of Probability

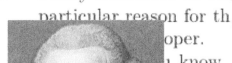

1600		
1654	Pascal & Fermat	
1657	Huygens	
1700		
1713	Bernoulli	
1718	De Moivre	
1764	**Bayes & Price**	
1774	**Laplace**	

Pierre-Simon Laplace

1800		
1837	Poisson	
1838	De Morgan	
1843	Mill	
1843	Cournot	
1849	Ellis	
1854	Boole	
1866	Venn	
1892	Peirce	
1900		
1921	Keynes	
1921	Knight	
1922	Fisher	
1926	Ramsey	
1926	Neyman & Pearson	
1928	Von Mises	
1937	De Finetti	
1949	Reichenbach	
1954	Savage	
1959	Popper	

LII. *An Essay to*
of Chances. By
by Mr. Price,
F. R. S.

Dear Sir,

d Dec. 23, 1763. I now
ur deceased friend
l well deserves to be
nearly interested in the
particular reason for th
oper.
u know,
much es
ich he h
subject
probabil
n that w

Richard Price

1/3

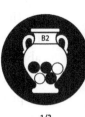

1/3

1/3

probability seems to have become so established that these earlier concepts were rarely mentioned explicitly.

During this critical transitional period, the concept of probability, defined as the *fraction of chances*, became solidified. This idea of probability as a fraction of some vaguely defined and metaphysical "chances" has been referred to by historians as *classical probability*. Concomitantly, the interpretation of this fraction of chances as the epistemic degree of certainty gained widespread currency. However, it would be a mistake to assume that probability was being applied much more broadly to civil and economic affairs. Its use was still restricted almost entirely to the narrow context of gambling in which it had originated. On the other hand, the potential to expand this new and mathematically tractable version of probability well beyond these bounds was starting to be recognized. Beginning in the early 1770s, Pierre-Simon Laplace would take the lead in this endeavor.

REVOLUTIONARY REVERENDS

Laplace was a towering figure who dominated the landscape of probability for 50 years. His monumental scientific and mathematical achievements earned Laplace the sobriquet of The French Newton. However, before we tackle the subject of Laplace's role in the evolution of probability, a slight detour is in order. A famous episode in England during the 1760s occurred that is usually considered an interesting sidebar, but may in fact have played an important role in the development of probability and statistics.

The protagonists in this little drama were two clergymen living in mid-century England. One was renowned in his time for many reasons, including his contributions related to probability and statistics, but he is almost entirely overlooked today. The other led a quiet and private life but has become quite notorious in ours, mainly for a single posthumous contribution to the theory of probability.

The Reverend Thomas Bayes

Although he is famous today for Bayes's rule, perhaps the best-known formula in the entire canon of probability, the eponymous Thomas Bayes

(1701–1761) cast almost no shadow during his rather uneventful life.[2] Very little is known about the details of his existence. His now-famous rule, or theorem, only came to light posthumously, thanks to the efforts of his friend, the Reverend Richard Price. Moreover, the essay in which the celebrated theorem was presented was ignored until it was rediscovered later, after a far more immediately influential version of essentially the same idea was independently proposed by Laplace.

The traditional rendition of the Bayesian story starts off with the demise of a little-known Protestant minister named Thomas Bayes in 1761. Among his papers were found some documents pertaining to obscure mathematical matters, in which Bayes, as an amateur mathematician, had been interested. In his will, Bayes had mentioned the Reverend Richard Price, "now I suppose preacher at Newington Green," to whom his papers should be sent. Price recognized the potential importance of Bayes's essay on probability and arranged for publication in the *Philosophical Transactions of the Royal Society.* The rest is silence.

In recent years, scholars have learned a bit more about this episode and about Bayes the man, but not very much. Thomas Bayes was born around 1701, but the exact date is uncertain. His father was a Presbyterian minister and came from a fairly well-to-do family of Sheffield, in the north of England. Their fortune had been derived from the cutlery business, for which Sheffield was renowned. At that time, those who professed religious views that were not sanctioned by the Church of England were called "nonconforming" or "dissenting" Christians. Dissenters were allowed to practice and preach but were denied certain rights, including the ability to attend Oxford or Cambridge. Consequently, Thomas was educated within the schools that were open to Dissenters at that time, and he matriculated at the University of Edinburgh in 1719.

While his course of study was designed primarily to prepare him for a career in the ministry, he must have displayed some talent for mathematics. At Edinburgh, Bayes studied under James Gregory (1666–1731), younger brother of David Gregory.[3] James had assumed the professorship of mathematics in 1692 after David left Scotland to set up shop at Oxford. From James Gregory, Bayes would undoubtedly have learned about Newton's theory of fluxions. Whether he was exposed to the doctrine of chances during his studies at Edinburgh is unknown.

Almost nothing of his life between school and 1733 is known. In that year (probably) he arrived in Tunbridge Wells, located 40 miles southeast of London, to become the resident Presbyterian minister. The town was at that time a popular vacation destination, attracting many summer visitors and known originally for its reputedly health-enhancing spa. He remained there for the remainder of his life, staying on even after he retired from the pulpit in 1752. Bayes was a rather uninspiring speaker, was not very active in the social sphere, despite the rather lively atmosphere of Tunbridge Wells, and led a quiet bachelor's life.

As for mathematical pursuits, we know that in 1736 he published (anonymously) a text on Newtonian calculus meant in part as a defense against the philosophical criticisms that had been leveled by Bishop George Berkeley (1685–1753) against the infinitesimal calculus.[4] Around this time Bayes may have met Lord Philip Stanhope (1694–1773), amateur mathematician and patron of the sciences, who encouraged Bayes's mathematical interests. In 1742, Stanhope was responsible for the election of Reverend Bayes to membership in the Royal Society. It is apparent from the wording of his nomination that Bayes was regarded as an accomplished mathematician[5]:

> The Revd Thomas Bays of Tunbridge Wells, Desiring the honour of being Elected into this Society, we propose and recommend him as a Gentleman of known merit, well skilled in Geometry and all parts of Mathematical and Philosophical Learning, and every way qualified to be a valuable member of the same.

While there is scant evidence of his active participation in the Royal Society, Bayes appears to have become an advisor to Stanhope and through him to others in the Earl's wide circle. In 1755, Bayes was asked to comment on a paper by Thomas Simpson, de Moivre's erstwhile admirer and sometime nemesis.[6] Simpson had tried to address an important practical problem—how can we best estimate the true value of some quantity based on several fallible measurements? This was a critical issue for astronomers, who were trying to determine the precise position of a star or some other heavenly object for which several independent observations had been obtained.

The conventional approach to such problems had been qualitative. The "best" measurement was selected based on a detailed analysis of the conditions and instruments that had been employed to produce the observation. However, some astronomers had begun to adopt a new practice of taking a mean, or average, of the several measurements rather than trying to decide subjectively which one was the most reliable. In effect, they were applying the principle of willful ignorance. At the time it was an open question whether it was better to apply expert judgment based on all the known facts or to *ignore* the myriad of unknown possible "causes" of measurement error?

Simpson was the first to link the problem of observational errors with the doctrine of chances. His paper was in the form of a letter addressed to Lord Macclesfield that was read to the Royal Society on April 10, 1755, and appeared later that year in the *Philosophical Transactions*. Here is how he framed the issue:

> It is well known to your Lordship, that the method practiced by astronomers, in order to diminish the errors arising from the imperfections of instruments, and of the organs of sense, by taking the Mean of several observations, has not been so generally received, but that some persons, of considerable note, have been of opinion, and even publickly maintained, that one observation, taken with due care, was as much to be relied on as the Mean of a great number.

> As this appeared to me to be a matter of much importance, I had a strong inclination to try whether, by the application of mathematical principles, it might not receive some new light; from whence the utility and advantage of the method in practice might appear with a greater degree of evidence.

From our vantage point, it is remarkable that this problem had apparently *not* previously been regarded as a mathematical question! Simpson was breaking new ground just by considering it in this light. He went on to offer a sophisticated rationale for preferring the statistical approach of averaging several observations. Essentially, he illustrated how, under certain assumptions, the average of the measurement errors becomes smaller as the number of observations grows larger. Focusing on the *errors* rather than on the value of the quantity to be estimated was an important conceptual breakthrough that would prove very fruitful.

Simpson's paper represents one of the earliest practical applications outside games of chance of a basic concept that would later be termed a *random variable*. A random variable is a quantity that can take on different possible values with certain probabilities. For example, the outcome of rolling a single die can be considered a random variable. So can the predicted price of a particular stock at some future date. Corresponding to each possible value of the stock, a probability can, in principle, be specified. The aggregate of all these probabilities constitutes the *probability distribution* of the random variable. A particular probability distribution can be characterized in many different ways, but the mean (average) value is the most common summarization.

Simpson conceived of the observational *error* (measured in seconds of arc) as an integer value between −5 and +5. Corresponding to each of these 11 possible values (including zero) of the measurement error he posited a particular probability. In effect, the measurement error was regarded as a random variable, and the set of 11 equal probabilities was its probability distribution. Applying the doctrine of chances, he found that the probability distribution of the mean of several errors tended to become closer to zero as the number of observations increased. Specifically, the mean of the errors had a greater probability of being within any specified distance of zero than the error for any individual observation. Therefore, the mean value of the observed positions would tend to become closer to the true position as the number of observations increased.

Simpson's discussion of his analysis illustrates beautifully the gradual transition of thought taking place between the older emphasis on *chances* and the emerging focus on *probability*. He seems to vacillate, invoking probability in the context of calculations but referring to chances and odds for the ultimate expression of his results. Here is how he explains that the probability that the error is less than two arc seconds is much higher when taking the mean than when using a single observation:

These particulars being premised, let it be now required to find what *probability*, or *chance* for an error of 1, 2, 3, 4, or 5 seconds will be, when, instead of relying on one, the mean of the observations is taken ...

To determine, now, the *probability* that the result comes within two seconds of the truth ... the *odds*, or proportion of the *chances*, will therefore be ... as 29 to 1, nearly. But the proportion, or *odds*, when a single observation is taken, is only as 2 to 1: so that the *chance* for an error exceeding two seconds, is not $\frac{1}{10}$ th part so great, from the mean of six, as from one single observation (emphasis added).

By probability he clearly intends the fraction of the chances, but referring to chances and odds was necessary to convey his meaning to the intended audience.

After agreeing to review Simpson's letter to Lord Macclesfield, Bayes must have been intrigued. His review indicated that he found the mathematical development to be quite correct. However, he raised a simple but important point about the generality claimed by Simpson for his conclusion. Simpson had argued that taking the mean was *always* likely to be the preferred approach. Bayes astutely observed that Simpson's conclusion depended on assuming that the measuring device was free from systematic bias:

> On the contrary the more observations you make with an imperfect instrument the more certain it seems to be that the error in your conclusion will be proportional to the imperfection of the instrument made use of. For were it otherwise there would be little or no advantage in making your observations with a very accurate instrument rather than with a more ordinary one, in those cases where the observation cou'd be very often repeated: & yet this I think is what no one will pretend to say.[7]

In other words, measurement accuracy depends not only upon the precision of the observational device or procedure, but also on proper calibration. Put simply, you need to be aiming at the right target. Simpson appreciated the wisdom of Bayes's remark, and in later writings amended his assumptions to exclude the case of a biased instrument.

It is possible that Simpson's paper was the stimulus for Bayes to think more deeply about matters of probability, leading to his famous essay. However, it seems more plausible that the essential ideas in the essay were being discussed by Bayes (and perhaps others) as early as the 1740s.[8] David Hartley (1705–1757) was a physician, philosopher, and founder of the "associationist" school of psychology. By around 1735, he had established a reputation in London as a respected medical practitioner and scientist and in 1736 he was elected to the Royal Society. In 1749, Hartley published a remarkable treatise combining philosophy and theology with a very thoughtful and imaginative account of psychological processes.

In his medical research activity, Hartley was one of the pioneers in appealing to statistical data, and was apparently familiar with de Moivre's *Doctrine of Chances*. Through the Royal Society, he was probably acquainted with de Moivre and with Thomas Bayes, who were also members. Hartley's writing about probability is revealing as a possible reflection of the general transition in the understanding of probability that was occurring in England at the time.

As I have mentioned, both de Moivre and Simpson had begun to think in terms of fractional probabilities, rather than chances or odds. However, neither of these mathematicians had particularly emphasized the possible link between this mathematical concept and the venerable epistemic connotation of probability. Writing in the 1740s, David Hartley saw clearly a connection between uncertainty in general and mathematical probability:

> If it be asked, upon what authority absolute certainty is represented by unity, and the several degrees of probability by fractions less than unity, in the doctrine of chances? Also, upon what authority the reasoning used in that doctrine is transferred to other subjects, and made general, as here proposed? I answer, that no person who weighs these matters carefully can avoid giving his assent; and that this precludes all objections. No skeptic would, in fact, be so absurd as to lay two to one, where the doctrine of chances determines the probability to be equal on each side; and therefore we may be sure that he gives a practical assent at least to the doctrine of chances.[9]

By the 1740s, the merging of probability as a degree of certainty and probability as a fraction of chances subject to the rules governing games of chance had apparently progressed to the extent of becoming self-evident, as it would remain for succeeding generations. Furthermore, another statement by Hartley refers to "an ingenious friend" who had communicated a solution to the "inverse problem" that, as we shall see, came to be known as Bayes's Theorem.[10] So, it is possible that Bayes's knowledge of probability and his ideas about the inverse problem may have existed for some time prior to his review of Simpson's letter to Lord Macclesfield.

The Reverend Richard Price

Richard Price (1723–1791) was virtually unknown in 1761, when he answered the call to examine the papers of his late friend, or at least acquaintance, Thomas Bayes. To statisticians who have heard the traditional story about Bayes's Theorem, Price is a rather shadowy figure, like an anonymous midwife who mediates the birth of the hero and then fades silently out of the story. Most statisticians would be surprised (as I was) to learn that Price in 1761 was destined to become one of the most famous men of the eighteenth century, and not just in England. Furthermore, a large measure of his prominence would flow indirectly from his knowledge of probability, stimulated by the encounter with Bayes's essay in 1761.

Who was Richard Price? His father, a Congregational minister in the Welsh city of Glamorgan, expected his son to follow in his ecclesiastical footsteps.[11] In 1739, after his father's unexpected death, Richard was sent to London to attend the Fund Academy, one of the schools established by the Dissenters to provide the higher education their children were barred from obtaining at the English universities. Besides preparation for the ministry, Price acquired a fairly extensive grounding in science and mathematics under the tutelage of John Eames (1686–1744), a disciple of Newton and member of the Royal Society. In fact, Eames was one of the signatories to the nomination of Thomas Bayes for membership in 1742.

After graduating and becoming ordained, Price moved to Stoke Newington, then a suburb of London. There he served as chaplain to the family of George Streatfield, and gave sermons as an assistant minister to several local congregations. In 1756, both Streatfield and a wealthy uncle of Price died, and each left him a generous bequest. This unanticipated bounty provided Price with sufficient resources to live comfortably and soon to marry his sweetheart, Sarah Blundell. The couple was happily married for the ensuing 30 years, despite Sarah's physical frailty and inability to have children. By all accounts, both Price and his wife were friendly, outgoing, and well liked. During most of their marriage they remained in Stoke Newington, where Price eventually became established as a full-time preacher.

While not particularly noted for his oratorical skills, Price was an excellent writer on both religious and secular matters. In 1758, he published *A Review of the Principal Questions and Difficulties in Morals*, the first of several publications (and numerous letters) that dealt with philosophical and theological matters.[12] Based on these writings, Price was awarded a Doctor of Divinity degree from the University of Edinburgh in 1768. These various written works reveal Price as somewhat of a contradiction, from our modern perspective.

On the one hand, he held fast to traditional ideas about Divine benevolence, literal salvation, and God's active role in shaping the world. On the other hand, his political and economic views were surprisingly modern, and even considered radical by his contemporaries. Moreover, he was in the vanguard of mathematical and scientific progress. The unifying theme in much of his thinking was the Newtonian belief in natural laws that could be understood by the employment of man's rational faculties. Price was a strong believer in individual liberty and freedom from repression, which he viewed as both morally right and confirmed by reason. One of his congregants was Mary Wollstonecraft (1759–1797), who gained fame as an early feminist. She was strongly influenced by Price's liberal philosophy.

As mentioned, in 1761 Price accepted the responsibility of editing the papers of Thomas Bayes. It has been speculated that Price's "editing" role may actually have been considerable. All we know for sure is what Price wrote in the introduction that he added, in which he was characteristically modest. "An Essay Towards Solving a Problem in the Doctrine of Chances" was finally submitted to the Royal Society by Price in 1763 and published in the *Philosophical Transactions* the following year.[13] Based on this work and perhaps other evidence of his mathematical ability, Price was elected as a member of the Royal Society in 1765. Meanwhile, Bayes's *Essay* appears to have elicited no significant interest at the time and was forgotten, although through Price it did indirectly contribute to the early development of actuarial science.

In 1764, Price was consulted by "three gentlemen" regarding a proposed plan of operation for the new Society for Equitable Assurance on Lives and Survivorships.[14] Founded 2 years earlier as the first mutual life insurance company, the Equitable was seeking methods for assessing risk, at a time when mortality data remained very sparse. Thus began a very fruitful long-term sideline for Price. He became a recognized expert on the financing of insurance, annuities, and various "friendly society" schemes to provide old-age and sickness benefits for workers and their families.

Price served as an advisor to the Equitable Society for many years, and in 1769 published *Observations on Reversionary Payments*.[15] This text eventually ran through seven editions and supplanted de Moivre's book as the classic source on actuarial methods. Price drew upon his mathematical background, including his knowledge of probability theory, to develop the most sophisticated analyses of annuities and other financial instruments to date. Furthermore, he developed new mortality data, finally rendering Halley's 1693 data from Breslau obsolete.

Price became interested in the subject of vital statistics not only for actuarial applications but also for political and philosophical reasons. He became a leading figure in the debate over the state of Britain's population. Price was among those who argued that the population was declining, and adduced statistical evidence supporting this (incorrect, as it turns out) position. He believed in the virtues of hard work and a simple agrarian lifestyle, and blamed luxurious living and increasing urbanization for the alleged population decrease.

Through his writings on financial, actuarial, and demographic matters, Price had by the 1770s become quite well known, and was regularly called upon by prominent politicians for advice. He had also developed a number of relationships in the scientific world. In particular, from 1766 on he was very close to Joseph Priestley (1733–1804), who is hailed as a pioneer of modern chemistry, and discoverer of oxygen, but was also active as a theologian, educator, and political philosopher.

Price was widely respected as kindhearted and magnanimous in his dealings, even in his philosophical disputes. He became personally acquainted with many of the leading progressive thinkers of the day, including the prison reformer John Howard (1726–1790), economist Adam Smith (1723–1790), and philosopher David Hume (1711–1776). He was generally well regarded, even by those, like Priestley and Hume, whose sometimes extreme views conflicted with his own religious beliefs. Price not only preached, but truly practiced, tolerance for free expression and participation in rational dialogue. So, it "was ironical that Price, so pacific and equable, had a genius for starting controversies."

Some of these unintended public imbroglios revolved around issues pertaining to political economy, such as whether or not Britain's population was truly in decline or how best to handle the mounting National Debt. However, in the mid-1770s international political events would catapult this mild-mannered intellectual to a much greater level of notoriety. Sometime around 1760, Price had become friendly with Benjamin Franklin (1706–1790), who was then living in London. Through Franklin, he came to know and admire many of the leading American political figures as they passed through England over the years, including John Adams (1735–1826), Thomas Jefferson (1743–1826), Thomas Paine (1737–1809), and Josiah Quincy, (1709–1784). As relations between England and the American Colonies deteriorated, Price became a strong supporter of the American cause, which he regarded as a beacon of divinely inspired light. He hoped that the example of a nation established on the ideals of liberty would inspire Britain and other countries to loosen the reins of political and religious intolerance.

On February 8, 1776, Price published a rather inflammatory pamphlet—*Observations on Civil Liberty and the War with America.*[16] He argued that American independence was not only morally justified, but would also benefit Great Britain in the long run. He even advocated the formation of a similar kind of confederacy among the states of Europe. The pamphlet sold out immediately, was reprinted several times within a few weeks, and sold over 60,000 copies in total. It set off a chain reaction of literary salvos pro and con, and may even have influenced the framers of the Declaration of Independence.

In the spring of 1777, Price wrote another pamphlet in which he made suggestions for dealing with the serious financial problems faced by the fledgling American republic.[17] A year later, he politely declined an invitation from the Continental Congress to come and assist personally in the new nation's financial administration. In the Congressional debates over the national debt and other problems relating to fiscal policy, Price was cited as a leading authority in such matters. For a man who had never set foot on American soil, Price was a most vocal and influential supporter of the American Revolution and the new nation it produced.

After the Revolutionary War, he continued an active correspondence with Franklin and many other prominent citizens of the new country who valued his advice and considered him a true friend. When the Bastille fell in France on July 14, 1789, Dr. Price believed that the cause of liberty had taken another major step forward. In November of that year, he gave an impassioned sermon that burnished his (unwanted) reputation as a flaming radical. However, his health was already beginning to decline, and he eventually died on April 26, 1791, too soon for him to witness the chaotic and tragic conclusion of the drama beginning to unfold in Paris, about which he had been so hopeful.

In a real sense, Price was a forgotten founding father of the United States. The esteem in which he was held by Americans in his time was evidenced by an extraordinary tribute received by Price in absentia in New Haven, Connecticut, in 1781. Two honorary doctorates were awarded that year at the Yale University graduation ceremony. One was given to General George Washington, Commander-in-Chief of the Continental Army and father of his country, the other to Dr. Richard Price of Newington Green, philosopher, preacher, actuary, and vicarious revolutionary.

The Famous Essay

It is a stretch to attribute much of Price's later fame to his role in editing Thomas Bayes's essay. However, this effort did lead almost immediately to membership in the Royal Society and to his early actuarial work, including the *Observations on Reversionary Payments*, which by the early 1770s had made him a respected authority on financial and statistical matters. However, as mentioned above, the direct effect of Bayes's essay on the wider world was essentially nil. Why was this work, destined to become so celebrated much later on, so completely ignored at the time?

Perhaps the best answer is that Bayes's innovations were both mathematically complex and completely original. They represented in several ways a radical shift in perspective for which his contemporaries were not yet ready. Fortunately, in Richard Price he had chosen a literary executor who could appreciate his insights and the subtlety of his reasoning. Unfortunately, today there is tremendous confusion about exactly what Bayes's Theorem really is, and what it was that Thomas Bayes can be said to have "discovered."

To understand the essence of Bayes's rule, consider the following simple problem. A single ball is to be drawn randomly from one of two urns, each of which contains 5 balls. Urn A contains 4 white balls and 1 black one; urn B contains 2 white and 3 black balls (see Figure 7.1). First one of the two urns will be chosen randomly, and then the ball will be drawn from that urn. Assume you are told that the probability is 1/3 that Urn A will be selected and is 2/3 that Urn B will be selected. You will not be allowed to see which urn is chosen.

Suppose that after the drawing you are informed that the ball is white. What is the probability that this ball came from Urn A? Note that *a priori* (beforehand) the probability of Urn A was 1/3. However, after seeing the white ball, you have additional information. How should this a posteriori

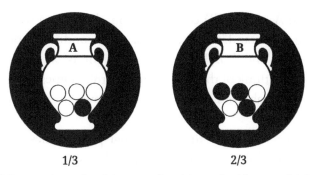

FIGURE 7.1 Example of the type of problem solved by Bayes's Theorem.

(afterward) knowledge affect the probability that Urn A was in fact the source? Since Urn A contains 4 white balls and Urn B only 2, it is obvious that the posterior probability must be greater than 1/3. But how much greater?

This is where Bayes's rule comes in. In essence, it formalizes the following intuitive reasoning. Since Urn B has an a priori probability of 2/3, we can imagine that there were actually two identical urns (Urn B1 and Urn B2) each of which contained 2 white and 3 black balls and had a selection probability of 1/3 (see Figure 7.2). So, between these three urns (all equally likely to be chosen) there would be 8 white balls in total (4 in Urn A, 2 in Urn B1 and 2 in Urn B2, all equally likely to be drawn. Because 4 of these 8 were from Urn A, the posterior probability that it was drawn from Urn A must now be 1/2 (see Figure 7.2). By the same logic, if the ball drawn had been black, the probability that the source was A would turn out to be only 1/7.

Bayes's rule is a general formula for computing unknown *conditional* probabilities. In our example, we could obtain the probability that the

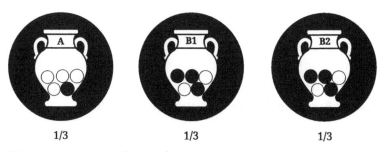

FIGURE 7.2 Essential logic of the solution provided by Bayes's Theorem.

source was Urn A (or Urn B) conditional on observing a white ball in a single drawing. The standard notation for these conditional probabilities would be $P(A|W)$ and $P(B|W)$, where the event W is the drawing of a white ball. We can think of these conditional probabilities as the "inverse" of the "direct" probabilities that are usually known, in this case $P(W|A)$ and $P(W|B)$.

In general, we will know the conditional probabilities of some *evidence* given the possible *sources* of the data.[18] We want to invert these to determine the inverse probabilities, the conditional probabilities of various sources *given the evidence*. Bayes's rule provides the link between the direct and inverse probabilities. However, there is a catch. To apply the rules, we must know the prior probabilities of the various sources. In our example these are $P(A)$ and $P(B)$.

As a simple practical example, suppose a doctor is trying to decide whether her patient suffers from a particular type of infection. Her diagnostic procedure can indicate the infection (correctly) with probability 90% if the infection is truly present. That is:

$$P(\text{test positive} \mid \text{infection}) = \frac{9}{10}$$

However, it will also (incorrectly) detect the infection with probability 10% when the patient is free of the infection:

$$P(\text{test positive} \mid \text{no infection}) = \frac{1}{10}$$

Suppose further that the doctor believes that 5% of her patients are actually infected:

$$P(\text{infection}) = \frac{1}{20}$$

If her patient tests positive, what is the probability that the infection is truly present? Applying Bayes's Theorem, we would find:

$$P(\text{infection} \mid \text{test positive}) = \frac{9}{28}$$

A simpler way to understand Bayes's Theorem is in terms of frequencies rather than probabilities. The psychologist Gerd Gigerenzer has shown that our minds have evolved to deal much more easily with information in the form of frequencies than probabilities.[19] This is not surprising since simple counting has been around for millennia, while mathematical probability is a very recent invention.

To understand how we could arrive at the correct answer via Gigerenzer's frequency approach, imagine there exists a hypothetical population of 1000 individuals, of whom 50 (5%) have the infection. The diagnostic procedure will find 45 (90%) of these. On the other hand, the procedure will also (falsely) incriminate 95 of the 950 (10%) disease-free individuals. So, the probability that a positive indication is truly an infection would be:

$$P(\text{infection} \mid \text{positive}) = \frac{45}{45 + 95} = \frac{9}{28}$$

Philosophical Significance

Most students of probability and statistics do not realize that Reverend Bayes derived this mathematical formula not for statistics, but in order to solve a particular philosophical problem of great importance. Here is how he stated this problem:

> *Given* the number of times in which an unknown event has happened and failed:
> *Required* the chance that the probability of its happening in a single trial lies somewhere between any two degrees of probability that can be named.

Bayes was after big game, nothing less than a general solution to the problem of *induction*—how can we generalize based on past experience? In particular, how can we draw credible inferences about the future based on events that have previously been observed?

His attempted solution was to formulate the problem in terms of conditional probabilities. Given that so many "happenings" and "failings" have been observed, what is the conditional probability that the true probability (on a single trial) is between any two specified limits? In our simple example, there are only two urns, and the proportion of white balls in each is assumed to be known. However, suppose that we know absolutely

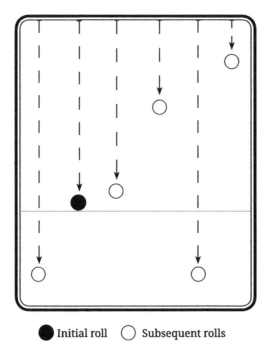

● Initial roll   ○ Subsequent rolls

FIGURE 7.3   Bayes's famous "billiard-table" model: The position of the horizontal line marked by the black ball's landing spot is analogous to the unknown probability on each Bernoulli trial. A "success" is deemed to occur each time one of the white balls crosses the horizontal line.

nothing about the urn from which the ball is to be drawn, except that it contains 5 balls, all of which are either black or white. Then there are six possibilities for the number of white balls that the urn might contain (0, 1, 2, 3, 4, and 5). Now suppose that we do not even know how many balls are in the urn. Then, in principle, the proportion of white balls could be any fraction between 0 and 1.

To deal with this general situation, Bayes replaced the conventional urn model with a different physical analogy. He imagined a rectangular table similar to a billiard table (see Figure 7.3). In a thought experiment, Bayes considered how the table could be divided randomly into two parts by rolling a ball and marking the ball's landing spot with an invisible line. The line would determine a fraction of the total length of the table. The black ball in Figure 7.3 represents this initial roll.

This fraction determined by rolling the initial ball represented the unknown probability associated with an underlying process that has generated some observed events. This ball would then be removed after its position was secretly marked. Then another ball, represented here by a white ball, would be rolled again several times. After each such roll, a record would be kept of whether or not it landed beyond the invisible line. Each such trial on which the ball rolled past the invisible line represented an occurrence of the event.

Using this billiard-table model of how the "happenings" and "failings" were being generated, Bayes asked the following question. Suppose that you were told only the number of times that a ball landed beyond the invisible line and the number it did not. In our illustration, there would be two happenings and three failings. What could you infer about the position of the line? In principle, this problem could be solved in the same way as the simple urn problem. However, instead of only two urns, each corresponding to a different prior probability, we would have an infinite number of possible prior probabilities. Each of these probabilities would be represented by one value of the line's location expressed as a proportion of the table's length ranging from 0 to 1.

Let us denote the probability of a happening in a single trial as p. Then, Bayes made the seemingly plausible assumption that essentially all values of p are equally likely. In his physical analogy, the invisible line might have an equal chance of lying anywhere on the table. However, obviously we cannot count all the possible points on a continuum. Bayes got around this difficulty by assuming instead that the prior probability that p will lie in any specified *interval* would be equal to the length of that interval. For example, the probability that p would lie between 0.25 and 0.40 would be 0.15. Statisticians would say that p has a *uniform distribution* over the interval [0,1]. This is the continuous analog of assuming that the two urns in our simple example each have a probability 1/2 of being selected.

Conceptually, this is easy to understand. However, it turns out that the mathematical analysis of this problem is formidable and requires the application of integral calculus. Even so, only a good approximation, not an exact solution, can be derived. Consequently, a practical solution to Bayes's problem would have to await twentieth-century computing power. Bayes and Price made valiant efforts to obtain a workable approximation, using the limited tools at their disposal. The mathematical complexity of the problem may be one reason why his basic insights did not immediately catch on. However, the unconventional *conceptual* framework that Bayes adopted was also very difficult for his readers to grasp.

Unlike de Moivre and Simpson, Bayes chose not to define probability in terms of the more familiar but ambiguous concept of chances. Rather, he interpreted probability in a way that would preclude philosophical problems, as Price explained:

> He has also made an apology for the peculiar definition he has given of the word *chance* or *probability*. His design herein was to cut off all dispute about the meaning of the word, which in common language is used in different senses by persons of different opinions ... Instead therefore, of the proper sense of the word *probability*, he has given that which all will allow to be its proper measure in every case where the word is used.[20]

This approach is strikingly modern. Whatever may be our interpretation of the *concept* of probability, a *measure* of this probability must adhere to certain mathematical principles, namely, the usual rules applying to games of chance.

In this way Bayes merged the epistemic sense of probability with de Moivre's mathematical definition as a fraction between 0 and 1. However, he jettisoned the underpinning of "chances" that had previously buttressed the epistemic interpretation of probability. "By *chance* I mean the same as probability," Bayes asserted. What exactly Bayes had in mind by this statement was not explained clearly by him, and is open to speculation. What seems clear is that Bayes's mathematical development required that prior and inverse probabilities be considered in some sense comparable. As a result, it became permissible to think about the probability of a probability! This mind-bending idea would have been (and was) unthinkable for Jacob Bernoulli, or even Abraham de Moivre.

As Price wrote in his introduction, neither of these giants had attempted to *invert* their laws of large numbers to derive a probability statement about the ratio of hidden chances. To apply the idea of probability, as they understood it, to these ratios would require some notion like the chances of chances. Such a recursion would have seemed to them incomprehensible. But by tossing out the baggage of chances, Bayes could begin to think of a probability as something primary. This reification of probabilities allowed him to conceive of *prior* probabilities for these probabilities of interest. Price tells us that Bayes's intention was to:

> find out a method by which we might judge concerning the probability that an event has to happen, in given circumstances, upon supposition that we know nothing concerning it but that, under the same circumstances, it has happened a certain number of times, and failed a certain other number of times. He adds, that he soon perceived that it would not be very difficult to do this, provided some rule could be found, according to which we ought to estimate the chance that the probability for the happening of an event perfectly unknown, should lie between any two named degrees of probability, antecedently to any experiments made about it; and that it appeared to him that the rule must be to suppose the chance the same that it should lie between any two equidifferent degrees; which, if it were allowed, all the rest might be easily calculated in the common method of proceeding in the doctrine of chances.

Statisticians have been wrestling with the consequences of what Price called this "very ingenious solution" ever since.

Particularly controversial has been the assumption of a uniform prior probability distribution for the probability of interest, p. The idea that we can represent complete ignorance about p by assuming all possible values to be equally likely is sometimes called *Bayes's Postulate*, but more often the *principle of insufficient reason* or (following Keynes) the *principle of indifference*. Bayes himself expressed reservations about this seductively simple solution. It had the huge advantage of allowing a computation of inverse probabilities. However, it seemed too facile. How can pure ignorance do so much? This question continues to haunt statistical theory to the present day.

Bayes's essay is modern also in another way that has been little noticed by historians. It may be the first true exposition framed completely in terms of what would become the modern *theory of probability*. Bayes trafficked in probabilities, not only for mathematical convenience, as de Moivre did, but also for the final statement of his results. He did not feel compelled to convert the probability back into odds, as his predecessors did. Nor did he refer to chances in his definition of probability.

Finally, as I mentioned, Bayes and Price were motivated by the problem of induction, which was a hot intellectual topic at that time. As early as 1740, Price had been greatly influenced by the writings of Bishop Joseph Butler (1692–1752).[21] Butler, in his *Analogy of Religion,*

Natural and Revealed (1736) had famously written: "But for us, probability is the very guide of life." Here he was using probability in the traditional sense of probability, not as a mathematical concept related to games of chance. He was arguing that human rationality can be applied to discover generally reliable, albeit imperfect, knowledge in an uncertain world. This "natural religion" based on observation could supplement the "revealed religion" of scriptures.

Taking issue with this optimism about the strength of inductive inference was the famous philosopher David Hume, who championed a *skeptical* philosophy in his *Treatise on Human Nature* (1739) and *An Enquiry Concerning Human Understanding* (1748).[22] By the 1760s, Price had come to know Hume personally, and he took seriously many of Hume's insights about the limitations of knowledge gained from experience. However, he was severely critical of Hume's ideas on some questions. Like Butler and David Hartley, Price was much more sanguine than Hume about mankind's justification for interpreting observed regularities in nature as causal, and he was less skeptical than Hume about the possibility of occasional miracles.

Hume had dealt with probabilistic reasoning at some length in his consideration of causality and induction. His concept of probability was very similar to the older, more qualitative probability that had motivated Jacob Bernoulli. Like Bernoulli, Hume thought of probability as a degree of justification for and against a proposition. Like Bernoulli, he assumed that both of these probabilities would be considered separately, and then compared, with the preponderance of evidence determining what was rational to accept.

When Richard Price stumbled upon his late friend's essay (or notes), he was greatly impressed by the potential philosophical implications:

> Every judicious person will be sensible that the problem now mentioned is by no means merely a curious speculation in the doctrine of chances, but necessary to be solved in order to provide a sure foundation for all our reasonings concerning past facts, and what is likely to be hereafter . . . it is certain that we cannot determine, at least not to any nicety, in what degree repeated experiments confirm a conclusion, without the particular discussion of the beforementioned problem; which therefore, is necessary to be considered by any that would give a clear account of the strength of *analogical* or *inductive reasoning*; concerning which at present, we seem to know little more than that it does sometimes in fact convince us, and at other times not;

In an Appendix, Price goes on to deal with the special situation in which a particular outcome has invariably been observed in *all* prior situations of the same type. Then Bayes's rule, he says, can inform us with precision what range of probabilities it is rational to hold after any number of such observations. As this number grows very large, the range becomes very narrow. However, he sagely cautions:

> What has been said seems sufficient to shew us what conclusions to draw from *uniform* experience. It demonstrates, particularly, that instead of proving that events will *always* happen agreeably to it, there will be always reason against this conclusion. In other words, where the course of nature has been the most constant, we can have only reason to reckon upon a recurrency of events proportioned to the degree of this constancy, but we can have no reason for thinking that there are no causes in nature which will *ever* interfere with the operations of the causes from which this constancy is derived, or no circumstances of the world in which it will fail. And if this is true, supposing our only *data* derived from experience, we shall find additional reason for thinking thus if we apply other principles, or have recourse to such considerations as reason, independently of experience, can suggest.

In the context of Price's debate with Hume about miracles, this passage is quite significant. Bayes had proved, Price believed, that even a very large body of evidence, all pointing in the same direction, cannot rule out the very remote chance of a miraculous occurrence. On the other hand, also contrary to Hume's arguments, there may exist "independently of experience" other reasons to convince us of law-like natural regularities.

Price believed that man's reason could often discern the underlying laws at work. Like Jacob Bernoulli, he regarded empirical frequencies as a default basis for probability estimation when there is "total ignorance of nature." However, inferring causality based on even a relatively small number of consistent observations might sometimes be justified on the basis that "operations of nature are in general regular."

Here Price and Hume disagreed. In essence, Price was emphasizing the potential value of considering all the relevant evidence, not just the historical pattern of events. Price's religious faith fueled his optimism that the laws of nature might often be deduced, even with limited empirical evidence. He believed Bayes had demonstrated that empirical data by itself could never prove the impossibility of a thing, even of a miracle. In summary, Price was optimistic that underlying causes could often be assumed, but that deviations from causal laws could very occasionally occur.

Hume, on the other hand, believed that *all* knowledge of causes must be inferred (imperfectly) from observed regularities. A miracle for him would represent a logical contradiction, since it would be the violation of causal laws, which were nothing more than accepted generalizations that by definition did not allow exceptions. Hume held that an enormous amount of prior empirical regularity (e.g., lead weights always fall, all men eventually die) could establish practical certainty of causation. However, he was extremely skeptical that any report of the miraculous suspension of such a law would ever be credible.

FROM CHANCES TO PROBABILITY

Pierre-Simon Laplace was the pivotal figure in the transformation of the doctrine of chances into the classical theory of probability. Unlike de Moivre and Bayes, he rose meteorically to great heights and his achievements were celebrated in his own time. He became the most famous scientist and mathematician of his era, maintaining this position for decades in spite of extraordinary political and social upheavals.

Before discussing Laplace's career and impact on the evolution of probability, I will outline some relevant currents of thought in and around France that shaped his perspective. As in England, de Moivre's *Doctrine of Chances* was recognized in continental Europe as the authoritative treatment of the mathematical aspects of games of chance. Moreover, the merging of probability as a fraction of chances with epistemic probability was beginning to occur. However, the mid-eighteenth century was a time of transition, and there was still some life left in Bernoulli's idea of quantifying probability as a general logic of uncertainty.

Two well-known mathematicians who, like Bernoulli, hailed originally from Switzerland wrote about the interpretation of probability prior to 1770: Gabriel Cramer (1704–1752) and Johann Heinrich Lambert (1728–1777).[23] Their theories both took as a starting point Jacob Bernoulli's logic of combining arguments. In a series of lectures in 1744 and 1745, Cramer offered a slightly amended version of Jacob's theory. In an article published in 1764, Lambert attempted to generalize and "correct" Bernoulli's mathematical rules for combining arguments. Recall that Jacob's rules for combining arguments had led to some awkward implications, and Lambert proposed an alternative approach to get around this problem.

Neither of these works focused on empirical frequencies or on games of chance. As far as we know, these efforts represent the last serious attempts prior to the twentieth century to frame a formal logic of uncertainty in any terms *other* than those derived from the doctrine of chances. In the 1740s and 1750s, it was still possible to mean by "probability" both a degree of certainty in a general way and the more restricted concept of a fraction of chances in games and a few actuarial applications. This somewhat ambiguous status of the term left open various possible lines of future intellectual development, but also engendered some confusion. It is particularly difficult for us, looking back, to make sense of some writing about probability during this period.

This confusing state of affairs is perhaps best exemplified in a long article entitled "*Probabilité*" (Probability) written by Denis Diderot (1713–1784).[24] Diderot was a well-known member of the *philosophes*, the leading intellectuals of the Enlightenment in France. Starting in 1750, Diderot and Jean le Rond D'Alembert (1717–1783) undertook one of the most ambitious intellectual enterprises of all time. As coeditors, the pair began to publish the *Encyclopédie* (Encyclopedia), a compendium of the world's knowledge that eventually included 28 volumes and over 70,000 articles, contributed by many experts in a wide variety of disciplines. The article on "*Probabilité*" was probably written in the early 1750s. The subheadings listed below the title were Philosophy, Logic, and Mathematics.

Diderot's discussion of probability was indeed a kind of fluid amalgam that seemed to gloss over a number of distinctions that would trouble later philosophers and mathematicians. Lorraine Daston, in her classic study of *Classical Probability in the Enlightenment*, sums up Diderot's presentation:

> The project, if not the results, of Part IV of the *Ars Conjectandi* won converts among philosophers as well as mathematicians, perhaps because the legal and mathematical probabilities of evidence were seldom distinguished. The 'Probabilité' article of the *Encyclopédie* illustrates to what extent the mathematical and legal senses of probability were still intertwined … Although the author was thoroughly conversant with Jakob Bernoulli's *Ars Conjectandi*, the article is more philosophical than technical. The article borrowed heavily from Part IV of the *Ars Conjectandi*, reproducing Bernoulli's general rules for weighing evidence and conjecturing, and interpreting Bernoulli's theorem as a demonstration that 'past experience is a principle of probability for the future; we have reason to expect events similar to those we have seen happen.'[25]

Diderot may seem to us somewhat incoherent as he attempts to explain the concept of probability in a way that does justice to both its older and newer formulations.

By the 1760s, the ambiguity reflected in Diderot's article had been largely resolved by a nearly complete fusing of the epistemic and mathematical connotations of probability. The archaic probability that Jacob Bernoulli had tried to mathematicize was receding from consciousness. Increasingly, the "logic" of uncertain inference (including induction from observations of nature) was conceived as obeying the same mathematical principles that governed games of chance.

The narrowing and sharpening of probability represented a double-edged sword. On the one hand, philosophical analysis became more limited in scope. On the other hand, the new probability concept paved the way for great progress in collecting and analyzing statistical information. At the time, the allure of potential benefits from applying probability to various practical problems was great. The *philosophes* were generally hopeful that scientific and social dividends would flow from the rational analysis of nature and society using this new calculus. But a few skeptics were more guarded in their enthusiasm.

One of those who raised red flags was Diderot's coeditor D'Alembert, an eminent mathematician, physicist, and philosopher. As scientific editor for the *Encyclopédie*, he authored two articles on games of chance that were published in the 1750s, and he may also have contributed to Diderot's lengthy article on probability. D'Alembert was a contentious sort, well known for engaging in heated controversies with other scientists and mathematicians. With respect to probability he was something of a contrarian. While he recognized the importance of the new probability theory, he expressed various reservations about the extent to which it could directly be applied to practical problems. Some of his ideas, especially in his early writing, appear simply muddled, while others display deep philosophical insight.

Diderot and D'Alembert were dominant figures in the European intellectual landscape, and their ideas would have been well known to the young Laplace. However, a more immediate source of inspiration for his interest in probability and its potential applications was D'Alembert's younger protégé Nicolas Condorcet (1743–1794), better known as the Marquis de Condorcet. Of noble birth, Condorcet studied under D'Alembert starting in 1759 and eventually achieved great renown as a mathematician, philosopher, and political theorist.

In 1773, Condorcet was appointed acting Secretary of the French Academy of Sciences, and he became the permanent Secretary 3 years later. This venerable institution had been founded in 1666, 4 years after the Royal Society of London. However, unlike its British counterpart, the French Academy had always enjoyed state sponsorship and funding, and had hosted eminent scientists from all over Europe. (Christiaan Huygens had been one of its founding members.) Condorcet's position permitted him to exert great influence over the scientific papers selected for publication in the Academy's journals.

Condorcet's interest in probability dates from the early 1770s, although his famous treatise on the application of probability to voting behavior was not published until 1785.[26] In December 1771, Condorcet received a letter from the virtually unknown Laplace, then 22 years old. It concerned a highly original mathematical paper on esoteric methods motivated by some problems related to the doctrine of chances. Laplace was at this stage seeking to launch a career in mathematics and science, and believed that Condorcet's support would be helpful to him. Condorcet was enthusiastic about possible contributions of the probability calculus to rational decision-making in the social, political, and judicial spheres.

In addition to his philosophical and scientific pursuits, Condorcet was actively involved in political affairs, and he rose to a position of great power and influence. In August 1774, Condorcet's close friend Anne-Robert-Jacques Turgot (1727–1781) was appointed Controller-General of France, a very powerful administrative position. Turgot had Condorcet appointed Inspector General of the Mint, a post he managed to hold for 17 years, even though Turgot fell from power in 1776. So, Condorcet's enchantment with probability was not only academic; he was intimately involved with issues of public policy to which he regarded probability as highly relevant.

It seems probable that Condorcet was the muse who stimulated Laplace to complete the conceptual transition from chances to probabilities that would transform human knowledge:

> There is no question but that the technical development that made the transition was his [Laplace's]. It does seem likely, however, that it was Condorcet whose

enthusiasm opened the prospect and pointed his talent toward the opportunity and the problems to be found in demography and statistics. Condorcet could not see very far into the problems. But he could see the subject; and he did see it; and he showed it to Laplace.

The French Newton

Pierre-Simon Laplace was born at Beaumont-en-Auge in the Normandy region of France on March 23, 1749.[27] His early life has not been well documented. His father may have been a cider merchant, who envisioned for Pierre-Simon a clerical career. In 1765, Laplace was sent off to the University of Caen to study theology. However, under the influence of two professors there, he soon turned from theology to mathematics. Armed with a letter of introduction, he ventured off to Paris in 1768 to study under D'Alembert, who at age 51 was at the height of his influence. After some initial skepticism, D'Alembert quickly became convinced of Laplace's extraordinary talent and agreed to tutor him. He also arranged for Laplace to obtain a teaching post at the *École Militaire* (Military School), the academy for training young cadets.

Before long, Laplace was cranking out a stream of original papers related to astronomy and mathematics. By 1773 this work, along with the sponsorship of D'Alembert and Condorcet, had secured him an appointment to the Academy of Sciences. As an associate member, he received financial support that allowed him to pursue full-time his various researches. Two of Laplace's earliest research reports concerned the doctrine of chances. One of these, delivered in 1774, was entitled "Memoir on the Probability of the Causes Given the Events." The essence of this work was similar to that of Thomas Bayes's posthumous essay, which was hardly known in England, let alone France. Laplace described his topic as:

> a question which has not been given due consideration before, but which deserves even more to be studied, for it is principally from this point of view that the science of chances can be useful in civil life.[28]

It is not clear whether Condorcet had in fact suggested this subject of inquiry, but he enthusiastically endorsed Laplace's contribution.

In an introduction to the published article, Condorcet wrote that the paper[29]:

> treats a branch of the analysis of chance, much more important and less known than that which forms the subject of the former Memoir; here the probability is unknown, that is to say the number of chances for or against a possible event is undetermined. It is known only that in a given number of experiments this event occurred a certain number of times, and it is required to know how from that information alone the probability of what is going to happen in the future can be stated. It is obvious that this question comprises all the applications that can be made of the doctrine of chance to the uses of ordinary life, and of that whole science, it is the only useful part, the only one worthy of the serious attention of Philosophers.

It is clear that both Condorcet and Laplace had somehow arrived at a "Bayesian" perspective about the importance of inverse probability and the method by which it could be calculated. Elaborating the mathematical and philosophical implications of this approach would become a leitmotif of Laplace's research for the rest of his long career.

Over the next 20 years, Laplace rose to a position of dominance in the French Academy of Sciences, and established his reputation in many scientific areas, especially mathematics and celestial mechanics. Laplace was very ambitious and not particularly modest about his abilities, often causing friction with some of his contemporaries. However, his intellectual superiority, coupled with political agility, stood him in good stead. In 1784, he took on an additional responsibility as an examiner at the Royal Artillery Corps, which brought him into contact with powerful political leaders in France. In this capacity in 1785, he first encountered a promising cadet by the name of Napoleon Bonaparte (1769–1821).

In 1787, Laplace began a fruitful collaboration with another of Europe's greatest mathematicians, Joseph Lagrange (1736–1813), who had recently arrived in Paris. The two geniuses shared many areas of interest and complemented each other well. While Lagrange's forte was mathematical theory, Laplace's mathematical brilliance was deployed mainly in order to solve practical problems.

The following year, at the age of 39, Laplace married Marie-Charlotte de Courty de Romanges, only 18 years old. Soon after, a son and daughter arrived. After a few quiet years, the Laplaces were caught up in the political turmoil engulfing France. They moved to a small town 30 miles outside Paris to evade the Reign of Terror in 1793, returning when it was safer in July 1794.

In 1795, the Academy of Sciences was reopened as the National Institute of Sciences and Laplace resumed his former responsibilities. Also in 1795, the Bureau of Longitudes was established, with Laplace and Lagrange as the only two mathematicians among its founders. This office was established in an attempt to revive French naval power in the wake of Britain's recent ascendance to mastery of the high seas. The Bureau was placed in charge of all institutions concerned with astronomical, geodesic, and related studies, including the Paris Observatory, of which Laplace became director. In 1796, he published the famous "nebular theory," an account of how he believed the solar system had formed from a cloud of rotating and cooling incandescent gas. His astronomical work led to an appointment as one of the 40 "immortals" of the *Académie Francaise*.

When Napoleon rose to power as First Consul of France in 1799, Laplace finagled an appointment as Minister of the Interior, but was replaced after only 6 weeks on the job. Like many master technocrats, Laplace lacked the pragmatic attitude required of a successful administrator. Bonaparte wryly observed about this episode:

> Geometrician of the first rank, Laplace was not long in showing himself a worse than average administrator; since his first actions in office we recognized our mistake. Laplace did not consider any question from the right angle: he sought subtleties everywhere, only conceived problems, and finally carried the spirit of 'infinitesimals' into the administration.[30]

Nonetheless, Napoleon appreciated Laplace's talents enough to appoint him a member, and later Chancellor, of the French Senate. Laplace received the Legion of Honor award in 1805. In that year he also helped to found the Society of Arcueil, an organization whose goal was to promote a more mathematical approach to science. As the leader of this group, he exerted great influence on the administration of scientific research and education throughout the country.

In 1812, Laplace published the first edition of his masterwork on probability, the *Theorie Analytique des Probabilités* (*Analytic Theory of*

Probabilities).[31] It contained a comprehensive overview of the mathematical theory of probability, including many of Laplace's groundbreaking original contributions. Most notably, the *TAP* included a full exposition of a result he had first presented 2 years earlier. Recall that in 1733, de Moivre had shown that the probability distribution for the total number of successes in any large number of Bernoulli trials could be closely approximated using the normal (bell-shaped) curve. I mentioned that this was the earliest version of what would much later be called the Central Limit Theorem.

Laplace went much further by generalizing this theorem. He was able to demonstrate that for virtually *any* random variables of practical importance, the probability distribution of the sum (or the average) of the values of the variables could be approximated by using the normal distribution. This mathematical *tour de force* was derived in the context of a theory of observational errors, which at that time was the main scientific application of probability theory. While this general version of the Central Limit Theorem is Laplace's most notable mathematical discovery related to probability theory, the *TAP* covered a vast terrain, well beyond anything that had gone before.

A second, and substantially expanded, edition of the *TAP* followed in 1814, with two further editions in 1820 and 1825. The Introduction to the 1814 edition was published separately as a *Philosophical Essay on Probabilities*.[32] This was a comprehensive nontechnical discussion of Laplace's conception of how the calculus of probability could be applied to a great many practical problems. Laplace regarded probability theory as not only a practical tool and mathematical discipline, but as the very essence of logical thinking about uncertain matters. In spirit he was very close to Jacob Bernoulli, whom he admired, except that by probability he meant specifically the new probability that conformed to the doctrine of chances. On the last page of his *Philosophical Essay* is his much-quoted remark that "the theory of probability is at bottom only common sense reduced to calculus."

Laplace was named a Count of the Empire 1806, and managed to weather Napoleon's inconvenient downfall in 1815. Indeed, he became the Marquis de Laplace in 1817 after the monarchy's restoration. Once again, he proved himself too useful to ignore and pliable enough to adapt to the political exigencies. He continued to be productive, although his reputation was somewhat tarnished by his blatant political opportunism over the years. His later years were also marred by the loss of his only daughter Sophie-Suzanne, who had died in childbirth in 1813. When the final edition of *TAP* was published in 1825, Laplace was 76 years old and fading. He died 2 years later.

Laplace's Philosophy of Probability

To the Marquis de Laplace many things were perfectly clear that to "lesser" minds were far from obvious. In his hands, the theory of probability became a powerful instrument. His dazzling mathematics, acute logic, and sublime self-assurance swept aside any objections to his ideas about probability. Before Laplace, probability was still somewhat ambiguous, and the mathematical doctrine of chances had not fully fused with the epistemic sense of probability. After Laplace, the merger was complete, a development that would have enormous repercussions, both practical and philosophical, over the next two centuries.

To understand Laplace's mature perspective we can turn to *A Philosophical Essay on Probabilities*. On the opening page he set out the broad scope of probability:

> I present here without the aid of analysis the principles and general results of this theory, applying them to the most important questions of life, which are indeed for the most part only problems of probability. Strictly speaking it may even be said that nearly all our knowledge is problematical; ... the principal means for ascertaining truth—induction and analogy—are based on probabilities; so that the entire system of human knowledge is connected with the theory set forth in this essay.[33]

Jacob Bernoulli might have been gratified that his program of extending probability to the moral and social sciences was finally being taken seriously. However, upon reading further, he would perhaps have been chagrined at the ease with which Laplace simply *assumed* that the laws governing games of chance were applicable to "the entire system of human knowledge." Moreover, Laplace's theories reflected an extreme of Enlightenment thinking that dispensed completely with a Divine role in the administration of natural law. When asked about this absence by Napoleon, Laplace is said to have replied: "I have no need for that hypothesis."

Laplace next stated his conception of a deterministic universe, arguing that blind chance, or fortune, is only "an illusion of the mind." He subscribed to *the principle of sufficient reason*, according to which "a thing cannot occur without a cause which produces it." Laplace interpreted this philosophical principle in its strongest form:

> We ought then to regard the current state of the universe as the effect of its anterior state and as the cause of the one which is to follow. Given for one instant an intelligence which could comprehend all the forces by which nature is animated and the respective situations of the beings who compose it—an intelligence sufficiently vast to submit these data to analysis—it would embrace in the same formula the movements of the greatest bodies of the universe and those of the lightest atom; for it, nothing would be uncertain, and the future, as the past, would be present to its eyes.[34]

This clockwork universe (without a clockmaker needed to maintain it) is the logical extension of Newton's discoveries.

Jacob Bernoulli had deliberately sidestepped the problem of explaining how chance could be reconciled with God's omniscience and omnipotence. For him it was enough to know that events unfolded *as if* they were random. De Moivre had avoided most metaphysical problems by dealing only with games of chance and actuarial problems. Laplace lived during the Enlightenment, when it was possible to aver that causal laws must be universal, that in principle every sparrow's fall could be ascribed to potentially knowable causes.

It is only our ignorance of these laws that creates an appearance of randomness. "Probability is relative in part to this ignorance, in part to our knowledge." Our knowledge is important because it frames for us the different chances, or *possibilities*, that might exist. "We know that of three or a greater number of events a single one ought to occur, but nothing induces us to believe that one of them will occur rather than the others." Knowing the possibilities is useful knowledge, but not sufficient to achieve certainty. "In this state of indecision it is impossible for us to announce their occurrence with certainty." Thus, probability is necessary to balance our knowledge and ignorance appropriately.

Laplace then launched into an exposition of the mathematical principles of probability. While he interpreted probability epistemically, as a measure of belief, he assumed (without explanation) that the usual rules of mathematical probability theory must apply:

> The theory of chance consists in reducing all the events of the same kind to a certain number of cases equally possible, that is to say, to such as *we may be equally undecided about in regard to their existence,* and in determining the number of cases favorable to the event whose probability is sought. The ratio of this number to that of all the cases possible is the measure of this probability, which is thus simply a fraction whose numerator is the number of favorable cases and whose denominator is the number of all the cases possible (emphasis added).[35]

Laplace slid back and forth between examples involving chance mechanisms (coins, urns, or dice) and practical applications of the theory (annuities, testimony, astronomy). However, he glossed over the question of exactly how the possible cases underlying the more complex natural and social phenomena resembled those in the games of chance.

This ambiguity did not seem to bother Laplace, but his failure to clarify this important issue would create many problems for others. There is a long leap between the "chances" in a lottery and those in a complex social process. I believe that Laplace's thinking may have been grounded in a conceptual framework in which metaphysical chances were meaningful, so that his readers would not be troubled by this ambiguity. Perhaps the chances for him were "obviously" metaphorical, since he believed the underlying unknown causes to be in fact strictly deterministic. So, probability assessments might vary, but mainly because different individuals would possess different *information* regarding the underlying causes: "In things which are only probable the difference of the data, which each man has in regard to them, is one of the principal causes of the diversity of opinions which prevail in regard to the same objects."

He then criticized irrational beliefs such as magic and astrology that emanate from blind superstition rather than observed data. Laplace seemed to imply that probability is based on a rational appraisal of chances that accounts for the available information pertaining to the hidden causes at work. In this way, the problem of induction is, in principle, reducible to a matter of deductive logic. However, he did not specify the precise manner in which this logic is to be implemented:

> The difference of opinions depends, however, upon the manner in which the influence of known data is determined. The theory of probabilities holds to considerations so delicate that it is not surprising that with the same data two persons arrive at different results, especially in very complicated questions.[36]

Fair enough. But what principles can guide us in our deliberations regarding probabilities implied by the available data? In particular, how can we assess whether the cases (chances) we have enumerated are really equally possible? "If they are not so, we will determine first their respective possibilities, whose exact appreciation is one of the most delicate points of the theory of chance."

He then tried to explain this point with a simple coin-tossing scenario. Suppose that we are allowed two tosses of a fair coin. If heads arises on the first toss, we win. If not, then we get to toss again, and win if a head occurs on this second throw. What is the probability of winning the game? In this situation, we might delineate three possible cases: HH, TH, and TT. Since two cases would result in success, we *might* believe the probability of winning to be 2/3. (Indeed, D'Alembert was initially confused about this before realizing the fallacy.) However, we all "know" that these cases are not equally likely. As Fermat had reasoned in 1654, we can imagine there are actually four chances that would be equally possible if we were to toss both coins, regardless of the outcome on the first toss. Three of these possible outcomes (HH, HT, and TH) are winners and one (TT) results in a loss, so the "correct" answer is 3/4.

This knowledge of the right answer derives from our understanding of the physical setup and resulting causal process in this simple case. Laplace used this simple example as a means of calling attention to the difficulty in practical problems of determining the equally likely chances. However, he did not offer much practical guidance when it came to situations in which the presumed underlying causal mechanism was not known. This "most delicate" problem had troubled D'Alembert deeply, and he remained somewhat skeptical about the ease with which mathematical laws of chance could be applied to the physical or social world. Laplace was mindful of his old mentor's philosophical reservations, but far less worried about their practical importance.

The Probability of Causes

By the 1750s the *fraction* of chances had become a natural way of measuring the probability of an event. This chance-based probability, which represented the appropriate degree of belief for events in games of chance, gradually came to be accepted as the sole way of thinking about epistemic probability more generally. Thus, mathematical probability came to assume the dual connotation of both a degree of certainty and a reflection of underlying causal structure in the real world, as perceived imperfectly through the veil of human ignorance.

Bernoulli's law of large numbers and de Moivre's improved approximation proved that the hidden ratio of chances could be discovered if the number of observations grew very large. Even a more modest number of observations would provide *some* indication of this ratio. However, neither Bernoulli nor de Moivre was able to imagine how to quantify the degree of certainty associated with an "estimate" based on a small sample. They were both wedded to the idea that practical applications of the doctrine of chances would require large enough samples to assure something like "moral certainty."

Bayes thought it might be possible to derive a precise inference about the underlying probability based on a much smaller sample. He devised a clever way of obtaining a probability statement about an underlying probability (fraction of chances). In order to do this, however, he had to adopt what Price called his "peculiar definition" of probability as meaning the same as chance. Then he could utilize the standard definition of conditional probability to obtain the desired inverse probability.

Bayes never referred explicitly to causes in his essay. However, in a "Scholium" Bayes did consider some broader philosophical implications of his analysis for the issue of causation. His work on probability was motivated by his interest in causal regularities. How much could be known about the chances for a thing to occur based only on the frequency of past occurrence? Moreover, Richard Price certainly had the philosophical implications in mind.

Laplace, on the other hand, was more confident and ambitious. He was explicitly concerned with the probability of causes very generally. He had no intention of sidestepping philosophical issues by simply treating chance and probability as identical, whatever they might really mean. So, Laplace could not find the "probability of causes" by straightforwardly applying de Moivre's definition of conditional probabilities. He needed to expand the theory of probability to encompass causal processes. This he accomplished by positing a new principle that he believed to be self-evident.

To understand Laplace's idea, suppose there are three possible causes: C_1, C_2, and C_3. The posterior probability of C_1 given the event E would be:

$$P(C_1|E) = KP(E|C_1)$$

That is, the posterior (inverse) probability of any cause such as C_1 given the event E would be proportional to the corresponding direct probability of the event given the cause. Here the proportionality constant K is necessary to make the sum of the inverse probabilities for all the possible causes add to 1. So,

$$K = \frac{1}{P(E|C_1) + P(E|C_2) + P(E|C_3)}$$

This new principle can be regarded as the special case of Bayes's Theorem when the three causes have equal prior probabilities (1/3 in this case). Laplace's rule produced the same mathematical result, but his logic was reversed. It seemed self-evident to Laplace that this fundamental principle should normally be assumed as the default, absent a reason to depart from it. That "unusual" case would happen when the various causes were known to be "unequally probable." In that special case, Laplace would weight the different possible causes in accordance with their unequal prior probabilities of happening.

Mathematically the resulting formula was identical to Bayes's Theorem, but the relevance to causation was more direct and "obvious" within Laplace's philosophical framework. Indeed, from his earliest paper on the probability of causes in 1774, the identification of "probabilities" with "causes" was evident:

> The uncertainty of human knowledge is concerned with events or with causes of events. If one is assured, for example, that an urn only contains white and black tickets in a given ratio, and one asks the probability that a ticket drawn by chance will be white, then the event is uncertain but the cause upon which the probability of its occurrence depends, the ratio of white to black tickets, is known.[37]

Bernoulli had regarded the ratio of chances as a reflection of some hidden causal process. Bayes preferred to evade the question of what exactly was meant by a probability. Laplace wrote as if the probability could be treated as somehow *equivalent* to a cause.

Insufficient Reason

Bayes explained in his Scholium the rationale for his proposal to treat all prior probabilities as equally probable. This idea later became known as the *principle of insufficient reason*. According to this principle, if we know absolutely nothing a priori about the probability p of a particular event, we should act *as if* the value of p has been determined, as in Bayes's analog, by metaphorically rolling a ball on a smooth surface and observing where it lands.

Bayes had offered a sophisticated mathematical rationale for why it *may* be reasonable to represent complete a priori ignorance by equal prior probabilities.[38] To him, it was not obvious that ignorance meant equal probabilities. He was not certain that his "billiard table" analogy could be fully justified. Laplace suffered no such compunctions. Rather than trying, like Bayes, to derive a solution using only the existing elements of the doctrine of chances, Laplace introduced a new principle, or axiom, into the theory of probability.

As I explained above, Laplace's new principle was framed in terms of causes rather than probabilities. However, he regarded causes and probabilities as effectively interchangeable. Therefore, it was quite natural for him to treat probabilities mathematically just like causes. If the probabilities associated with the unknown causes were unknown, then there would be no sufficient reason to regard these probabilities as being unequal. So, the principle of insufficient reason should, he thought, be applied to any unknown probabilities: "When the probability of an event is unknown we may suppose it equal to any value from zero to unity." Here, however, Laplace's failure to define precisely what the underlying cases, or chances, really represent would run into difficulties.

To avoid confusion, it is important to realize first that Bayes's Theorem as a mathematical formula is almost trivial to derive from basic axioms of mathematical probability. Contrary to much misunderstanding, there has never been any dispute about the formula itself.[39] Moreover, there are many practical situations in which its use is entirely uncontroversial. Consider the problem of medical diagnosis discussed previously. Often the "base-rate" at which a disease is prevalent in the population is fairly well known. For example, the probability that a randomly selected individual has the disease might be 0.05, or 5%. Furthermore the respective conditional probabilities of detecting the disease given that it is or is not present may also be known.

When these prior probabilities are known, Bayes's Theorem tells us how to put these pieces of information together to obtain the posterior (inverse) probability that a patient has the disease given that she tests positive. The difficulties arise when the prior probabilities are unknown or subject to disagreement. In particular, what is reasonable when we lack *any* information upon which to specify the prior probabilities? It is this typical situation that has generated the most heated controversies pertaining to so-called Bayesian analyses. So, the papers by Bayes in 1763 and Laplace in 1774 were more important for the philosophical Pandora's Box they opened up than for their mathematical content.

The principle of insufficient reason seems plausible if we are dealing with a well-defined set of concrete possible events, such as the possible outcomes in a game of chance. In the absence of any evidence to the contrary, each outcome can be assumed equally possible. This is certainly a reasonable position to adopt, at least as a practical expedient. For instance, if I come to a fork in a trail, and have no idea which way to go, I may as well just flip a coin to decide. If the alternatives are specific hypotheses regarding possible causes, then we can in principle apply the same logic. We can list the possibilities and decide whether there are any relevant distinctions among them that would lead us to expect one rather than another.

However, when the assumed alternatives are mathematical probabilities, it is not clear that the same logic necessarily pertains. Probabilities *in the abstract* are simply numbers that have no context or meaning. The only way to judge the relative likelihood of occurrence for any such number would be to translate it somehow into a concrete cause, or causal processes. So, our uncertainty about probabilities regarded as naked numerical values entails much more ambiguity than our uncertainty about causes. As a result, applying the principle of insufficient reason directly to probabilities rests on a much weaker rationale than applying it to causes.

The principle of insufficient reason applied to probabilities assumes there is a one-to-one correspondence between causes and probabilities. However, since the nature of these underlying causes is completely unknown, there is no way to decide rationally whether this makes sense. This basic conundrum can be illustrated by a simple example. Suppose we know that there exist three possible causes that might have given rise to an event: C_1, C_2, C_3.

Assume first that the probabilities for the event given these three causes, respectively, are 1/8, 1/4, and 1/2. Then, by the principle of insufficient reason, our prior probabilities must be

$$P(C_1) = P(C_2) = P(C_3) = 1/3$$

Equivalently, we would have

$$P(1/8) = P(1/4) = P(1/2) = 1/3$$

However, suppose that the probability of the event given C_1 is actually 1/4 rather than 1/8. Then, we would have

$$P(1/4) = 2/3$$

$$P(1/2) = 1/3$$

Although the three possible *causes* would each have the same prior probability of 1/3, the two possible probability values would have unequal prior probabilities. So, applying the principle of insufficient reason to the two possible probability values would be arbitrary and misleading. We have no way to know whether or not it is reasonable to assume there is a one-to-one correspondence between possible probabilities and possible causes.

The same issue arises when we consider a continuum of possible probability values, as in Bayes's framework. It may seem natural to apply the principle of insufficient reason to the values of probabilities. However, we could equally well apply the principle to any other mathematical function of the probability, such as the logarithm. Indeed, we could apply the principle of insufficient reason to the *odds* rather than the probabilities. After all, probability has only recently supplanted the much older concept of odds as a standard way to represent uncertainty. We must remember that a mathematical probability is only one possible way to measure our uncertainty about a specified event. Applying the principle of insufficient reason to this particular measure can have different consequences than applying it to some other valid measure.

A Coincidence?

Condorcet referred to Bayes's essay in an introduction to one of Laplace's memoirs published in 1781. It is generally believed that Laplace must have learned about Bayes's essay around that time and was therefore unaware of it when he wrote his landmark paper on the probabilities of causes in 1774. In his *Philosophical Essay* Laplace mentioned that he admired Bayes's analysis, but found the approach a bit peculiar. Laplace quizzically remarked that Bayes found "the probability that the possibilities indicated by past experience are comprised within given limits; and he has arrived at this in a refined and very ingenious manner, although a little perplexing."[40]

As I mentioned previously, Bayes's essay was believed to have exerted no immediate influence on later developments in probability and statistics. Laplace's work on inverse probability a decade later, which *did* have great influence, was directly stimulated by Condorcet, who had a strong interest in the application of probabilistic ideas to social and political affairs. But here we have a mystery. Was Laplace truly unaware of Bayes's ideas when he conceived his own version of inverse probability? Is it possible that some hint of what Bayes had accomplished had somehow made its way across the Channel and stimulated Laplace's thinking?

Before we dismiss this speculation as entirely fanciful, let us consider that there was a substantial commerce of ideas between the leading intellectuals of England and France. It therefore seems plausible that Condorcet could have read David Hartley's *Observations on Man*. Recall that Hartley had written of his ingenious friend, probably Bayes, who had solved the problem of inverse probability. Hartley had suggested that this result might allow us to "determine the proportions, and by degrees, the whole nature, of unknown causes, by a sufficient observation of their effects."[41] Indeed, there seems to be an uncanny similarity between Laplace's formulation in 1774 and Hartley's discussion in 1749.[42] So, one possibility is that Condorcet had alluded to Hartley's "Bayesian" ideas when he was first stimulating the young Laplace's interest in the probability of causes.

Another possible agent for the transmission of Bayesian thinking across the Channel was the ubiquitous Richard Price. Price's philosophical writings were well known on the Continent. In 1767, Price had published a treatise entitled *Four Dissertations*, which included a discussion of the problem of induction in response to Hume's famous argument against belief in miracles.[43] In a very lengthy footnote, he had referred to Bayes's essay, described the general idea, and provided some examples. Furthermore, we know that Price met the Abbé Morellet (1727–1819), who had visited England in the summer of 1772, right around the time that Laplace began thinking seriously about probability.[44,45]

Morellet was one of France's most prominent *philosophes* and a close friend of Turgot, whom Condorcet had met around this same time. Morellet had written about political economy and was interested in Price's views about the population question. At a dinner in London attended by Price, along with Benjamin Franklin, Joseph Priestley, and other luminaries, Morellet found the conversation "instructive and varied." It is certainly possible that Price discussed his views on Hume and the potential importance he ascribed to the Bayes essay. If so, the general idea of inverse probability may have been conveyed to Condorcet by Morellet, who had returned to Paris in the fall of 1772. I hope that further scholarship will eventually reveal whether some link between Bayes and Laplace actually may have existed.

CHAPTER 8

BABEL

Mathematical probability as we know it arose somewhat fortuitously. It gradually supplanted a much older and more ambiguous sense of probability that had prevailed for many centuries. This new mathematical probability grew directly out of the mathematics of games of chance, and was thus not possible until, in the mid-1650s, a critical mass of mathematical talent happened to be focused, albeit momentarily, on such games. It was then not until the 1680s that Jacob Bernoulli first conceived of probability as being calibrated on a scale between zero and one, and 1718 before another lone genius, Abraham de Moivre, defined probability as *a fraction of chances.*

This classical definition of probability was still not firmly established until Pierre-Simon Laplace promoted its broader appreciation and application in the late 1700s. By around 1800, this version of probability had become the "obvious" way to think about uncertainty. When an outcome (or conclusion) was uncertain, it was *as if* the result was chosen by chance, as by a lottery or similar random mechanism. That is, we could regard the outcome as being determined by a *metaphorical lottery*. The laws of nature would of course determine the outcome, but our limited knowledge about

Willful Ignorance: The Mismeasure of Uncertainty, First Edition. Herbert I. Weisberg.
© 2014 John Wiley & Sons, Inc. Published 2014 by John Wiley & Sons, Inc.

the underlying causal processes would place us in the position of a spectator who observes a game of chance. So, Laplace could assert famously that probability is the measure of our ignorance. By this, he meant that probability is the means of quantifying our partial knowledge based on our degree of ignorance about the true causes.

This metaphorical lottery concept eventually became the basis for what is now called *classical probability*. Gradually, however, the explicit analogy to games of chance became superfluous, retained only as a ritualistic observance. Every textbook on probability theory written prior to the twentieth century began with the formal definition of probability as a fraction of chances. However, the subsequent mathematical development would dispense entirely with any reference to the underlying chances. The mathematical laws of probability became perceived as self-evident and were justified by an appeal to common sense. Based on these seemingly universal laws, Laplace and his followers erected an elaborate intellectual edifice with very broad applicability. The theory of probability was rightly regarded as a major achievement of the Age of Reason.

What happened next, however, was unexpected. Shortly after Laplace's death in 1827, the structure of classical probability came tumbling down, much like the Tower of Babel and for a similar reason. The proponents of classical probability were guilty of overreaching, and their hubris was punished by a strong backlash. Over time, probability as a universal language of uncertainty became fractured into many differing interpretations of what probability "really" meant:

> It is unanimously agreed that statistics depends somehow on probability. But, as to what probability is and how it is connected with statistics, there has seldom been such complete disagreement and breakdown of communication since the Tower of Babel. There must be dozens of different interpretations of probability defended by living authorities, and some authorities hold that several different interpretations may be useful ... Considering the confusion about the foundations of statistics, it is surprising, and certainly gratifying, to find that almost everyone is agreed on what the purely mathematical properties of probability are.[1]

This stunning reversal would have astonished Jacob Bernoulli. Probability as a fraction of chances had become *obvious*, while the odds, chances, and expectations from which probability was originally derived had lost much of their intuitive appeal. As a result, no one was quite sure what this word "probability" really meant.

Laplace's classical probability seems to us quaint and outmoded. What are these possible "chances" or equally possible cases, and how do we know they are really equally possible? Is it not circular to define probability as a fraction of chances? But such questions are naïvely predicated on a literal interpretation of the lottery metaphor. Even sophisticated philosophers have fallen prey to this common misconception[2]:

> The fact, Φ, that the rear tires are completely bald, confers 60% probability on having a flat before reaching Massachusetts. It is a mere myth that Φ should break down into a set of cases Φ_1, which entail getting a flat tire and another set Φ_2, entailing the opposite. We certainly know of no such decomposition and have no good reason to think there is one. Yet the myth that every problem in probability can be reduced to a set of favourable and unfavourable cases persisted for centuries.

Hacking here seems to be saying that classical probability referred to a set of actual chances. For instance, there might be 60 future possible eventualities that would entail a flat tire and 40 that would not.

Was this a myth, or a useful metaphor? I am quite confident that Bernoulli, de Moivre, and Laplace did not interpret the concept of equally likely cases literally, except possibly for games of chance. Framing our probabilities as if they are similar to fractions of chances in a metaphorical lottery does not imply we believe there are actual chances. Rather, we have a degree of uncertainty that can be described by such a hypothetical fraction. Recall that Bernoulli had explained that virtually *any* event "can be conceived as divisible with regard to the number of cases in which it can be gained or lost, happen or fail to happen."[3]

Because the event "can be divided in this conceptual way," it is only the *ratio* of the chances for happening to the chances for failing that matter. Bernoulli was the first to realize that if we conceived of things, such as the weather, *as if* such cases did really exist, we could learn about the corresponding ratio of hypothetical cases from empirical data. Although Laplace was maddeningly vague about his interpretation of the equally likely cases, I believe he had something similar in mind. Nowhere except in relation to games of chance or lotteries did he ever spell out what the cases actually were or how they might be counted. Moreover, he certainly understood that probability dealt only with the ratio of chances, never their absolute number: "The preceding notion of probability supposes that, in increasing in the same ratio the number of favorable cases and that of all the cases possible, the probability remains the same."[4]

THE GREAT UNRAVELING

Classical probability eventually reached its zenith during the early nineteenth century. Laplace and his followers had crafted a coherent, and seemingly airtight, system for thinking about uncertainty. Until around 1840, this system remained unassailable, and its scope of application gradually expanded. About that time, the general consensus about the meaning of probability began to break down. This occurred not primarily because classical probability was deemed defective *per se*, but rather because the ambitions of those applying this probability theory were too grand. In particular, the promise of being able to resolve difficult social and political issues through mathematical analysis was deemed unrealistic.

Laplace, initially inspired by Condorcet, had been optimistic about the ability of probability theory to place the "moral sciences" on a more scientific and rational footing. In his *Philosophical Essay*, three chapters were devoted to such applications.[5] These concerned the credibility of testimonies, the decisions of assemblies, and the judgments of tribunals. For example, Laplace was very concerned about the optimal number of jurors in a legal trial and the strength of the majority that should be required to condemn an accused person (e.g., 7 votes to convict out of 12 or 8 out of 10, etc.).

His followers, including most notably Siméon Poisson (1781–1840), drove the mathematical analysis of these issues to great lengths.[6] These efforts reached their culmination in Poisson's famous and controversial monograph (*Research on the Probability of Judgments in Criminal and Civil Matters*), published in 1837. However, the proposal of submitting such delicate considerations to a precise mathematical calculus provoked a strong reaction. In 1843, the philosopher John Stuart Mill famously condemned such applications of probability as the "opprobrium" of mathematics.[7]

Landmarks of Probability

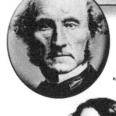

1600

1654	Pascal & Fermat
1657	Huygens

Siméon Denis Poisson

1700

1713	Bernoulli
1718	De Moivre

1764	Bayes & Price
1774	Laplace

Augustus De Morgan

John Stuart Mill

1800

1837	**Poisson**
1838	**De Morgan**
1843	**Mill**
1843	**Cournot**
1849	**Ellis**
1854	**Boole**
1866	**Venn**
1892	**Peirce**

Robert Leslie Ellis

1900

1921	Keynes
1921	Knight
1922	Fisher
1926	Ramsey
1926	Neyman & Pearson
1928	Von Mises
1937	De Finetti
1949	Reichenbach
1954	Savage
1959	Popper

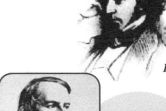

George Boole

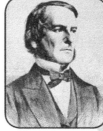

John Venn

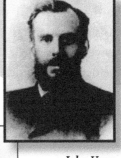

Charles Sanders Peirce

A particular target of criticism was the theory of inverse probability, which had been proposed by Bayes and Laplace. Recall that Laplace had advocated the principle of insufficient reason: when we are completely ignorant, we should assign an equal degree of probability to each of the possible causes. Laplace went even further by equating each possible a priori value of the unknown probability with a distinct cause. Applying the principle of insufficient reason to underlying causes, he could supply a priori probabilities that would then be modified by empirical observations, using what we now call Bayes's rule. In this way, an inverse probability distribution for the unknown probability could be obtained.

Laplace's approach led him to derive a general rule for estimating the probability that a particular event will occur after a succession of occurrences and nonoccurrences. For example, suppose that all we know is that in a series of encounters between two top tennis players, Player A has won six matches and Player B has won two. What is the probability that Player A will prevail the next time they meet? Using inverse probability and the principle of insufficient reason, Laplace could calculate the answer to be 7/10. More generally, if an event (say, Player A wins) has occurred n times and failed m times, Laplace's famous Rule of Succession would estimate the probability of the event on the subsequent trial as

$$P(E) = \frac{n+1}{n+m+2}$$

Of particular significance is the special case when all of the previous trials have resulted in the event's occurrence. A frequently mentioned example was the probability that the sun will rise tomorrow, given that it has done so a great many times in succession so far. If n is the number of successive events observed, then the probability of an occurrence on the next possible occasion would be

$$P(E) = \frac{n+1}{n+2}$$

Of course, there are many possible arguments against such a facile application of probability theory, and Laplace himself would undoubtedly have applied his formula rather judiciously. Nonetheless, the idea that our ignorance itself could be harnessed to power the engine of inductive inference seemed too good to be true, rather like the dream of a perpetual motion machine.

Although the mathematical rules and usefulness of probability had been firmly established, the philosophical foundation of this concept began to be questioned. Probability still retained the formal definition of being a fraction of chances, but the intuitive understanding of "chances" so familiar to Huygens and Bernoulli had faded. By Poisson's time, probability was at least as "real" as the metaphysical chances on which it was, in theory, based. But without the intuitive "ratio of chances" conceptualization that had motivated Bernoulli and Huygens, probability lacked a firm foundation. Difficult questions began to be posed about the true meaning of probability.

These questions have been discussed and debated ever since. There have been a great many attempts by mathematicians, philosophers, statisticians, and scientists to pin down this elusive concept.[8] For the most part, the various proposals have laid primary emphasis on one or another of four common intuitions about probability.

- Probability pertains to a relative *frequency* of occurrence.
- Probability is a *logical* relationship between evidence and belief.
- Probability measures a *subjective* degree of belief.
- Probability is a measure of the *propensity* to occur.

From the classical (metaphorical lottery) perspective, these are four aspects, or connotations, of probability. Each aspect is consistent with and implied by the fundamental analogy between something uncertain and the outcome of an idealized game of chance. Defining probability in terms of any one of these connotations promises greater clarity but seems in some way inadequate.

PROBABILITY AS A RELATIVE FREQUENCY

One of the earliest proposals to define unambiguously the true meaning of probability was put forward by an English mathematician named Robert Leslie Ellis (1817–1859) in an essay read to the Cambridge Philosophical

Society in 1842.[9] "On the Foundations of the Theory of Probabilities" was published in 1849. In it, Ellis suggested a radically new interpretation of Jacob Bernoulli's law of large numbers. Recall that Bernoulli in Part Four of the *Ars Conjectandi* had, in effect, been the first to prove that the observed frequency of an event in a large number of trials would eventually converge toward the true underlying ratio of chances.

Bernoulli believed his proof provided a rigorous justification for adopting the long-run observed frequency as an approximation to the true underlying degree of belief, or probability. Ellis lived in a time when the concept of hidden cases, or chances, had become rather nebulous. Meanwhile, mathematical probability had become intuitively meaningful. Additionally, there was a lot more actual data available, so that it was easier to imagine frequencies of events in a large number of trials. Ellis believed that these observable frequencies constituted the natural foundation for the concept of probability. He interpreted the vaunted laws of large numbers proved by Bernoulli, de Moivre, Laplace, and Poisson as mere tautologies:

> If the probability of a given event be correctly determined, the event will, on a long run of trials, tend to recur with frequency proportional to this probability. This is generally proved mathematically. It seems to me to be true *a priori*.

His main argument was that this frequency in a long run of independent trials is in fact what we really *mean* by a probability:

> When on a single trial we expect one event rather than another, we necessarily believe that on a series of similar trials the former event will occur more frequently than the latter. The connection between these two things seems to me to be an ultimate fact ... the evidence of which must rest upon an appeal to consciousness.... after giving a painful degree of attention to the point, I have been unable to sever the judgment that one event is more likely to happen than another, or that it is to be expected in preference to it, from the belief that on the long run it will occur more frequently.

For Ellis, and for many who followed in his tracks, the notion of a long-run frequency in a potentially observable series of trials was both intuitive and logically defensible. For them, recourse to some vague metaphysical notion of equally likely "chances" was not persuasive. Why not simply dispense with such a fiction and define an event's probability to be its proportion of occurrences in a long series of similar occasions?

Independently, and almost simultaneously, a very similar idea occurred to the French economist and philosopher Antoine Augustin Cournot (1801–1877).[10] In his *Exposition of the Theory of Chances and Probabilities* (1843), Cournot distinguished between an objective version of probability and a subjective one. Objective probabilities, reflected in observable frequencies, "have an objective existence, which gives a measure of the possibility of things." These he contrasts with subjective probability, which are "relative in part to our knowledge, in part to our ignorance, and which vary from one individual to another, according to their capacities and the data provided to them." Thus began a long conversation that has persisted to the present day regarding the subjective and objective aspects of probability.

Two decades later, John Venn (1834–1923) expanded upon the idea of objective probability in his *Logic of Chance*, published in 1866.[11] Venn asserted that the word "probability" is best reserved for a particular kind of use. Probability for him represented an efficient way to describe or summarize a complex empirical reality. John Maynard Keynes a half-century later summarized Venn's theory:

> The two principle tenets, then, of Venn's system are these—that probability is concerned with series or groups of events, and that all the requisite facts must be determined empirically, a statement in probability merely summing up in a convenient way a group of experiences. Aggregate regularity combined with individual difference happens, he says, to be characteristic of many events in the real world.... As our knowledge regarding the class as a whole may give us valuable guidance in dealing with an individual instance, we require a convenient way of saying that an individual belongs to a class in which certain characteristics appear on the average with a known frequency ... The importance of probability depends solely upon the actual existence of such groups ... and a judgment of probability must necessarily depend for its validity upon our empirical knowledge of them.[12]

In this view, probability is explicitly objective in nature, rather than conceptual, and is a literal, if approximate, statistical summary of empirical reality.

As Keynes noted, this perspective has the virtue of avoiding metaphysical ambiguities but at the cost of severely restricting the meaning and usefulness of probability:

> It is the obvious, as well as the correct, criticism of such a theory, that the identification of probability with statistical frequency is a very grave departure from the established use of words; for it clearly excludes a great number of judgments which are generally believed to deal with probability.... Venn's theory by itself has few practical applications, and if we allow it to hold the field, we must admit that probability is *not* the guide of life, and that in following it we are not acting according to reason.

Venn's hard-headed *frequentist* alternative was widely regarded as a salutary antidote to the excesses of Laplace and Poisson. For example, to assign a probability to the event that a tribunal would reach a correct decision was nonsense, according to Venn's point of view. Where could we obtain data pertaining to the probability that an individual judge would rule correctly?

The spirit of Venn's frequentism has animated most statistical analyses ever since. Most statisticians believe that their subject deals with summarizing and analyzing patterns in large aggregates of observations or measurements. Their concerns are pragmatic, and their implicit philosophy tends to be positivistic. Early in the twentieth century, frequentist probability attracted champions among positivistic philosophers of science, most notably Richard von Mises (1883–1953) and Hans Reichenbach (1891–1953).

Von Mises saw probability as a form of applied mathematics applicable to "mass phenomena" in the same way that differential and integral calculus are necessary to describe the laws of physics.[13] The essence of a mass phenomenon was "unlimited repetition" of a particular kind of uniform occurrence:

> The rational concept of probability, which is the only basis of probability calculus, applies only to problems in which either the same event repeats itself again and again, or a great number of uniform elements are involved at the same time. Using the language of physics, we may say that in order to apply the theory of probability we must have a practically unlimited sequence of uniform observations.

Central to his conceptualization was the idea of a *collective*. A collective "denotes a sequence of uniform events or processes which differ by certain attributes."

> All the peas grown by a botanist concerned with the problem of heredity may be considered as a collective, the attributes in which we are interested being the colors of the flowers. All the throws of dice made in the course of a game form a collective, wherein the attribute of the single event is the number of points thrown. Again, all the molecules in a given volume of gas may be considered as a collective, and the attribute of a single molecule might be its velocity. A further example of a collective is the whole class of men and women whose ages at death have been registered by an insurance office.

Von Mises adopted the motto: "First the collective—then the probability." He tried to explain what he meant more precisely:

> We will say that a collective is a mass phenomenon or a repetitive event … for which there are sufficient reasons to believe that the relative frequency of the observed attribute would tend to a fixed limit if the observations were indefinitely continued. This limit will be considered *the probability of the attribute considered within the given collective* … 'The probability of winning a battle', for instance, has no place in our theory of probability, because we cannot think of a collective to which it belongs.

It is evident that for von Mises the "scientific," as opposed to colloquial, meaning of probability pertained to objective facts about the real world. He believed that certain mass phenomena could be identified that corresponded more or less closely to the idealization of a collective. To the extent that a designated collective in the real world satisfied his definition of a collective, the usual rules of mathematical probability would be applicable.

Like his predecessors, such as Ellis and Venn, von Mises took as a given that the sequence would approach a fixed limiting value of the relative frequency in a long run; it was not something that needed to be proved. Once a sequence of observations was properly defined, they thought, the proportion of events in this extended sequence was by definition the probability. However, von Mises recognized something more that needed to be considered to avoid an essential ambiguity. As an example of the problem, he discussed a series of road markers consisting of small stones placed at intervals of exactly 1/10 of a mile and a large stone placed at each mile mark. He noted that, on such a road, the fraction of large stones observed after several miles would be approximately 1/10 and would approach this fraction more and more closely as we proceed. He contrasted this situation to that in a game of chance:

> After having just passed a large stone, we are in no doubt about the size of the next one; there is no chance of its being large. If, however, we cast a double 6 with two dice, this fact in no way affects our chances of getting the same result in the next cast. Similarly, the death of an insured person during his forty-first year does not give the slightest indication of what will be the fate of another who is registered next to him in the books of the insurance company, regardless of how the company's list was prepared.

Accordingly, von Mises posited that a collective must be a sequence of observations that satisfy a condition of complete lawlessness, or randomness. Here, von Mises confronted head-on one of the essential aspects of ambiguity inherent in (additive) mathematical probability by virtue of its metaphorical lottery origins. He made a heroic attempt to eliminate, or at least minimize, this ambiguity by introducing the *principle of the impossibility of a gambling system*. He regarded a sequence to be random if there was no possibility of identifying any subset of observations whose limiting frequency differed from that characterizing the whole sequence.

Identifying such a subset of observations would allow cherry-picking of a favorable subsequence in betting against someone who accepted the odds associated with the entire sequence. This principle of the excluded gambling system had for him a status akin to that of the principle of conservation of energy for the physicist. It was his sole justification for treating the outcomes of mass phenomena like genetic variability or life expectancy as probabilistic:

> The whole financial basis of insurance would be questionable if it were possible to change the relative frequency … by excluding, for example, every tenth one of the insured persons, or by some other selection principle. The principle of the impossibility of a gambling system has the same importance for the insurance companies as the principle of the conservation of energy for the electric power station: it is the rock on which all the calculations rest.

Later critics have adduced many problems with a frequentist interpretation along the lines laid out by von Mises and the positivistic philosophy upon which it was based. Three particular issues have received the most attention.

- The meaning of randomness
- The reference class problem
- The problem of the single case

I will briefly consider each of these issues from the metaphorical lottery perspective.

The Meaning of Randomness

Pure randomness can never be defined unambiguously, because absence of any possible pattern cannot be made precise. On the other hand, randomization, as what happens approximately when a well-designed "random" mechanism is employed, is easy enough to grasp conceptually. Modern frequentists, starting with von Mises, have often appealed to practical experience to support the existence of randomness, as *exemplified* by well-constructed games of chance.

The lack of a successful gambling system in any real-world situation, such as insurance, means that the relevant causal process is very similar to that in an idealized lottery. But the precise nature of this similarity cannot be spelled out explicitly. We are left, as always, with the idea of an analogy between some real-world process and a game of chance. All gambling systems fail precisely *because* the process is in certain relevant respects *just like* an idealized game of chance. So, defining randomness in terms of such failure is ultimately circular; it all boils down to an analogy with a game of chance.

On the other hand, it has been argued that a pragmatic definition of randomness might be adequate for practical purposes. Suppose we can specify some observable property of a process or an actual sequence that would allow it to be considered effectively random. Such a "pseudorandom" sequence would certainly be satisfactory for many practical purposes, such as selecting a representative sample from some population or assigning treatments in a clinical trial to compare alternative treatments. In fact, computer algorithms that generate such pseudorandom sequences are employed routinely for such purposes.

Should we perhaps define a collective to be a sequence in which pseudorandomness of some sort prevails? That would solve the philosophical conundrum, as some have suggested, but would be rather contrived. It is not what we intuitively mean about randomness. This problem was recognized by other philosophers, including Hans Reichenbach. His proposal was to define randomness relative to our ability to detect a pattern[14]:

> Random sequences are characterized by the peculiarity that a person who does not know the attributes of the elements is unable to construct a mathematical selection by which he would, on an average, select more hits than would correspond to the frequency of the major sequence ... . In this form, the impossibility of making a deviating selection is expressed by a psychological, not a logical, statement; it refers to acts performed by a human being. This may be called a psychological randomness.

For instance, consider a very long sequence that contains half zeroes and half ones. You cannot see this sequence but are allowed to specify any pattern of your own, and will receive a point for each time your value matches that of the unknown sequence. Then the unknown sequence would be deemed "psychologically random" if no human being could concoct a system that would in the long run allow her to obtain more than 50% of hits.

Writing in 1949, Reichenbach could not envision the possibilities that have become open to a human aided by a high-speed computer. Perhaps he would have attempted a definition of "digital randomness" limited by the computational capabilities of digital computers. In the end, I feel confident that no such "rigorous" definition of randomness is possible. Rather, we must accept that pure randomness is merely an idealization of that which can occur in an actual game of chance.

To be random is to lack any pattern or order, but what do we mean by order? So, the idea of randomness is intuitively meaningful but ultimately ambiguous, much like causation. Nevertheless, like the tangent line to a curve, a purely random process seems to "exist" as a kind of limit. We can obviously construct *approximately* random mechanisms (e.g., dice) that are certainly good enough artificial randomizers for most practical purposes. So, it is not difficult for us to imagine a perfect lottery, for example, as an idealization that can only be approached but never completely realized.

The Reference Class Problem

The question of which reference class to adopt has always been awkward for frequentists. On the one hand, they perceive probability as an objective aspect of the real world. On the other, they recognize that there are many possible reference classes to which an individual event might be assigned. The choice of reference class is somewhat arbitrary and subjective, at the discretion of the person making the probability assessment. How can these divergent perspectives possibly be reconciled?

Consider the problem faced by a surgical candidate, Jane, and her physician. There are many factors that might be considered relevant to the outcome of her contemplated operation. Which of these should be taken into account in specifying Jane's "real" probability of a successful outcome? Of these, which can *in fact* be taken into account because there is pertinent data? Von Mises did not have much to say about such situations. He seemed content to restrict "scientific" probability to those few "mass phenomena" in which it was apparent that the outcomes would occur effectively at random. Presumably, the aggregate of all surgical operations like Jane's would not qualify as a collective in his sense.

Reichenbach, like many other frequentists, was not satisfied with such a narrow view of the scope of probability. So, he grappled with the reference-class problem and adopted a more pragmatic position than von Mises. He believed that the reference class should be chosen to admit as many cases "similar" to the one in question as possible but no more. Similarity was defined in terms of "relevant" characteristics of the situation. In other words, we must strive to account for what is truly relevant and to ignore all else. In that way, our probability is relative to a "homogeneous" reference class. This homogeneous class is conceptualized as the broadest class within which there are no relevant differences among its members.

Furthermore, Reichenbach was aware that in practice, our data pertaining to potentially relevant factors is always limited. So, even if we can delineate in theory the relevant factors, we may not have sufficient data to adjust for them. For example, Jane's age and state of health are obviously relevant, but the available statistics might not be broken down by these factors. Even if we possess some relevant data, the number of previous cases in each of the subclasses may be inadequate for precise estimation of probabilities. Reichenbach recommended that we rely on the "smallest" class about which we have "adequate" statistics. This makes sense conceptually perhaps but remains quite ambiguous.

The Problem of the Single Case

Closely related to the reference class problem is the problem of the single case. From a frequentist perspective, probability is a property of the entire reference class. Only secondarily and figuratively can we refer to the probability of a unique event: "First the collective—then the probability." From this perspective, the probability of a particular event is merely a shorthand for the long-run frequency of occurrence that is approached in the limit. It has a sort of "as-if" quality; we speak about the probability of a particular event, but we always have in mind a class of events.

Von Mises was completely untroubled by the inapplicability of probability to unique events. He stated explicitly that probability as applied to an individual event was meaningless. Other frequentists have been less doctrinaire. They accept the basic idea that probability must refer to some kind of sequence of homogeneous occurrences, either actual or conceptual, but seek a bridge to the more colloquial usage of the word.

PROBABILITY AS A LOGICAL RELATIONSHIP

A contemporary of Robert Leslie Ellis, Augustus De Morgan (1806–1871), took a very different tack regarding probability. De Morgan was a professor of mathematics at University College in London who was best known for his pioneering work on symbolic logic. Unlike Ellis, De Morgan basically subscribed to the "classical" interpretation of probability bequeathed by Laplace and Poisson. He shared their belief that probability was a measure of our ignorance about the true state of affairs.

For De Morgan, probability had no necessary connection with real frequencies of repetitive phenomena, but pertained merely to our mental grasp of the real world. In an influential essay published in 1838, he situated probability squarely within the realm of logical analysis: "I throw away objective probability altogether, and consider the word as meaning the state of mind with respect to an assertion, a coming event, or any other matter on which absolute knowledge does not exist."[15,16]

For De Morgan, probability was much broader in scope than it was for Ellis or Venn; it could be applied to any assertion or event. However, De Morgan gave little guidance concerning how he believed the "state of mind" about an assertion or event might be obtained. He regarded probability as based upon a *rational* opinion, such as that which would be entertained by someone (presumably an educated Victorian Englishman) who could correctly interpret all available information. Undoubtedly, this sort of appeal to an ideal standard of rationality was more persuasive in 1838 than it would be for us today. Even so, De Morgan's concept represented only a beginning that would soon be fleshed out by others.

Perhaps the quintessential rational man of the nineteenth century was George Boole (1815–1864). Most famous today as the eponymous inventor of Boolean algebra, he made substantial contributions to several areas of mathematics and logic. Indeed, he is largely responsible for the fact that we consider logic today to be fundamentally mathematical in nature. Unfortunately for him, however, his logical acumen was apparently more theoretical than practical.

One day, while walking the two miles from home to his class at the University of Cork, in Ireland, where he had taught for many years, Prof. Boole was caught in a sudden downpour. Soldiering on, he proceeded to lecture for a full hour while remaining in his soaking garments. Upon returning home, he became seriously ill and was confined to bed. To compound matters, according to lore, his devoted but misguided wife, apparently subscribing to the "hair of the dog" theory of medicine, decided to pour cold water over him periodically. Alas, this regimen proved a dismal failure, and probably contributed to the good professor's untimely demise.

A decade prior to this unfortunate incident, Boole had published his masterpiece: *An Investigation of the Laws of Thought* (1854).[17] Boole created symbolic logic in order to express rigorously how we ought to reason about the relationships among statements that can be true or false. Given a specified set of premises, how should we logically infer that a particular conclusion is true or false? Probability theory, on the other hand, concerned how we should think rationally when our knowledge was incomplete: "Probability is expectation founded upon partial knowledge."

Like De Morgan, Boole asserted that probability pertained to a rational state of mind about some event or proposition. However, just as logic concerned relationships among propositions about events, not actual events themselves, so probability also dealt with propositions:

> Although the immediate business of the theory of probability is with the frequency of the occurrence of events … the theory of probabilities must bear some definite relation to logic. The events of which it takes account are expressed by propositions; their relations are involved in the relations of propositions. Regarded in this light, the object of the theory of probabilities may be thus stated: Given the separate probabilities of any propositions to find the probability of another proposition.[18]

Boole was emphasizing here the epistemic aspect of probability, somewhat echoing Jacob Bernoulli's ideas. Indeed, like Bernoulli, Boole explicitly stated that probability statements must rest on the evidence available:

> *Probability*, in its mathematical acceptation has reference to the state of our knowledge of the circumstances under which an event may happen or fail. With the degree of information which we possess concerning the circumstances of an event, the reason that we have to think that it will occur, or, to use a single term, our *expectation* of it, will vary.[19]

In this passage, he seems to have in mind some way of combining "arguments" along the lines suggested in Part Four of *Ars Conjectandi*. However, there is a critical difference. Writing 200 years after the seminal correspondence between Pascal and Fermat in 1654, Boole can only mean by probability "the ratio of the number of cases favorable to that event, to the total number of cases favorable or contrary, and all equally possible." He construes the mathematical laws of this classical probability to be in fact the "laws of thought" that should govern our rational deliberations. In this respect he is closer in spirit to Laplace, for whom probability embodied "common sense reduced to calculus."

To grasp Boole's logic we must understand what he considered to be the scope of probability and the kind of evidence on which it can depend.

In order to be the basis of rational expectations regarding events, this evidence must either be "deduced from a knowledge of the peculiar constitution of things" or "derived from the long-continued observation of past series of their occurrences and failures." By the former, he meant such considerations of symmetry as prevail in games of chance; by the latter, he meant statistical evidence based on empirical data.

In contrast with frequentists like Ellis and Venn, however, Boole was not *defining* the probability as an actual, or even hypothetical, frequency. For him, probability was essentially a measure of the rational grounds for belief. Thus, knowledge of symmetry or of statistical frequencies could sometimes provide the evidential basis, or at least some substantial part of it. Moreover, *only* when our evidence has this character, according to Boole's thinking, can we truly be said to have a *rational* expectation.

By adopting this stance, Boole narrowed the scope of probability just as surely as the frequentists had. For example, the probability that France would invade Holland would have had no meaning for him, unless some series of situations could be invoked as a logical reference class. Moreover, purely personal opinions about an event that were not grounded in symmetry considerations or statistical frequencies were effectively barred from his theory. In essence, Boole was completely in accord with Jacob Bernoulli when it came to situations in which any relevant information about individual circumstances (such as our surgical candidate Jane's state of health) was lacking. However, the broader concept of epistemic probability familiar to Bernoulli had by his time lost all meaning.

An important corollary of Boole's position was his strong rejection of Laplace's principle of insufficient reason and its implications. Recall that for Laplace, the starting point for many analyses was an a priori distribution of ignorance. All possible values of an unknown probability could be deemed equally probable if we had no "sufficient reason" to believe otherwise. This a priori supposition could then be combined with the likelihood provided by observed data using Bayes's Theorem to derive the inverse probabilities (probabilities of causes).

As mentioned previously, by 1854 the bloom had already faded from this rose, thanks to skeptics like John Stuart Mill who felt that Laplace and Poisson had gone much too far. Laplace's famous Rule of Succession was subjected to particular derision. Boole held that a firm basis for probability judgments, related to symmetry or statistical frequencies, was necessary.

So, he could not tolerate ignorance *per se* as such a basis. Commenting on the Rule of Succession, he noted:

> It has been said that the principle involved … is that of the equal distribution of our knowledge, or rather of our ignorance—the assigning to different states of things of which we know nothing, and upon the very ground that we know nothing, equal degrees of probability. I apprehend, however, that this is an arbitrary method of procedure.[20]

Remember that Boole had defined probability as a fraction of favorable cases among a total number of cases, *all equally possible*. Laplace might have argued that absent knowledge to the contrary, all cases can be regarded as equally possible. This was very convenient, but not good enough for Boole, who demanded some positive grounds upon which to base an assumption of equally possible.

Boole's perspective on probability was highly influential and the first of many attempts over the ensuing 150 years to cast probability as a logical relationship. Some advocates of the logical interpretation have been closer in spirit to the frequentists, emphasizing the importance of a long series of similar events as the primary source of evidence in practical applications. These have tended to be unsympathetic to the principle of insufficient reason. Others have been more open to the principle and "Bayesian" analysis more generally.

Indeed, Boole's most immediate successor in the logical school of probability held quite a different view of Laplace's controversial proposal.[21] William Stanley Jevons (1835–1882) began as a professor of logic and moral philosophy and ended as a professor of political economy. Like Boole, Jevons believed that probability belonged "wholly to the mind" and dealt with our "quantity of knowledge" about something. He even rejected "belief" altogether as a word much too nebulous to be scientifically useful. Probability "does not measure what the belief is, but what it ought to be."

Had he managed to survive his ill-fated drenching episode to read these central tenets in Jevons's *The Principles of Science* (1873), Boole would certainly have agreed. However, Jevons parted company with Boole when it came to the logical basis for probability assessments.[22] Jevons swallowed wholeheartedly Laplace's theory of inverse probability. To apply the inverse method in practice, Laplace's principle of insufficient reason was, according to Jevons, a useful expedient. He admitted it to be somewhat arbitrary, as alleged by Boole and others, but defended its utility on pragmatic grounds.

The idea of probability as a branch of logic has continued to attract advocates down to the present day. Many different theories along these lines have been propounded, varying widely in their details.[23] However, nearly all of these doctrines have had one critical aspect in common: they assume the usual mathematical version of probability.[24] With one major exception, proponents of logical probability have adhered to the restriction that probability must satisfy the Kolmogorov axioms. The one great thinker who adopted a much broader view of the subject is all but ignored today, although his economic theories remain very influential. Indeed, it is in the context of economics that his aphorisms about uncertainty are often quoted.

Keynesian Probability

John Maynard Keynes (1883–1946) is perhaps the most well-known economist of the twentieth century. His early intellectual development and career, starting with his membership in a genius cluster that developed around Cambridge University in the early 1900s is well chronicled. This extraordinary group included such luminaries as Bertrand Russell (1872–1970), Alfred North Whitehead (1861–1947), Lytton Strachey (1880–1932), G.E. Moore (1873–1958), G.H. Hardy (1877–1947), and E.M. Forster (1879–1970). During the years 1906–1911, Keynes was developing his theory of probability as a branch of logic that could deal with situations in which the evidence was not fully conclusive, but rather entailed some degree of uncertainty.

Keynes was a rising star in the intellectual firmament, and his book was much anticipated. However, owing to the Great War and his civic responsibilities, it was not until 1921 that *A Treatise on Probability* was finally published. The philosopher C.D. Broad (1887–1971) captured in his review the initial enthusiasm with which the *Treatise* was greeted: "I can only conclude by congratulating Mr. Keynes on finding time, amidst so many public duties, to complete this book, and the philosophical public on getting the best work on Probability that they are likely to see in this generation."[25] However, the mathematical development and practical applications of probability soon took center stage. Keynes's ambitious and profound philosophical contribution is almost entirely unknown to practicing statisticians and scientists today.

A substantial portion of the *Treatise* is taken up with a kind of symbolic logic somewhat similar to that developed by Russell and Whitehead in their famous *Principia Mathematica*, which was being composed around the same time. Of much greater practical importance, however, was his extensive discussion of the philosophical underpinnings of inductive logic. Keynes took a very broad view of probability, which he conceived as pertaining to "the various degrees of rational belief about a proposition which different amounts of knowledge authorize us to entertain."

Keynes regarded ordinary mathematical probability as an important aspect of the logical relations between uncertain propositions, but only applicable under certain limited conditions. In this respect, his notion of probability harked back to the kind of probability envisioned by Jacob Bernoulli, whom he considered "the real founder of the classical school of mathematical probability." Like Bernoulli, Keynes emphasized what he termed Bernoulli's second axiom, which he interpreted as meaning "that in reckoning a probability we must take everything into account."

Keynes followed Boole in that his concept of probability was thoroughly epistemic; probability pertained to propositions, not to events *per se*. A fundamental idea for Keynes was that the probability of any *hypothesis* must be conditioned on the available *evidence*, whatever that evidence might be. Given the evidence, our knowledge may assume a variety of different forms, and may authorize a merely qualitative or sometimes a quantitative probability assessment. For some propositions, our relevant information may be so limited that a probability cannot even be said to exist at all.

For example, suppose that someone is asked about the probability that Brazil will win the next soccer World Cup. Both the magnitude of such a probability and its precision would vary widely across individuals. At one extreme, a person might have only the vaguest of conceptions, not even amenable to quantification. At the other extreme, a soccer aficionado might be aware of many relevant factors, including recent performance by Brazil's team, injuries to key players, and the odds currently being offered in Rio de Janeiro.

The distinction between a hypothesis whose probability is unknown and one whose probability is nonexistent, or indeterminate, was critical for Keynes.

> I am here dealing with a probability in its widest sense, and am averse to confining its scope to a limited type of argument. If the opinion that not all probabilities can be measured seems paradoxical, it may be due to this divergence from a usage which the reader may expect ... I maintain, then, in what follows, that there are some pairs of probabilities between the members of which no comparison of magnitude is possible; that we may say, nevertheless, ... that the one is greater and the other less, although it is not possible to measure the difference between them; and that in a very special type of case ... a meaning can be given to a numerical comparison of magnitude.[26]

From this perspective, an assessment of probability can be expressed as a number between zero and one in the usual manner *only* under special conditions that Keynes attempted to spell out.

One such fundamental condition is that the base of evidence assumed relevant to a proposition and its contrary must be the same. Otherwise, comparing the probability of a statement and its contrary would not be meaningful. Recall that Jacob Bernoulli discussed, in Part Four of his *Ars Conjectandi*, a situation in which the probability of an event was 3/4 and its contrary 2/3. Keynes recognized that to avoid such a possibility would require the tacit assumption that both probabilities were based on the same body of evidence:

> Some probabilities are not comparable in respect of more or less, because there exists more than one path, so to speak, between proof and disproof, between certainty and impossibility; and neither of two probabilities, which lie on different paths, bears to the other and to certainty the relation of 'between' which is necessary for quantitative comparison.

In other words, if there is ambiguity about the situation under consideration, we cannot determine uniquely how "far" from certainty to place a particular outcome. Only if we can eliminate such ambiguity can our degrees of uncertainty be ranged on the single dimension of doubtfulness, so that various degrees of evidentiary support can be compared directly.

Keynes recognized that a *numerical* probability was conceptually based on some notion of a fraction of equally possible cases. But to be deemed equally possible, the cases must first of all be comparable. So, in principle, we would need to establish somehow that all the cases can be arrayed along the same evidentiary "path." Laplace's principle of insufficient reason held that we could always assume equal probabilities absent any sufficient reason to the contrary. Keynes found this unsatisfactory, especially in the important context of unknown prior probabilities. Keynes pointed out that applying this principle when we are truly ignorant about prior probabilities required some positive justification.

Beyond this general philosophical objection, he discussed a number of logical paradoxes that could arise when attempting to apply the principle of insufficient reason. For example, recall the confusion of Jean le Rond D'Alembert, Laplace's mentor, regarding the probability of obtaining heads at least once when allowed two tosses of a coin that can land heads (H) or tails (T). He observed that there are three possible outcomes: H on the first toss, T on the first and H on the second, and T on both. Therefore, D'Alembert at first believed that the probability was 2/3 of winning. He was later embarrassed to admit his error, after he realized that these three outcomes were not equally likely, so the true probability must be 3/4. This example was mentioned by Laplace in his discussion of the "delicate" considerations that can be entailed in probability theory.

What Laplace had no way to fully appreciate was the degree of delicacy that was truly involved. Classical probability essentially defines probability as a fraction of imaginary chances in a metaphorical lottery. However, the precise properties of this probability can depend on exactly how we conceive of this metaphorical lottery, and there may be different ways to do this. For example, Bayes imagined a probability as the fraction of the distance traveled by a ball on a smooth table relative to the table's length. Laplace, on the other hand, envisioned a lottery in which an unknown proportion of tickets were winners. Both "models" of reality are conceivable, but their consequences are not always identical!

Keynes considered the case in which we select a ball from an urn in which there are a given number of balls, some black and some white, in an unknown proportion.[27] Suppose we are interested in the proportion of white balls in the urn. The usual assumption is that all the possible (i.e., conceivable) *proportions* are equally likely. Keynes discussed the situation in which there are four balls in the urn. Suppose first we assume that there are five equally possible values for the number of white balls: 0, 1,

TABLE 8.1   Keynes's Urn: Possible *Constitutions* vs. Possible *Numbers* of White Balls

Constitution	Ball 1	Ball 2	Ball 3	Ball 4	Number White
1	W	W	W	W	**4**
2	W	W	W	B	**3**
3	W	W	B	W	**3**
4	W	B	W	W	**3**
5	B	W	W	W	**3**
6	W	W	B	B	**2**
7	W	B	W	B	**2**
8	W	B	B	W	**2**
9	B	W	B	W	**2**
10	B	B	W	W	**2**
11	B	W	W	B	**2**
12	W	B	B	B	**1**
13	B	W	B	B	**1**
14	B	B	W	B	**1**
15	B	B	B	W	**1**
16	B	B	B	B	**0**

2, 3, and 4. This assumption corresponds to a method that first selects a number between zero and four at random, and then places that number of white balls and the rest black in the urn. However, there is another equally logical way to express our ignorance.

Each of the four balls in the urn can be either black or white. Imagine that the balls are selected and placed in the urn one at a time, and the color determined by tossing a fair coin. Then, there would be 16 possible *constitutions* of the urn, as shown in Table 8.1. Suppose we consider all 16 constitutions equally likely. Then, the probabilities of the different *proportions* would not be equal. For example, the probability of getting zero white balls would be 1/16, but the probability of getting two would be 3/8. Conversely, if we chose to regard each proportion as equally probable, then the constitutions would not be equally likely.

Which assumption is correct? If we mean which is the "real" probability, there is no unique answer. In an actual situation in which a real urn had been filled with real balls, there would in fact be a definitive answer; the probabilities would depend on exactly how the balls were selected and placed in the urn. But in the abstract scenario, as usually described, we are not given these details. We may not even know the number of balls, let alone the procedure for filling the urn. So, there is an inherent ambiguity in the determination of these probabilities.

Nonetheless, Keynes drew a distinction that he believed could often help to avoid such ambiguity. He suggested that the principle of insufficient reason, which he preferred to term the *principle of indifference*, can only generate a paradox when the presumed equally likely events are not *elementary units*:

> The examples in which the Principle of Indifference broke down had a great deal in common. We broke up the field of possibility, as we may term it, into a number of disjunctive judgments.... The paradoxes and contradictions arose, in each case, when the alternatives, which the Principle of Indifference treated as equivalent, actually contained or might contain a different or an indefinite number of more elementary units.

Applying this insight to the four-ball urn example, Keynes concluded that the approach based on constitutions was potentially acceptable, while the one based on the proportions was not.

Keynes's notion of "elementary units" contains the germ of an important idea, although difficult to apply. Mathematical probability is always rooted conceptually in the analogy to a metaphorical lottery in which one among some number of possible chances, or eventualities, is being chosen at random. Thus, applying this conceptual model to an actual situation in which the various eventualities are actually specified may not make sense if some of these eventualities can be regarded as *compound* in nature.

In D'Alembert's coin-tossing problem, the compound nature of one eventuality (heads on the first trial) seems evident to us. Fermat was the first to suggest that it could usefully be viewed as two outcomes (HT, HH) among the four that could possibly occur (HT, HH, TH, and TT). But when we enter the domain of real-world problems, the precise meanings of "elementary" and "compound" are quite ambiguous. Keynes went on to discuss how, once a set of alternatives has been established, we ought to judge whether the principle of indifference is warranted:

> The principle states that 'There must be no known reason for preferring one of a set of alternatives to any other.' What does this mean? What are 'reasons,' and how are we to know whether they do or do not justify us in preferring one alternative to another? I do not know any discussion of Probability in which this question has been so much as asked.

He proceeded to explain what he believed to be the essential consideration that must be entailed in a rational judgment of indifference.

Any relevant information pertaining to the alternatives must be equally balanced. For example, in the case of two possible alternatives:

> There must be no *relevant* evidence relating to one alternative, unless there is *corresponding* evidence relating to the other; our relevant evidence, that is to say, must be symmetrical with regard to the alternatives, and must be applicable to each in the same manner. This is the rule at which the Principle of Indifference somewhat obscurely aims.

Determining the relevance of our evidence requires "a series of judgments of relevance not easily reduced to rule."

In other words, the formulation of a numerical probability via the principle of indifference entails *judgment*. But the grounds for such judgment must depend on some understanding of what the possible events are. If the nature of these possibilities is completely unknown, then our uncertainty contains too much ambiguity to support any numerical probabilities. In particular, if all we know is that *any* numerical probability is *conceivable*, we really know nothing at all upon which to form our judgments. So, Keynes effectively rejected Laplace's principle of insufficient reason in the case of complete ignorance about prior probabilities, but endorsed it in the case that there is actual evidence about a set of possible probabilities that is equally balanced.

PROBABILITY AS A SUBJECTIVE ASSESSMENT

Both frequentists and proponents of logical probability were concerned primarily with what we *ought* to believe about an uncertain event or proposition. How could our measure of belief be concordant with the evidence that was available? In this sense, probability was impersonal, based upon some actual or perceived aspect of the real world (observed frequency, evidence, etc.) and a rational inference regarding the implications of this aspect. However, in the 1920s this fundamental presumption began to be called into question.

During the "Roaring Twenties" much received wisdom was being questioned. In the wake of unprecedented chaos occasioned by the Great War, many traditional assumptions and values, along with the social institutions they supported, no longer seemed so secure. Relativity was in the air, from physics to morality. So, it was perhaps inevitable that objective and rational foundations for probability would come under fire.

Another Cambridge Prodigy

In a response to Keynes's *Treatise*, his younger compatriot Frank Plumpton Ramsey (1903–1930) offered a radically new perspective on probability. Ramsey was a multifaceted genius whose life was tragically cut short by complications of surgery. In addition to his influential papers on probability, Ramsey derived an important result in combinatorial mathematics known as Ramsey's theorem. He also made major contributions to mathematical economics, including the Ramsey model and the theory of Ramsey pricing. In philosophy, he authored several original publications and translated the famous *Tractatus Logico Philosophicus* of Ludwig Wittgenstein (1891–1951) from German to English.

In 1926, Ramsey produced an essay on "Truth and Probability." He began by attacking the notion that there could exist the kind of logical relation that Keynes had posited between evidence and belief: "There do not seem to be any such things as the probability relations he describes."[28] Keynes was in fact a colleague, supporter, and admirer of Ramsey; he was apparently not insulted, and wrote a glowing eulogy after Ramsey's shocking demise.

Ramsey's attack was actually more narrowly targeted than is often believed. Ramsey was not disputing all of Keynes's insights regarding probability as it pertained to inductive inference in scientific analysis. However, he took Keynes to task for attempting to locate his theory within the framework of pure logic. Ramsey argued that the *logic* of partial belief ought to be much more limited in scope. Ordinary logic, he observed, dealt with consistency between assumed premises and the conclusions that were entailed by them. Similarly, a logic of partial entailment should delineate only what conclusions were not *inconsistent* with the premises that one held to be true, that is, one's beliefs. From this narrower perspective, any other principles that constrained rational belief, such as standards for scientific inference, would fall outside the province of logic *per se*.

Ramsey also objected to Keynes's notion that some probabilities were unknown, or only partially known. He believed that probability, as a numerical measure of belief, always existed for any individual, but that "beliefs do differ in measurability." He regarded the problem of elucidating these subjective probabilities as a psychological problem. Armed with such an operationally defined measure of the degree of belief, we might be able to decide whether any particular set of beliefs is rational (consistent).

In his essay, Ramsey sets about establishing the desired method by starting from the principle that someone's beliefs can be inferred by observing his actions. He then goes on to develop a sophisticated theory that allows him to define probability in terms of betting behavior, but to evade problems related to the diminishing marginal utility of money. In essence, he posits the existence of some "ultimate goods" as the currency for his proposed bets. Ramsey defines probability in terms of an individual's certainty equivalents for various proposed bets.

For example, suppose I am offered an award of 50 ultimate goods units (UGU). Alternatively, I can receive an amount of 150 UGU if it rains tomorrow or zero if it does not. Then if I am indifferent between these alternatives, it means that my degree of belief that it will rain must be 1/3. Ramsey proves that in order to be internally consistent, my degrees of belief elicited in this manner must satisfy certain rules, and these turn out to be none other than the usual laws of mathematical probability!

> If anyone's mental condition violated these laws, … He could have a book made against him by a cunning better and would then stand to lose in any event.… the laws of probability are laws of consistency, an extension to partial beliefs of formal logic, the logic of consistency.

Here we have a complete separation between probability and the real world. For Ramsey, probability can refer to any logically consistent set of beliefs, however misguided. The truth of these beliefs and their justification on the basis of evidence are irrelevant.

The only restriction imposed is that one's probabilities must not permit others to hedge their bets in such a way as to guarantee them a profit. For example, suppose we consider the situation discussed by Jacob Bernoulli in which the argument for a certain event implied a probability of 2/3, while the argument for the contrary implied a probability of 3/4. Then, if

TABLE 8.2   Example of a "Dutch Book"

	E Happens	E Fails
Bet $400 on E @ 2:1 odds	Win $800	Lose $400
Bet $300 against E @ 3:1 odds	Lose $900	Win $300
Net payoff:	**Lose $100**	**Lose $100**

we interpret these as subjective mathematical probabilities, a Dutch Book could be made against a person holding these beliefs.

Such a person would presumably be willing to *offer* odds of 3:1 that the event *will not* occur (Bet 1), because that would be a fair bet for someone who had a subjective probability of 3/4. Similarly, he would be willing to *accept* odds of 2:1 that the same event *will* occur (Bet 2). Then this discrepancy allows for the possibility of arbitrage (see Table 8.2). Suppose that I wager $400 that the event will occur and accept the 2:1 odds. Then I will gain $800 if the event occurs, and will lose $400 if it does not. However, suppose that I also bet $900 that the event will *not* occur, and offer 3:1 odds. Then I will lose my $900 if the event occurs, but will win $300 if it does not occur. Regardless of the actual outcome, I stand to lose $100.

Ramsey is often cited as the originator of the idea that probability is *always* subjective, or *personal*, in nature. But Ramsey did not reject the notion of a more objective interpretation of probability outside of formal logic. He stated that there is a "lesser logic" of consistency and the "larger logic" of discovery. Within this larger inductive logic, he believed that empirical evidence, and especially observed frequencies, had an important role to play, although he regarded Keynes's attempts to elucidate this role as inadequate.

Ramsey's understanding of probability in the realm of the larger logic seems to recognize the classical concept of a metaphorical lottery: "partial belief involves reference to a hypothetical or ideal frequency ... belief of degree $\frac{m}{n}$ is ... the kind of belief most appropriate to a number of hypothetical occasions otherwise identical in a proportion $\frac{m}{n}$ of which the proposition in question is true." The frequency and subjective interpretations of probability he regards as the "objective and subjective aspects of the same inner meaning."

Ramsey thus appears to recognize that the essential core of probability is the analogy with a lottery. Each occasion is like a single drawing from a collection of identical hypothetical occasions. Once this conception of a metaphorical lottery is accepted, it is understood that observed frequencies as potentially relevant evidence and personal degrees of belief are both "aspects of the same inner meaning."

Subjectivity Italian Style

As I suggested above, during the 1920s the idea of relativity was *au courant*. So we should not be surprised that almost simultaneously with Ramsey's writing about probability, another young genius was independently formulating a remarkably similar point of view. Like Ramsey, Bruno de Finetti (1906–1985) believed that probability prescribed how an individual should act *relative to* his or her own belief structure. But, he went even further. Unlike Ramsey, he did not feel the need to distinguish the lesser logic of consistency from the larger logic of induction.

De Finetti was born in Innsbruck, then part of the Austro-Hungarian Empire, but lived most of his life in Italy. His father was an engineer, and young Bruno was destined and educated to become one as well. However, after this formal training, his interests turned to mathematics, and especially to probability and statistics, in which he eventfully achieved worldwide renown, coupled with considerable controversy. Beginning in the late 1920s, de Finetti published several papers that dealt with the mathematical and philosophical aspects of probability. This work culminated in his masterful 1937 essay on "Foresight, Its Logical Laws, Its Subjective Sources."[29]

Like Ramsey, de Finetti held that the laws of mathematical probability were standards of consistency, or *coherence*. Like Ramsey, he believed that potential betting behavior could provide an operational basis for measuring subjective probabilities. But de Finetti went further. He asserted that the *only* valid way to interpret probability was as a purely subjective degree of belief. He asserted that there exist:

> rather profound psychological reasons which make the exact or approximate agreement that is observed between the opinions of different individuals very natural, but that there are no reasons, rational, positive, or metaphysical, that can give this fact any meaning beyond that of subjective opinions.

De Finetti offered a series of arguments to buttress his contention that all meaningful probability statements are at base subjective. Consider, for example, the widespread convergence of belief regarding the probability that a die will land on 6. We all accept the value of 1/6 because of the symmetrical construction of the die and, perhaps, our experience playing games that employ dice. Like David Hume, his philosophical hero, de Finetti did not concede that this probability is demonstrably connected to the causal structure of reality. He rejected both the frequentists' objective relative frequencies and the logicists' necessary relationship between evidence and rational belief.

Within de Finetti's dogmatically "relativistic" framework, the importance of inverse probability, as originally proposed by Bayes and Laplace, emerged in a new guise. He offered a sophisticated rationale for utilizing Bayes's Theorem as the basis for all practical applications of probability theory, including statistical inference. Recall that Bayes's Theorem allows us, in principle, to make (posterior) probability statements about some quantity such as an unknown probability or the unknown mean value of some variable in a certain population. However, we need two pieces of information: (a) the conditional probability distribution of the data, given each value of the unknown quantity and (b) the prior distribution of the unknown quantity.

De Finetti asserted that *all* probabilities were properly regarded as subjective degrees of belief, so that a prior probability was just a measure of someone's belief. Furthermore, he turned the tables on traditional views by "proving" that *objective* probabilities were, in a sense, illusory. We could, he believed, justify the use of Bayes's Theorem as a statement about the relationship between prior (he called them *initial*) subjective probabilities and posterior (*final*) subjective probabilities without alluding to any objective probabilities at all!

Consider a coin with an unknown probability of Heads (H) that is tossed three times, resulting in HTH. In this classical application of Bayes's Theorem, the unknown probability of H is understood to be a real property of the coin toss. In de Finetti's view, this "objective" probability is a metaphysical abstraction that has no meaning. All that is needed to obtain a valid posterior probability is an assumption that he termed *exchangeability*. Exchangeability is a property not defined in relation to some unobservable equally possible chances, but is directly related to potentially observable events or quantities (random variables).

In our example, there are three possible outcomes in which H occurs exactly twice (HHT, HTH, THH). In this simple case, the various coin tosses would be considered exchangeable (for me) if my subjective probability depended *only* on how many times H and T occur. For example, the three possible outcomes (HHT, HTH, THH) would have (for me) the same probability. In other words, I make no distinction between the particular coin tosses; the only characteristic I consider relevant to the probability of a sequence is how many times H and T each occur. It is completely irrelevant which specific trials result in H and which result in T.

De Finetti showed that under this exchangeability assumption, Bayes's Theorem must be used to obtain final subjective probabilities, given the initial probabilities and observed data. Furthermore, the laws of large numbers derived by Bernoulli, Laplace, de Moivre, and Poisson could essentially be reinterpreted as properties of subjective probabilities. No other definition of probability is necessary to establish these time-honored results. For instance, the approach of the relative frequency in a very long sequence of trials to the "true" probability is meaningless in de Finetti's scheme. It is quite natural to talk *as if* such a true probability exists, but this usage is just a manner of speaking.

De Finetti's logic may seem compelling, but it rests on a critical premise regarding human psychology. Like Ramsey, de Finetti assumed that degrees of belief are well ordered enough to be elicited by observing betting behavior. Keynes might have argued that in most cases our actual beliefs are quite vague and that forcing them into the mold of coherent mathematical probabilities is artificial. De Finetti had faith in our ability to frame subjective numerical probabilities upon which we would be willing to bet. Where would such probabilities come from? How precisely do they measure our belief structures? Are they any less metaphysical than the "objective" probabilities he denigrates?

De Finetti's brilliant concept of exchangeability was intended to exclude metaphysics by dealing only with observable outcomes. However, it seems to contain within it a hidden assumption. A series of exchangeable observations, such as three consecutive tosses of a coin, is characterized by the property that the observations are indistinguishable: the order in which they are observed is irrelevant. This is in fact the assumption of willful ignorance. That is, there is no basis on which to differentiate among the various observations, just as if they were selected from a metaphorical lottery.

Subjectivity and Statistics

For about 20 years, de Finetti's views were not widely known and exerted little practical influence. However, in the 1950s, a brilliant mathematical statistician named Leonard J. (Jimmie) Savage (1917–1971) rediscovered and expanded upon de Finetti's pioneering work. Savage believed that a subjective interpretation of probability was the most suitable foundation upon which to base the theory of statistical inference.

Savage's views were summarized in *The Foundations of Statistics* (1954).[30] This work is often credited with initiating a revival of interest in Bayesian methods within the field of statistics. At the time of the book's publication, Bayes's Theorem was well established as a mathematical truism and widely used for certain types of problems. However, these applications were almost exclusively those in which the prior probability distribution had an obvious frequentist interpretation. For example, in a manufacturing process, the percentage of defective items expected in a given batch might have a probability distribution that was roughly known from historical experience.

On the other hand, in most applications of statistical inference, there was little or no basis upon which such an "empirical" prior distribution could be based. From the dominant frequentist viewpoint, the use of subjective prior distributions was completely anathema. In the late 1960s, when I entered graduate school, Bayesian statistics was regarded almost as a kind of quackery. This attitude has certainly changed over time, but even today the use of Bayesian methods remains somewhat controversial in many scientific applications.

Savage, like de Finetti, contended that all probabilities were essentially subjective, although he preferred the term *personal*. So, the subjective Bayesian approach of starting with a personal prior distribution and then conditioning on observed data was, for him, quite natural. To deny the inevitable subjectivity inherent in statistical analyses, Savage believed, was simply unrealistic. In holding this opinion, however, Savage differed slightly from de Finetti in one important respect. Savage placed great emphasis on the premise that data analysis was a method of reaching optimal *decisions*. Since these decisions were ultimately intended to achieve the "personal" aims of individuals or institutions, he regarded statistical analysis as a branch of decision theory.

In the 1950s, the centrality of decision-making in statistical theory was becoming widely accepted among statisticians of all stripes, especially in America. The potential role of "statistical decision theory" in certain business and engineering applications began to gain traction. However, reliance on subjective probabilities in general, especially in scientific work, was quite limited. Moreover, the extreme mathematical complexity of implementing the necessary Bayesian analysis posed a major obstacle that was not overcome until the advent of modern high-speed computing capabilities.

PROBABILITY AS A PROPENSITY

By the early 1920s, the importance of probability as an essential aspect of our scientific descriptions of physical reality had become increasingly evident. In physics, statistical mechanics, which describes the observable properties (e.g., heat and energy) of enormous aggregates of molecules was well established, and Brownian motion had recently been explained by Einstein in statistical terms. In biology, the pioneering studies of Gregor Mendel (1822–1884) came to light and led to a probabilistic theory of genetic inheritance. Then, studies of radioactive decay showed that this phenomenon followed probabilistic laws very precisely.

Finally, quantum theory suggested that physical reality at the subatomic level seemed to be *intrinsically* probabilistic. Despite the best efforts of Einstein and others to prove that God does not play dice with the universe, randomness could not be explained away. Laplace's fiction of a hypothetical all-knowing intelligence that could predict everything became passé.

These dramatic developments in the sciences prompted philosophers to ponder anew just what probability really means. In what precise sense does an atom of carbon-14 have a 50% probability of decaying within 5730 years? What does it mean to say that the position of an atom can only be described by a probability distribution? The frequency, logical, and subjective interpretations of probability all seemed somehow inadequate to fully express the nature of these phenomena. So, the notion began to emerge that probability, at least in these scientific contexts, might have another aspect, that of a *propensity*.

An Unorthodox Thinker

The concept of probability as a propensity was foreshadowed by the highly original and somewhat quirky American scientist and philosopher, Charles Sanders Peirce (pronounced like "purse"). C.S. Peirce (1839–1914) grew up in Cambridge, Massachusetts. His father, Benjamin Peirce (1809–1880), was an eminent scientist and mathematician, who taught at Harvard University for nearly 50 years. In addition, he played a leading role in the United States Coast Survey, a predecessor of today's National Oceanic and Atmospheric Administration. In this role, Peirce senior made many practical mathematical and statistical contributions, including an important paper in 1852 on how to deal with anomalous observations, which we would call outliers today.

Benjamin Peirce and his wife, Sarah Mills Peirce, had four sons and a daughter. Charles, who was a child prodigy, may have been the most precocious, but was the black sheep of the family.[31] Unlike his brothers, all of whom followed conventional and highly successful career paths, C.S. Peirce marched to the beat of his own drum. He made many significant contributions to several fields, including mathematics, logic, psychology, biology, and geodesy. However, he may be best known today as a founder of the philosophy of pragmatism, along with William James (1842–1910) and John Dewey (1859–1952). His broad interests and highly original thinking made Peirce a fascinating figure, but his free-spirited antics caused him much personal grief.

For example, a promising academic career was derailed in 1884, when it became known that he had been living with a woman 20 years his junior while still legally married (albeit separated from his wife for 7 years). Johns Hopkins University, where he had been teaching logic and mathematics since 1879, refused to renew his contract and effectively blacklisted him. For much of his later career, he worked for the Coast Survey, thanks initially to his father's influence. However, it was not always smooth sailing, and Peirce's independence got him into hot water. In the end, his refusal to comply with a request to revise a major report on gravitational fields led to his dismissal.

The following description by a contemporary suggests how Peirce's unique combination of creativity and eccentricity could both delight and exasperate those around him:

> His dramatic manner, his reckless disregard of accuracy in what he termed 'unimportant details,' his clever newspaper articles ... interested and amused us all.... He was always hard up, living partly on what he could borrow from friends, and partly on what he got from odd jobs such as writing book reviews ... He was equally brilliant, whether under the influence of liquor or otherwise, and his company was prized by the various organizations to which he belonged; and he was never dropped from any of them even though he was unable to pay his dues. He infuriated Charlotte Angas Scott by contributing to the New York Evening Post an unsigned obituary of Arthur Cayley in which he stated upon no grounds, except that Cayley's father had for a time resided in Russia, that Cayley had inherited his genius from a Russian whom his father had married in St. Petersburg.[32]

Here was another kindred spirit of Gerolamo Cardano.

Peirce was apparently the first to suggest that probability was not just a matter of our ignorance regarding underlying causes. Rather, there was an inherently unpredictable, or random, aspect to reality. He coined the term *tychism* to describe this aspect of his philosophy, which was complex and continually evolving, but always entailed a belief in something akin to free will. At any rate, he clearly rejected the idea that all physical, biological, and psychological phenomena could ultimately be reduced to rigid mechanical laws.

His most famous discussion of probability describes the notion of a predisposition, rather like a personal habit, that exists as a kind of potentiality. As an example he explains what it means for a thrown die to have a probability of 1/3 to result in a 3 or 6:

> The statement means that the die has a certain 'would-be'; and to say that a die has a 'would-be' is to say that it has a property quite analogous to any *habit* that a man might have.... and just as it would be necessary, in order to define a man's habit, to describe how it would lead him to behave and upon what sort of occasion— albeit this statement would by no means imply that the habit *consists* in that action—so to define the die's 'would-be,' it is necessary to say how it would lead the die to behave on an occasion that would bring out the full consequence of the 'would-be'; and this statement would not of itself imply that the 'would-be' of the die consists of this behavior.[33]

There is a lot to ponder here.

A World of Propensities

Peirce's idea of probability lay fallow for half-a-century. Then, in the 1950s it was reincarnated as the *propensity* interpretation of probability by Karl Popper (1902–1994), a giant of twentieth-century philosophy of science. Popper became most famous for his theory of *falsifiability*.[34] He held, essentially, that scientific theories gained credibility only by withstanding challenges that might have proved them false. Thus, the method of building support for a scientific hypothesis was one of "conjecture and refutation."

The stiffer the challenge, the more "corroboration" there would be if the hypothesis could not be dislodged. Thus, Newton's theory of universal gravitation explained a great deal and withstood all challenges for over 200 years. It remained true for most practical purposes even after being dethroned by Einstein's general relativity in 1916. Einstein's theory, in turn, has been the reigning champion for nearly a century and seems likely to endure for a while longer.

Early in his career, Popper subscribed to the frequentist interpretation of probabilities, developing his own particular spin on it. Then, in the early 1950s he became disenchanted with his earlier views, mainly because they could not deal with "singular events." He found the frequency approach unsuitable for expressing the kind of uncertainty about physical events that quantum theory posited to be irreducible, even in principle. To cope with such phenomena, Popper proposed to introduce a modification he termed the "propensity interpretation."

Popper's modification transfers attention from a sequence of observations to a set of generating conditions for such a sequence:

> The frequency interpretation always takes probability as relative to a sequence which is assumed as given; and it works on the assumption that a probability is *a property of some given sequence*. But with our modification, the sequence in its turn is defined by its set of *generating conditions*; and in such a way that probability may now be said to be *a property of the generating conditions*.[35]

Popper's basic idea of probability as propensity continued to evolve within his general philosophical framework and has influenced many others. There are currently many prominent philosophers who include a propensity aspect in their thinking. On the other hand, most practitioners, such as statisticians, engineers, and social scientists, are almost entirely oblivious to these developments. For the most part, only philosophers of science and some thoughtful physicists worry about what the probabilities that play such a prominent role in quantum theory "really" mean.

Popper himself, in his later years, found the notion of propensities increasingly central to his world view. In *A World of Propensities* (1990), he gravitated toward an almost mystical understanding of probability. He saw propensities as physical realities, "as real as forces, or fields of forces." Just as a force field defines a potential for movement of an object, a propensity can frame the possible outcomes of virtually anything.

He saw propensity as proscribing the limits within which free action could occur, and actions in turn changing the propensities:

> In our world, the situation and, with it, the possibilities, and thus the propensities, change all the time. They certainly may change if we, or any other organism, *prefer* one possibility to another; or if we *discover* a new possibility where we have not seen one before. Our very understanding of the world changes the conditions of the changing world; and so do our wishes, our preferences, our motivations, our hopes, our dreams, our phantasies, our hypotheses, our theories. ... All this amounts to the fact that *determinism is simply mistaken*; ... This view of propensities allows us to see in a new light the processes that constitute our world, the world process. The world is no longer a causal machine—it can now be seen as a world of propensities, as an unfolding process of realizing possibilities and of unfolding new possibilities.[36]

The propensity view of probability derives from a philosophy that focuses on the dynamic unfolding of phenomena. Potentialities, predispositions to *become* (Peirce's would-be's), are taken to be fundamental, and fixed things or objects are derivative and secondary.

Like the frequency theory, the propensity interpretation of probability intends to describe an objectively existing reality. For example, purely epistemic probabilities, such as my assessment of who will win a future election or football game, are not considered; the theory is not meant to encompass all possible applications of probability. In particular, if we wish to consider the probability that a past event actually occurred, it is hard to see how the propensity theory would apply.

The primary motivation for the propensity theory was to reconcile the notions of *causation* and *uncertainty*. This need became acute with the advent of quantum physics. No longer could probability be explained away as just a function of ignorance about true underlying deterministic causes. The traditional view of causes as deterministic just does not work in quantum physics, which provides an amazingly precise description of reality. So, if probabilistic uncertainty exists in a pure form at the quantum level, why should intrinsic uncertainty not also exist in some form as an aspect of macro phenomena as well? Peirce would presumably have applauded these developments.

Regardless of the philosophical value of propensities as a conceptual framework, I believe this perspective has much practical value. In the biological, economic, social, and psychological sciences, to say nothing of everyday life, it may be fruitful to think of causation on a continuum. At one extreme, there are universal regularities, causal "laws" in the conventional sense. At the other, there is complete lack of predictability, or apparent randomness. Various observable processes can be regarded as somehow intermediate between these extremes.

The propensity interpretation captures an aspect of the metaphorical lottery model that is left out by the subjective, frequency, and logical theories. These other perspectives all fail to suggest a clear sense of how a singular potential event is somehow being impelled into being under certain conditions. Propensity theory reminds us that this "would-be" may be real, but in a way that challenges traditional views of reality.

CHAPTER 9

PROBABILITY AND REALITY

Uncertainty entails two different aspects, or dimensions. We can be uncertain either because we harbor positive doubt about something or because we interpret the situation to be ambiguous. Probability in the broadest sense relates to our uncertainty generally. However, in the face of substantial ambiguity, quantifying our full uncertainty may be difficult or impossible. Since Bernoulli's day, there have been just a few serious attempts to develop a calculus of uncertainty that accounts for potential ambiguity.

Several noted economists, starting with Keynes and Frank Knight, have called attention to the limitations of standard probabilistic models to deal with the uncertainties of economic systems. In the 1960s, Daniel Ellsberg (yes, *that* Daniel Ellsberg, for those of us old enough to remember the Pentagon Papers affair) raised a stir by describing a "paradox" that challenged standard economic theory. The accepted wisdom among economists was that individuals and companies were rational in the sense of attempting to optimize expected values, as defined by mathematical probability theory. Ellsberg argued that the ambiguity pertaining to a situation ought to be taken into account in decision-making.[1]

The latest in this tradition of highlighting the limits of probabilistic models is Nassim Nicholas Taleb, whose jeremiads have indeed proved

---

Willful Ignorance: The Mismeasure of Uncertainty, First Edition. Herbert I. Weisberg.
© 2014 John Wiley & Sons, Inc. Published 2014 by John Wiley & Sons, Inc.

prophetic in light of the financial collapse that began in 2007.[2] Taleb credits the iconoclastic genius Benoit Mandelbrot (1924–2010) as his inspiration. Mandelbrot developed a typology of varieties of randomness and argued that real-world economic phenomena could not be well described by the ordinary limited form of randomness implicit in our usual mathematical models based on the theory of probability.[3]

A few statisticians and mathematicians also began to explore some alternative mathematical versions of probability beginning in the 1960s. They have attempted to account for some types of ambiguity by developing various types of "nonadditive" probability. Art Dempster and Glenn Shafer initiated a theory of *belief functions*, often called Dempster–Shafer theory.[4] These efforts, in which as a graduate student I played a small supporting role, can be considered a revival of the grand designs of Jacob Bernoulli, Johann Lambert, and others over two centuries earlier.[5] In addition, computer scientists have tried to incorporate some consideration of ambiguity by proposing *possibility theory*, an offshoot of "fuzzy logic," introduced by Lofti Zadeh.[6]

So far, none of these unconventional mathematical systems has really caught on. The usual version of mathematical probability has become so entrenched that it has made it difficult to imagine any alternatives. Other proposals, whatever their theoretical merits might be, face an enormous barrier to entry. We have come to equate uncertainty with mathematical probability and ceased to take seriously questions regarding ambiguity that Keynes and others addressed a century ago. As a result, discussions about the relation of probability to the real world have been drastically narrowed. The two main "schools" of probability interpretation today essentially ignore this problem entirely.

The frequency theory forecloses ambiguity by defining probability directly in terms of potentially observable sequences of actual occurrences. The subjective approach sidesteps the issue by assuming that a rational individual is capable of resolving any ambiguity in the process of framing a probability. How he manages to accomplish this feat is a personal matter. Frequentists thus assume that the relationship of probabilities to reality is limited, but direct and obvious; subjectivists assume that this relationship does not matter. Both perspectives fail to grasp the essentially metaphorical nature of mathematical probability.

THE RAZOR'S EDGE

On the one hand, probability exists only in our minds (or in a certain sense in our computers as well) as a construct to help cope with uncertainty. As a purely mental phenomenon, probability is completely free-floating, not intrinsically tethered to the real world in any sense. On the other hand, probability is useless if it is completely divorced from reality. So, we may be tempted to conceive probability as a literal *representation* of observable phenomena in the outside world. In particular, we may link it directly to recorded frequencies of occurrence.

However, these "frequencies" do not exist objectively, ready-made for discovery. They are mental constructs forged from the raw material of sense impressions and past experience. What exists in our nervous systems is not some kind of photographic image of a collection of external objects. Rather, conceptualizations arise in our consciousness as our brains go about their real business of regulating and maintaining our bodily systems and functions.

So, were de Finetti and Savage indeed correct that probability can only be interpreted as personal, or subjective? Well, yes and no.

> We are faced with a formidable snag because it seems that the only alternative to a view of the nervous system as operating with representations is to deny the surrounding reality. Indeed, if the nervous system does not operate—and cannot operate—with a representation of the surrounding world, what brings about the extraordinary functional effectiveness of man and animal and their enormous capacity to learn and manipulate the world? If we deny the objectivity of a knowable world, are we not in the chaos of total arbitrariness because everything is possible?
>
> This is like walking on the razor's edge. ... We must learn to take the middle road, right on the razor's edge.[7]

In the context of probability, we must transcend the two partial perspectives of objective and subjective probabilities.

We can accept that the potential for complete arbitrariness exists, but acknowledge that this cannot be the whole story. Our assessments of probability, like all of our cognitions, can adapt to an external environment. Neuroscientists Humberto Maturana and Francisco Varela

(1946–2001) have used the term "structural coupling" to describe this congruence between internal and external reality.

In this light, each human being's subjective probabilities are aspects of that person's individual conceptualization of reality. However, the utility of these probabilities for each of us will depend on the structural coupling that happens to exist between our personal probabilities and the external environment. Probability can thus be considered objective to the extent that a "strong coupling" exists. By the strength of coupling I mean the extent to which the internal and external realities are synchronized or coordinated, so that they form a relatively stable system.

For instance, imagine that you are sitting comfortably and reading this book. Suddenly, you hear a very loud *bang*. Instantaneously, your startle response kicks in, precipitating a number of preprogrammed reflexive reactions. Your senses are oriented to determine the source of this disturbance, and your body is ready for fight or flight. During the eons when hominids were evolving, this extreme reaction was undoubtedly highly adaptive. In a sense, the noise was interpreted to mean there was a high "probability" of danger.

There was a strong coupling between this probability assessment and the external environment, since loud noises were often accompanied by serious threats. In this sense, the probability was objectively correct, although it did not necessarily imply any conceptual understanding of the actual situation. Flashing forward several million years, we still retain a vestige of this primitive probability assessment. However, in most cases today, the loud noise does not indicate any significant danger. So, our response, while it is not entirely inappropriate, is in most circumstances is an overreaction. In this sense, the coupling between the internal "probability" and the external reality is much more attenuated.

This idea of structural coupling offers a broader perspective on the apparent contradiction between objectivity probability and subjective probability:

> If we are able to keep our logical accounting in order, this complication vanishes; we become aware of these two perspectives and relate them in a broader realm that we establish. … Imagine a person who has always lived in a submarine. He has never left it and has been trained how to handle it. Now, we are standing on the shore and see the submarine gracefully surfacing. We then get on the radio and tell the navigator inside: 'Congratulations! You avoided the reefs and surfaced

beautifully. You really know how to handle a submarine.' The navigator in the submarine, however, is perplexed: 'What's this about reefs and surfacing? All I did was push some levers and turn knobs and make certain relationships between indicators as I operated the levers and knobs. It was all done in a prescribed sequence which I'm used to. I didn't do any special maneuver, and on top of that, you talk to me about a submarine. You must be kidding!'[8]

WHAT FISHER KNEW

Early in the twentieth century, a great scientist and mathematician revolutionized our basic understanding of the physical world; his name was Albert Einstein. At roughly the same time, R. A. Fisher revolutionized our understanding of quantitative data and its possible applications. Like Einstein, Fisher was recognized for his unique mathematical and conceptual gifts. However, also like Einstein, he spent much of his later years wandering in a kind of scientific wilderness, unwilling to follow wholeheartedly the trails being blazed by his followers.

Fisher's achievements were informed by his understanding that mathematical probability rested ultimately on a simple analogy to a metaphorical lottery. This metaphorical-lottery idea of probability facilitated some of his deepest insights. During the last 200 years, no major figure besides Fisher has so clearly articulated the metaphorical-lottery interpretation of probability, with all its built-in ambiguity. However, he was unable to communicate his insights successfully.

Fisher's view of probability was first stated in one of his earliest papers and was reiterated in one of his last ones. Here is his remarkable initial formulation in 1922:

> When we speak of the *probability* of a certain object fulfilling a certain condition, we imagine all such objects divided into two classes, according as whether they do or do not fulfil the condition. This is the only characteristic in them of which we take cognisance. For this reason probability is the most elementary of statistical concepts. It is a parameter which specifies a simple dichotomy in an infinite hypothetical population, and it represents neither more nor less than the frequency ratio which we imagine such a population to exhibit.[9]

Probability is something that is "imagined" and refers to an "infinite hypothetical population" of objects. This population is simply the set of equally likely chances or cases familiar to Bernoulli, de Moivre, and Laplace. We can also think about them in certain contexts as occasions, situations, or eventualities. The condition to be fulfilled is often the occurrence of a specified event or outcome.

Fisher described the outcome condition (event) as the sole characteristic that we consider. Here, he essentially invoked the idea of willful ignorance. A statement about probability implicitly treats the objects under consideration as indistinguishable *except for* the particular condition of interest (the outcome). Thus, the occurrence or nonoccurrence of the outcome condition is regarded as if it is determined by a random draw from the hypothetical infinite population.

Fisher introduced this definition and explanation in order to justify the conception of a hypothetical infinite population. From this perspective, the observed statistical data are then viewed as:

> a random sample from the totality of numbers produced by the same matrix of causal conditions: the hypothetical population which we are studying is an aspect of the totality of the effects of these conditions, of whatever nature they may be. The postulate of randomness thus resolves itself into the question, 'Of what population is this a random sample?' which must frequently be asked by every practicing statistician.[10]

Fisher's novel conceptualization of data as being derived from a hypothetical infinite population became a central feature of statistical theory.

The notion of a hypothetical infinite population underlying an observed set of observations was extraordinarily fruitful. For the first time, the real object of a statistical analysis was identified as some *parameter* (proportion, mean value) that was clearly distinguished from the observable data. Prior to Fisher, this distinction between a *sample* of observations and an underlying *population* had never explicitly been formulated. Fisher saw that to make valid scientific inferences, we must regard each observation as an independent draw from a lottery whose fixed distribution of possible outcomes is determined by "the same matrix of causal conditions." This draw is random in the sense that relative to whatever hypothetical population (or causal matrix) we have in mind, it is *just like* a selection from an idealized lottery.

Like many powerful instruments, however, this new tool needed to be handled with care. It is always possible to regard a set of data as a random sample, but a sample of *what*, exactly? Calculating a mean value for a sample of students' test scores tells us something useful about a hypothetical population of students who are *similar to those tested*. However, this caveat is usually paid only lip service. In statistical texts, very little is written about the issue of "external validity," which relates to how the results may generalize to a broader population. The focus is almost entirely on the sampling variability, which can be calculated mathematically, rather than the reference class, which must always entail an element of judgment.

Fisher understood the importance of specifying the reference class. However, this critical question regarding the hypothetical infinite population typically was suppressed and virtually forgotten in applications. Contrary to Fisher's statement, it was in fact almost *never* explicitly asked by *any* practicing statistician. This oversight was rarely consequential, however, because in the early applications of statistical inference, such as survey research and experiments in agriculture and industry, the relevant reference class was usually obvious and uncontroversial. If a new type of fertilizer proved superior to a conventional one in testing on plots of land near London, it most probably would work equally well (under broadly similar conditions) in Dublin, Des Moines, or New Delhi.

Near the end of his life, Fisher again tried to explain his concept of probability. Here is perhaps his clearest articulation of how probability pertains to an *analogy* between an imagined lottery and a real-world happening:

> Probability statements do not imply the existence of any such population in the real world. All that they assert is that the exact nature and degree of our uncertainty is just *as if* we knew it to have been chosen at random from such a population. The subject of a probability statement if we know what we are talking about is singular and unique; we have some degree of uncertainty about its value, and it so happens that we can specify the exact nature and extent of our uncertainty by means of the concept of Mathematical Probability as developed by the great mathematicians of the 17th century Fermat, Pascal, Leibnitz, Bernoulli and their immediate followers.[11]

Fisher suggested (correctly, I believe) that probability only became *possible* because of the model provided by games of chance:

> It was unknown to the Greeks, and to the Islamic mathematicians of the Middle Ages. It owes its emergence, I suppose, to the high prestige of the recreation of gambling among the nobility of France and England, and to the existence of technology advanced enough to supply apparatus of gambling, dice, cards, etc. with a precision sufficient to justify the calculations of the mathematicians.[12]

That the origins of modern probability did not appear before the seventeenth century is no mystery; the necessary and sufficient conditions simply did not exist previously:

> The type of uncertainty which the new concept was capable of specifying with exactitude was that which confronts a gambler in a game played fairly, with perfect apparatus. The probability statements refer to the particular throw or to the particular result of shuffling the cards, on which the gambler lays his stake. The state of rational uncertainty in which he is placed may be *equated* to that of the different situation which can be imagined in which his throw is chosen at random out of an aggregate of throws, or of shufflings, which might equally well have occurred, though such aggregates exist only in the imagination.[13]

Remarkable! This could have been written by Jacob Bernoulli.

Fisher emphasized that some act of the *imagination* is necessary to *equate* the occurrence of an actual event to a random selection from some aggregate of possible eventualities. A mathematical probability is, as he had written originally in 1922, "neither more nor less" than the fraction of chances in an imaginary population. So, although the metaphorical lottery is from one point of view merely a mental contrivance, it is intended to reflect our uncertainty pertaining to events in the real world. The manipulator of probabilities is like the submarine navigator, twiddling his knobs and levers, but wending his way safely through the reefs.

Much like Jacob Bernoulli, Fisher was widely misunderstood. Many believed that he was essentially a frequentist, because of his insistence that probability was intrinsically connected to scientific understanding based on empirical data. Others saw elements of subjectivism in his assertions that probability related to degrees of belief. Few appreciated that his thinking was also colored by aspects of logical probability as espoused by Keynes. Fisher attempted the high-wire act of maintaining his balance on the razor's edge. His exposition of probability as essentially metaphorical was completely out of step with his times. Those around him could not comprehend such a view; they attempted to interpret his words through the distorting lens of one or another limited interpretation of probability.

Fisher appreciated the inevitable tension between knowledge and ignorance embodied in every probability statement:

> It has often been recognized that any probability statement, being a rigorous statement involving uncertainty, has less factual content than an assertion of certain fact would have, and at the same time has more factual content than a statement

of complete ignorance. The *knowledge* required for such a statement refers to a well-defined aggregate, or population of possibilities within which the limiting frequency ratio must be exactly known. The necessary *ignorance* is specified by our inability to discriminate any of the different sub-aggregates having different limiting ratios, such as must always exist.[14]

For concreteness, he discussed the case of throwing a certain die. In what sense would the value 1/6 for rolling an "Ace" (i.e., an outcome of 1) apply specifically to any particular throw? The necessary and sufficient condition, according to Fisher, is that we conceptualize *this* throw as indistinguishable from any other among a set of hypothetical future throws that might occur. That is, we *willfully ignore* any characteristic of this throw that might enable us to specify a relevant subset to which it belongs:

> Before the limiting ratio of the whole set can be accepted as applicable to a particular throw, a second condition must be satisfied, namely that before the die is cast no such subset can be *recognized*. This is the necessary and sufficient condition for the applicability of the limiting ratio of the entire aggregate of future throws as the probability of one particular throw. On this condition we may think of a particular throw, or a succession of throws, as a *random* sample from the aggregate, which is in this sense homogeneous and without recognizable stratification.[15]

The reference to a limiting ratio in a succession of throws may appear to situate Fisher in the frequentist camp, but that is not so. Remember Fisher's assertion that probability, if properly understood, pertains to each individual trial. Therefore, the fraction of aces, say, in a sequence of future throws is a *consequence* of the causal process that generates each of the throws, not a definition.

Like Laplace, Fisher insisted that every probability statement depends on both the *knowledge* and *ignorance* that we bring to bear. Thus, the relationship of probability to reality is subtle and complex. Like any mental model, a statement of probability can be more or less congruent with reality, but is never (except perhaps in the realm of quantum physics) absolutely true or false. It is only true or false relative to a given body of logic, knowledge, and evidence that can hardly ever be made fully explicit. Its value ultimately resides in how well it can inform our decisions and actions. What Keynes famously said about economics, both he and Fisher would, I believe, have agreed applies also to probability theory: "It is a method rather than a doctrine, an apparatus of the mind, a technique for thinking, which helps the possessor to draw correct conclusions."[16]

WHAT REFERENCE CLASS?

To apply probability in the real world, we must implicitly or explicitly have in mind a reference class of possibilities, or chances. In games of chance, the reference class is generally straightforward and uncontroversial. In certain practical applications, this is also the case. For instance, there is a branch of statistical theory that pertains to sample surveys. In conducting a survey, it is typical to draw a random sample of respondents from a well-defined finite population, or *sampling frame*. For example, this sampling frame might be the eligible voters in the United States prior to an upcoming presidential election.

In scientific applications, the reference class is rarely spelled out as such, but nonetheless will often be tacitly understood. For example, suppose a meteorologist forecasts that the probability is 50% that at least 0.1 inch of rain will fall on any given day in June in a certain locale. There is little ambiguity here; the reference class consists of all possible future June days. I can imagine a lottery in which out of a large number of such days, exactly 50% will involve at least 0.1 inch of rain, and any particular future day can be regarded as if it were selected at random from this aggregate.

In many situations, however, the reference class being assumed may not be so obvious. Suppose that the weather forecaster claims that the probability of rain *tomorrow* is 50%. Think for a few moments about what this statement really means. Can you express your understanding precisely without any reference to some class of future todays? If so, then you will have accomplished something remarkable. Even the complex combination of mathematical modeling and expert judgment that generates a meteorologist's 50% probability is in essence just a fancy way of estimating the percentage of rainy tomorrows within a reference class of days that are considered similar to today.

As discussed in the previous chapter, there are always many possible reference classes to which a specified situation can be referred. Selecting a reference class is a matter of judgment. Once the class is determined, we may then be able to find some relevant data to estimate the probability of a particular outcome in the specified situation. In our example of weather forecasting, imagine that we observe the results of many past occasions on which a forecast of 50% probability of rain was made by a certain meteorologist named Sarah. Then, the relative frequency of rainy days on such occasions should be close to 50%. Suppose that in this sense Sarah is found to be highly accurate, or in statistical jargon, well-calibrated. Does that suggest that Sarah has found the correct reference class for such days?

Suppose that Joe, another meteorologist, has been able to discern a recognizable *subset* of the days to which Sarah has assigned a 50% chance of rain. Using additional data and a different statistical model, he has identified two separate subclasses. In half of the days, he predicts the probability of rain to be 10%, while in the other half he predicts 90%. In a purely statistical sense, his predictions may be no more accurate than hers. However, they are clearly much more *useful*; they provide a much better guide for appropriate actions, such as whether to wear a raincoat or carry an umbrella.

A more extreme probability expresses less uncertainty about the outcome. It is more precise in the sense of predicting whether the event will occur *on a particular occasion*, such as tomorrow, than an equally accurate prediction that is nearer to 50%. More generally, a probability that deviates substantially from some typical value tends to provide a more useful basis for action. A method of statistical estimation that can *discriminate* well between events that have relatively high and relatively low probabilities has more "certainty" in a sense that is not captured by the standard measure of mathematical probability.

In some way that is hard to define, a more refined reference class that provides better discrimination resolves some aspect of ambiguity. It generally accomplishes this by taking into account more (or better) data. Keynes attempted to express this idea by the concept of the *weight* of evidence upon which a probability was being predicated. However, he admitted to great difficulty in making this notion precise.

Like Jacob Bernoulli, Keynes construed the assessment of probability as a balancing of evidence. He understood that mathematical probability was incapable of expressing some essential element of our uncertainty:

> The magnitude of the probability of an argument ... depends upon a balance between what may be termed the favourable and the unfavourable evidence; a new

piece of evidence which leaves this balance unchanged, also leaves the probability of the argument unchanged. But it seems that there may be another respect in which some kind of quantitative comparison between arguments is possible. This comparison turns upon a balance, not between the favourable and unfavourable evidence, but between the *absolute* amounts of relevant knowledge and of relevant ignorance respectively.[17]

The balance between favorable and unfavorable evidence pertains to the dimension of *doubtfulness* about a statement versus its contrary. This is the ordinary realm of mathematical probability. The absolute amounts of relevant knowledge and ignorance entail considerations of *ambiguity*. Because the arguments pro and con may rest on different types or amounts of evidence, they would not be directly comparable.

Bernoulli referred to the "probative force," and I tried to explain his logic by introducing my two glasses filled with liquid. The weight of favorable evidence was represented by the height of liquid in one glass, and unfavorable evidence by the height in the other. The height in each glass would indicate the amount (weight) of relevant knowledge supporting the corresponding argument. The empty space would represent the amount of the remaining ignorance. Neither Bernoulli nor Keynes could fully articulate this elusive concept of the weight of evidence, but that does not make their intuitions any less important.

Whatever the weight of an argument or evidence might mean, some such concept seems relevant to specifying a useful reference class. The more we know about the situation giving rise to the event in question, the more artfully we can define the reference class. Thus, a more seasoned meteorologist may be more capable than a neophyte of framing a useful reference class. Keynes warned us against the seductions of mindless reliance on statistical frequencies as the sole basis for probability assessments:

Bernoulli's second axiom, that in reckoning a probability we must take everything into account, is easily forgotten in these cases of statistical probabilities. The statistical result is so attractive in its definiteness that it leads us to forget the more vague though more important considerations which may be, in a given case, within our knowledge. To a stranger the probability that I shall send a letter to the post unstamped may be derived from the statistics of the Post Office; for me those figures would have but the slightest bearing on the question.[18]

Awareness that mathematical probability rests on an analogy has the virtue of directing conscious attention toward the reference class. For a set of observed data, we are forced to reflect on Fisher's neglected question: "Of what population is this a random sample?" On the answer to this question hinges the applicability of probability statements, and of statistical analyses, to the real world.

The task of identifying an appropriate reference class for the problem at hand cannot be relegated to a computer, nor can it be solved with mathematical equations. It requires judgment based on substantive knowledge, and also on the purpose for which the probability is being used. Ultimately, the responsibility for defining the reference class lies not only with the person who is most knowledgeable, but also with the one who must bear the consequences for the implications of this choice. Thus, Jane and her doctor must jointly weigh the evidence not only about the frequencies of success that have been observed in various populations, but also about the relevance of these statistics to the unique event that her potential surgery would be.

Fisher, like Keynes, understood that determining a reference class from which the case in hand could be regarded as a random representative was fundamental. He articulated three requirements that are necessary for a valid statement of mathematical probability[19]:

(a) A conceptual Reference Set, which may be *conceived* as a population of possibilities of which an exactly known fraction possess some chosen characteristic. …

(b) It must be possible to assert that the subject of the probability statement belongs to this Set. To the mathematician this may seem trivial, though obviously a necessity. Tasks of identification, however, belong to the scientist, and may require his full attention. … This second requirement puts our probability statement into the real world.

(c) No subset can be *recognized* having a different probability. … This is a postulate of ignorance …

In other words, a proper statement of mathematical probability requires only an analogy to a metaphorical lottery. However, any *particular* such lottery will be apt only to the extent that the particular event or statement in question is actually a member of this class. By putting the probability statement into the real world, Fisher meant the "conceptual reference set" would in fact apply to the individual event in question. For example, if we conceive of Jane as a patient with a particular condition, she must actually have this condition, or else the probability would be irrelevant for her.

An excellent example of the potential ambiguity about the reference class, even in an artificially simple setting, is furnished by the game of poker. For instance, in the currently very popular game of Texas hold'em, each player is dealt two "hole cards" facedown. Then five cards are dealt faceup, one at a time, with rounds of betting as each card is revealed. These five up-cards are available in common to each of the players to use along with her hole cards to make up a five-card hand. The key to a player's strategy is her assessment of the other players' hole cards and their chances of winning relative to her own.

At one level of analysis, the obvious reference class is the set of all possible two-card hands that each player might have. There are 1326 possibilities. This reference class is about as objective as you can get, so probabilities based on it are effectively real. However, the actual probability estimation does not depend very much on these objective probabilities. That is because the players can take much more information into account:

> A good poker forecast is probabilistic. It should become more precise as the hand is played out, but it is usually not possible to predict exactly which of the 1,326 hands your opponent holds until the cards are revealed particularly if your opponent is skilled and is deliberately behaving unpredictably.

> Indeed, information is so hard to come by in Texas hold'em that skilled players begin to make estimates about their opponents' range of hands even before any of the cards are dealt. ... through players' past histories with one another—or, failing that, what amounts to ethnic profiling. ... Once the game begins, these crude assumptions are supplanted by more reliable information: how the player has played previous hands at the table that day and how she is playing this one. The process is fundamentally and profoundly Bayesian, with each player updating their probability assessments after each bet, check, and call.[20]

Nate Silver is here using the term "Bayesian" rather loosely here to mean a strategy that updates probabilities as new data arrive.

In fact, the problem faced by the players is much more complex than any purely mathematical analysis, because there is substantial ambiguity about an appropriate reference class that underlies these subjective assessments. In order even to frame the uncertainty as a mathematical probability, each player must resolve the ambiguity in the situation substantially. Success will depend in large part on skill in sifting through the welter of potential information to focus on those factors that are critically relevant to this problem.

When there is substantial ambiguity as in a game of poker, we can, like the submarine navigator, operate our probability "instruments" in many different ways. But avoiding the reefs will require that our procedures be sufficiently attuned to reality. As Fisher noted, this requires expertise from outside the realm of mathematics to attain. Two famous artificial puzzles can help to illuminate the issues. In each case, our intuitions can easily be led astray by the ambiguity of the situation described.

The Monty Hall Problem

Perhaps the most famous math puzzle involving probability is the Monty Hall Problem, so named because it was inspired by a popular TV game show, "Let's Make a Deal," hosted by Mr. Hall. The problem was brought to popular attention in 1990 by Marilyn vos Savant (reputedly the woman with the highest IQ score ever measured) in her column "Ask Marilyn," published in Parade Magazine.[21] It has been a favorite brain teaser ever since.

On the TV show, the contestant was shown three closed doors. Behind one of these doors was a car, and behind the other two a goat. The contestant initially chose one of these doors and could win what was behind that door. However, before opening that door, Monty opened one of the other closed doors. If a goat was revealed, the contestant was offered the option of switching from her initial choice to the remaining closed door.

If you were playing the game and Monty showed you a goat, would you elect to switch or to hold on to your original door? The answer, of course, depends on the probability of finding the car behind your initial door rather than the remaining closed door. Does switching increase, decrease, or leave unchanged this probability? With only the information given, this question is ambiguous: you do not know how exactly the game show host selects the door to open. As we will see, this ambiguity matters a great deal.

TABLE 9.1   **Monty Hall Game Version 1 Initially**

Your Door	Door Not Opened	Door Opened	Probability
Car	Goat	Goat	1/3
Goat	Car	Goat	1/3
Goat	Goat	Car	1/3

One way to think about this question is to observe that after the host has revealed a goat behind one of the three doors, there would be only two doors remaining. Therefore, you might think (like most people at first) that your chances of winning would be 1/2 whether or not you switched. So, it would make no difference. Indeed, this *could* be a valid conclusion if a certain scenario truly described how the game actually worked.

Suppose that Monty did not really know (or care) which door hid the car. In that case, he would presumably choose which door to open completely at random. However, there would be a chance that the car would be behind the door that he opened. In that case, it is not clear what would happen. Perhaps you would be allowed to switch to this door. This is really a moot point because in the problem as described, a goat happens to appear behind the open door.

We can represent this version of the game by Table 9.1. At the outset of the game, there were three equally likely possibilities, as shown. After the goat has been revealed, however, you are in a different situation. You have eliminated one of the three possibilities, the one in which Monty *would have* shown you the car. So, there remain two equally possible cases, and your winning probability is 1/2, whether or not you decide to switch (see Table 9.2). This logic justifies the common intuition that switching makes

TABLE 9.2   **Monty Hall Game Version 1 After Goat Revealed**

Your Door	Door Not Opened	Door Opened	Probability
Car	Goat	Goat	1/2
Goat	Car	Goat	1/2
Goat	Goat	Car	0

**TABLE 9.3   Monty Hall Game Version 2 Initially and
After Goat Revealed**

Your Door	Door Not Opened	Door Opened	Probability
Car	Goat	Goat	1/3
Goat	Car	Goat	2/3
Goat	Goat	Car	0

no difference. In this case, seeing the goat is informative and changes the initial probabilities. The probability that the goat is behind your initial door increases from 1/3 to 1/2.

Remember, though, that this logic was based on the assumption that Monty did not know (or care) which door he opened. On the actual TV program, Monty Hall did know and did care. As Monty freely admitted in an interview, he always knew where the car was and was sure to open a door that would reveal a goat. So, the game could be correctly described not by Table 9.1, but rather by Table 9.3.

Actually, there were only two possibilities. Regardless of which door hid the car, that door would never be opened. The true probability that Monty would open the door to reveal a goat was 100%!

So, Monty's "clue" was completely uninformative. All Monty was revealing was that one of the two doors hid a goat, which you already knew. The probability of winning the game in no way hinged on seeing the inevitable goat behind the door Monty opened. Given your preferred strategy (hold or switch), the probability of winning remained the same after the clue as before. But this probability was not 1/2! Rather it was either 1/3 (hold) or 2/3 (switch). So, it was truly always better to switch.

The moral here is that there is no such thing as *the* probability of winning. *Your* probability depends on your conceptual model of reality (metaphorical lottery). To be unambiguous, this conceptual model must include a detailed specification of the *protocol* according to which the game is being played.[22] The protocol is the set of rules and procedures that govern the situation. In an artificial scenario, such as a game of chance, this protocol can in principle be specified exactly. In other situations, we can conceptualize the world *as if* it is a complex game with an unknown protocol. Our mathematical models attempt to describe the workings of this underlying protocol, at least approximately. The practical usefulness of any particular model of reality depends on how faithfully it represents what Fisher called the true "matrix of causal conditions."

Knowing the true protocol would be like having our metaphorical submarine's navigational systems perfectly coupled with the external conditions. In this simple case of a game show, we know the relevant causal matrix with great specificity. So, we know the real protocol, and can prove the clear superiority of switching. In most practical applications of probability theory and statistical analysis, this kind of inside information is rarely available. In such situations, the probability may be truly ambiguous.

A POSTULATE OF IGNORANCE

The Monty Hall Problem illustrates how unraveling an apparent paradox hinges on being able to state clearly the protocol underlying the situation. However, there is another aspect of this puzzle that is also instructive. We must evaluate and compare two different strategies for playing the game: hold or switch. We must decide what we will do after we have obtained some additional information. Our decision will be based on our assessment of certain probabilities *after* we have obtained this information. In the parlance of probability, it is *conditional* on the observed information.

Conditional Probabilities

I have alluded previously to the notion of *conditional probability*. The basic idea is straightforward. Suppose that we know some characteristic of an uncertain event or statement. For example, we are trying to predict whether Lenny, who is currently 65, will survive for at least another 10 years. However, we know also that Lenny is a life-long heavy smoker. Then, the appropriate reference class for him is not men of his age in general, but such men who also have a similar smoking history. The probability limited to this subset of individuals is the conditional probability given this characteristic.

In the metaphorical lottery that underlies any statement of mathematical probability, an event A corresponds to some subset of the total possibilities (chances). Similarly, another event B corresponds to some other subset. But if we know that event B has occurred (or will occur), then the appropriate reference class for A shrinks to include only the chances that correspond to B. The conditional probability is then the fraction of these B chances that are also A chances. For example, out of 1000 possible chances for men aged 65, suppose that 900 (90%) entail surviving for at least another decade. However, suppose that 200 of these 1000 cases correspond to heavy smokers, and that 150 (75%) of these 200 smokers will survive for 10 years.

$P(A)$, the unconditional probability of survival, would be 90%, but $P(A|B)$, the conditional probability, would be only 75%. This conditional probability derives from the number of chances that correspond to the compound event of surviving for 10 years and being also a heavy smoker (150 in this case), relative to the total number corresponding to being a heavy smoker (200). In mathematical notation:

$$P(A|B) = \frac{P(A \cap B)}{P(B)}.$$

This reads: "The conditional probability of A given B is equal to the probability of both A and B, divided by the probability of B."

As a mathematical relationship, the interpretation of this definition is clear. However, confusion can arise in translating this concept into practical application. In particular, in specifying (or estimating) the probability of a certain event (A), when is it appropriate to condition on another event (B)?

In theory, we should condition when knowing B has occurred would be *relevant* to the occurrence of A in Fisher's sense. By relevant, he meant that our probability of A would change, depending on whether or not B occurs. In probability theory, to be relevant, B must have the property that the conditional probability given B (or given not-B) must differ from the unconditional probability, that is,

$$P(A|B) \neq P(A)$$

In the lingo of probability theory, we say that A and B are not *independent* events.

This formal property is all that mathematical probability can tell us, and is useful as far as it goes. However, there is an important distinction that is not addressed within the framework of mathematical probability theory *per se*. In the example of Lenny the smoker, we assume that the conditioning event B (Lenny is a heavy smoker) is true. In this case, there is no theoretical reason *not* to condition on it. Similarly, for any other potentially relevant characteristic of Lenny, the only objections to conditioning would be practical; we may not have sufficient statistical data to estimate the conditional probability very well.

Suppose, however, that we know B is relevant, but are unsure whether or not in fact B is true. Should we assign a probability of 90% or 75% to Lenny's survival chances? Perhaps we should choose some intermediate value. The important point is that Lenny's situation is ambiguous. In general, if our uncertainty is too ambiguous to determine unequivocally whether B is true, then there is no "correct" answer. So, we must resolve this ambiguity before being able to frame a mathematical probability.

Predicting Unique Events

"The subject of a probability statement if we know what we are talking about is singular and unique," said Fisher.[23] He then tried to articulate the conditions necessary for a proper statement of probability pertaining to such a unique event. Recall his postulate of ignorance quoted above: "No subset can be *recognized* having a different probability." What exactly did he mean by "recognized" in this context?

Fisher went on to explain by alluding to the situation of attempting to obtain an Ace when rolling a single die:

(i) The subset of throws made on a Tuesday is easily recognizable, it has, however, the same probability as the whole set and is therefore irrelevant.

(ii) The subset of throws of odd numbers (1, 3, 5) is obviously relevant, since all Aces are odd numbers; this subset is, however, unrecognizable before the die is cast.

(iii) A parapsychologist claiming the gift of precognition might recognize a subset in which the Ace is foreseen. If the gift is veridical, the proportion of Aces in this subset must exceed one in six. In such a case, the subset will supersede the original set as the basis of the probability statement. If, however, experience shows that the proportion is just one in six as it would be without precognition, the subset is recognized to be irrelevant, and the original set is reinstated.

Fisher was saying in (i) and (ii) that for a subset of possibilities to be useful, it must be both relevant and known to occur *before* the outcome is observed. By relevance, he meant that the conditional probability of the event given that it is in this subset must be different from the unconditional (overall) probability. So, throws on a Tuesday fail the relevance criterion because the probability of an Ace remains 1/6. But, the subset of odd-numbered outcomes is potentially relevant because the conditional probability would be 1/3. However, in (ii) he asserted that we must know *in advance* that a member of the subset will actually occur. So, the set of odd numbers, to which an Ace certainly belongs, does not qualify because we do not know that an odd number will occur.

To a frequentist, the "true" probability is a real (and fixed) aspect of a long series of potential throws. It is conventional to treat this probability as pertinent to each individual throw, but for the frequentist this is just a manner of speaking. The probability is an objective property of the die, assuming it is thrown in the usual manner under normal conditions. So, any sort of "recognition" on the part of anyone would be irrelevant to the probability. Moreover, Fisher's reference to the hypothetical parapsychologist's claims would be totally incomprehensible.

An advocate of the subjective probability interpretation would view Fisher's formulation in a rather different light. To such a person, the probability that the next trial will result in an Ace can be any number between 0 and 1. What specific information goes into her subjective assessment of this probability is up to her. So, the possible relevance (for her) of being thrown on a Tuesday, for example, would be entirely personal.

So, what was Fisher really trying to say? I believe he was attempting to express an important and largely overlooked distinction. A legitimate probability statement has both an objective and a subjective aspect. On the objective dimension, it refers to a certain reference class (in his terminology the reference set), of possibilities to which the uncertain event at issue is *believed* to belong. This subjective belief determines whether the probability assessment will be conditional on this reference class, which may be a subset of some larger class. So, *recognizability* pertains to the subjective aspect of probability.

On the other hand, the recognizable subset might be correct or not; that is, it may be in accord with reality or not. The *relevance* of this subset is an aspect what philosophers call the *ontological* realm. As such, it can potentially be confirmed or refuted. For example, my reference class for Lenny can be the set of 65-year-old men. However, if it turns out that Lenny is actually 70 years old, this class is simply wrong. As Fisher said, defining the reference class places the probability assessment *into the real world*.

Furthermore, the probability statement assumes that there is *no relevant subset* of the reference class. That is, we are unaware of any information that would lead us to refine our probability assessment. Once we *recognize* any such subset, we must (if we are being rational) adjust our probability by conditioning on it. In effect, we would adopt a more specific, or narrower, reference class. To recognize such a more specific reference class, means that *we accept it to be relevant for practical purposes*. That is, we are prepared to act as if this subset is relevant. This recognition is a subjective matter that depends on our personal judgment and available evidence. It falls within the *epistemological* realm.

Consider, for example, Lenny's medical history. This information would clearly be relevant to his survival probability. However, if we truly knew nothing about this history, we would perforce ignore it. Fisher noted that there are many such hidden factors (and associated relevant subsets) that *might* in reality exist. So we face a conundrum. In order to frame a probability statement, we must *ignore* the existence of such relevant subsets. Thus, as Fisher indicated, recognizability entails a postulate of ignorance.

Fisher understood that every probability statement implicitly relates to a reference class, and every reference class reflects a personal judgment, whether acknowledged or not. We must take only certain aspects of our knowledge about the world into account, and willfully ignore others. In nearly every instance, there will be *some* possibly relevant information or belief that comes to mind. We are rarely, if indeed ever, operating in a complete informational vacuum. So, we must at some level of consciousness scrutinize our knowledge and beliefs in order to decide how much ignorance is warranted. Where should we draw the line between our knowledge and belief, on the one hand, and our acceptance of ignorance, on the other?

Our answer to this critical question determines whether we should condition on this characteristic. But the answers may not be obvious. The essential point is that any probability is relative to a particular state of knowledge. The probability statement is made possible only because we are willing to assume (for the present) that beyond the boundaries of this knowledge lies *terra incognita*. Once we admit into evidence some additional information whose validity or relevance is uncertain, our sense of uncertainty becomes fuzzier.

In the extreme, when we have no knowledge about a particular event, a mathematical probability does not exist at all. In a remarkable passage that Fisher found quite "illuminating," Keynes explained how we often err by saying that a probability is *unknown* when we really mean that a mathematical probability cannot be specified at all:

> Do we mean unknown through lack of skill in arguing from evidence, or unknown through lack of evidence? The first alone is admissible, for new evidence would give us a new probability, not a fuller knowledge of the old one; we have not discovered the probability of a statement on given evidence, by determining its probability in relation to quite different evidence … For it is not *this* probability that we have discovered, when the accession of new evidence makes it possible to frame a numerical estimate.[24]

Similarly, imagine that we originally frame a probability based on some particular reference class, and later refine this class. The probability relative to this new reference class is not simply a new and improved version of the same probability. Rather, it is a *different* probability, one that conforms to our updated state of knowledge. For example, we may discover that Lenny has diabetes. In that case, our new probability would take this factor into account. However, the validity of our old probability is not impugned in any way, merely supplanted by a new probability.

The idea that there always exists some unique *true* probability waiting to be revealed is a myth shared by the frequentist and the subjectivist. To the frequentist, this probability resides "out there" in the real world. To the subjectivist, it lies "in there," buried within the individual's psyche. However, since the mathematical probability is part of a personal thought process about the world, it has no independent existence apart from the conceptual framework in which this thought process is embedded. Specifically, it depends on precisely how the implicit metaphorical lottery is being *conceived* at any given moment in time.

From this perspective, the core insights of both the frequency and subjective theories of probability are valid but incomplete. Von Mises, the archetypical frequentist, argued that "collectives" characterized by complete *impossibility of a gambling system* provided a rigorous foundation for probability. But there is *always* a possible gambling system, except perhaps in the quantum mechanical realm, and someone else may be privy to it, even if we remain blissfully ignorant. This is obviously true in games of chance, and less obvious but still true in other situations.

Meanwhile, according to Savage and de Finetti, the pioneer subjectivists, all probabilities are psychological in nature, nothing more than measures of our personal beliefs. That is fine, but on what grounds can we be sure that our beliefs can be properly expressed as mathematical probabilities? If they do take this special form, then what reference class has implicitly been invoked?

Inside Information

Conceptually, we can say that one evaluation of a probability is better than another when it is closer to reality, and is therefore a preferable guide to behavior. Of course, in most practical applications of probability, it is very difficult to spell out what it means for an evaluation to be closer to reality. So, we can rarely know for certain whether one probability assessment was better than another, even after the outcome becomes known.

Remember how Las Vegas George deployed his technology in such a way that the results of all his spins appeared (and in fact *were*) completely random. There was no way that anyone could detect his cheating by observing the pattern of outcomes produced by his roulette wheel. After extensive analysis, a disciple of Von Mises would be unable to discern the existence of a gambling system, and from his (limited) perspective, he would be correct. Of course, George would see things in a much different light.

He would perceive the true "causal matrix" generating the observed outcomes, which would involve two steps. First, there would be a process to decide whether or not to utilize his device on any particular spin. Second, for each spin George controlled, there would be a process to specify which slot was targeted. In our example, George arranged for each of these choices to be random. For George's employers (or the Von Mises disciple), these two steps would be invisible, and the spins would appear perfectly normal. However, *in reality*, they would be anything *but* normal. Most importantly, the *potential* would exist for anyone who knew what was really going on to make a lot of money.

The subset of controlled spins would comprise a relevant subset that was also recognizable to George. For any member of this subset, he could predict in advance the exact outcome. This *inside information* about the causal process generating the results would allow him to condition on the relevant information that was hidden from others. In effect, George would be operating on the basis of a set of conditional probabilities rather than the standard probabilities. For this relevant subset of the spins, the uncertainty would be completely eliminated. However, for his employers, each of the 38 possible outcomes on these same spins would have an equal chance of occurring.

In a similar way, knowing the true protocol in the Monty Hall Problem would allow the player to determine whether or not Monty's clue was relevant in Fisher's sense. Under the protocol that actually governed the TV game, Monty always opened a door that hid a goat, rather than selecting a door at random. Therefore, we could know that the probability was zero that opening this door would reveal the car. Consequently, the subset of games in which a goat would be revealed was *not* a relevant subset. In fact, it was not a subset at all. In contrast, if Monty truly opened a door at random, this subset *would* be relevant. In that case, seeing a goat would provide useful information, because it would change the probabilities. In essence, the confusion about the actual TV game arises because we assume that Monty's clue is relevant, when in fact it is not.

The Two Envelope Problem

Now let us consider another well-known puzzler. This one may at first seem simpler than the Monty Hall Problem, but is actually quite subtle, and potentially very instructive. It illustrates how the real probability can depend on the underlying protocol, which may be far from obvious. As in the Monty Hall Problem, you are imagined to be playing a game. You are shown two envelopes and informed that each contains a check for some amount of money. However, you are also told that *one of the checks is for exactly twice as much as the other.*

You can select either Envelope 1 or Envelope 2 and open it. After seeing the amount, you have the choice of keeping that check as a prize or of switching to the other envelope. Should you hold or switch? This problem has occasioned a lot of head-scratching by mathematicians, statisticians, and other experts in probability theory.[25] It is easy to become confused if we are not careful to have the actual protocol in mind.

On the one hand, it may seem obvious that your knowledge about the contents of the two envelopes is perfectly symmetrical. So, you have an equal probability of winning the larger amount, regardless of which envelope is first selected. Observing the amount in one of the envelopes does nothing to change this. You are simply choosing between two unknown but fixed amounts, so your expected value for the game must be the average of the two amounts. In general, suppose that the total amount of both the checks is T. Then we would know that one check must be for T/3 and the other for 2T/3. Your expected value would be the average, or T/2. For example, if the value of T is $90,000, then one envelope must contain $30,000 and the other $60,000, so your expectation would then be $45,000.

On the other hand, consider the following counterargument. After you observe the amount in one envelope, say Envelope 1, you realize that the amount in Envelope 2 must be either twice this amount or half. But you have no basis for deciding which possibility is true. For example, suppose you discover that there is a check for $40,000 in Envelope 1. Then, the amount in Envelope 2 must be either $20,000 or $80,000. If you switch, your expected reward will increase from $40,000 to $50,000, which is the average of these two possible prizes. In general, suppose you observe a value V in the envelope opened. Then, no matter what value V you see, your expected value for switching will be 5V/4. So, you should always switch. Right?

Hold on just a minute. Suppose you had chosen Envelope 2 first. Would not the same logic work equally well in reverse? Of course it would. So, regardless of which envelope you happened to choose first, you should switch to the other. But if you can always gain by switching, then if you play repeatedly, your long-run average amount for always choosing the envelope that is opened would be less than that for always choosing the remaining one. This logic contradicts the argument that the amounts in the two envelopes must be subject to exactly the same probability distribution. What is going on here? (Before reading on, you may wish to ponder this conundrum for a while on your own.)

To unravel this paradox, consider an alternative possible way the game could be played. Imagine that you are playing a computerized version of the Two Envelope game. You are first presented with two virtual "envelopes" and can choose one to open. You find that it contains V dollars. You are then offered the option of switching to a second envelope that will contain either V/2 or 2V dollars. Now, there are two possible situations that you may be facing. One possibility is that the amount in the other virtual envelope has already been fixed, as in the usual Two Envelope problem. In that case, it makes no difference whether you hold or switch. However, it is also possible that the amount in the second envelope will not be determined until *after* you have opened one of the two envelopes.

In that situation, you would not really be choosing between two predetermined amounts T/3 and 2T/3 after T had already been fixed. Rather, you would be choosing between $T = V + V/2$ and $T = V + 2V$ after V has been fixed. This differs from your situation in the usual version of the Two Envelope problem, since the real value of T would not be fixed *before* you observe V. Confusion arises because these two versions are perceived as identical, although the implicit protocols are very different.

If you really did not know whether the prize in the second envelope had already been determined before the first was opened, you could not say whether or not switching would always be advantageous. Information about the true underlying protocol is the kind of "evidence" upon which Keynes believed any probability assessment must be predicated. In his view, the true expected payoff of each strategy would be "unknown" in the sense of being undefined (ambiguous).

LAPLACE'S ERROR

Consider some situation that will occur in the near future about which you are certain. For concreteness, I assume you are absolutely sure that the color of your bedroom will not have changed when you wake up tomorrow morning. When that moment arrives, you will be able to verify whether or not this prognostication was correct. On the other hand, a situation lacking in certainty is quite different. For example, you may be unsure whether or not it will be raining when you awaken tomorrow. Suppose you remember that just before you retired for the night, a forecast on the local news indicated a 70% chance of rain. You wake up and find that the day is sunny and clear. In what sense, if any, can we say whether or not this prediction was correct?

Strictly speaking, a probability statement is incapable of being falsified. No matter what the outcome, it *could have* occurred and it *could have* failed to occur. On the other hand, suppose as here that we assigned a relatively high probability to the observed outcome, but it failed to occur, or conversely a low probability but it did occur. Then, in some respect and to some degree, we may feel that the assigned probability was wrong. Moreover, if the forecast had indicated a 90% chance of rain, you would consider it to have been even *more* wrong.

As I explained, this "paradox" of probability arises because we fail to keep our logical accounting in order. The probability was based on a judgment relative to our prior understanding of the situation. Whether the event actually occurs depends on the real protocol, or matrix of causal conditions. There is no *necessary* relationship between these different perspectives. Is there, though, a sense in which a probability statement is truly right or wrong? What *can* we say about the validity of the 70% probability of rain?

Laplace believed in a fully deterministic universe that was, in principle, completely comprehensible for a being of sufficient intelligence. Therefore, the true causal conditions *could* be known so precisely that chance would not really exist. Human uncertainty resulted, he believed, from our imperfect knowledge of these conditions. In a game of chance, the true protocol could be specified very precisely. This specification would depend on our knowledge about the outcome of any particular play of the game. The protocol would in effect define the different cases that could occur with equal possibility on any given play. The probability of any outcome, such as winning the game, would be the fraction of all the cases that correspond to this outcome.

In an ideal game of chance, the nature of the possible cases is exactly known, and the reasons for considering them equally possible are compelling. Therefore, as a practical matter, it is only possible to conceptualize the situation in one way. Our uncertainty pertaining to any particular outcome derives only from our *doubt* about whether or not it will occur. Probability is a measure of this doubt. In most situations, however, our uncertainty encompasses a degree of *ambiguity* as well as doubt. Even in the contrived scenarios of the Monty Hall and Two Envelope games, uncertainty about the underlying protocol would make it impossible to define uniquely the probabilities involved.

Jacob Bernoulli had implicitly attempted to deal with ambiguity as well as doubt in his system. Laplace, on the other hand, simply assumed away ambiguity as if the true nature of the situation could always, in principle, be clearly specified. So, he slid seamlessly in his discussion from games of chance to such matters as mortality tables, judicial decisions, and legal testimony. Regrettably, he never clarified exactly how he could justify this transition, and perhaps he never recognized that a serious issue existed. It was this failure that led to the criticisms of Laplace's grandiose aspirations for mathematical probability.

For Laplace, there was a *true* probability of rain, just as there was a true probability of 2/3 that a player "in the know" would win the Monty Hall game. A forecast of 70% for rain tomorrow might be construed to be accurate in the same sense as the probability of drawing a white ball from an urn containing seven white and three black balls. This probability was conceived by Laplace as applicable to the given situation that existed when the forecast was made, albeit in light of the relevant information available at the time. It represented the proper balance between our knowledge and our ignorance about the situation.

The problem here is that the precise nature of this situation and the information about it may be far from obvious. Our understanding of the world, at least in science, no longer assumes a privileged point of view from which everything could theoretically be known. Since Einstein, we cannot even define space and time as absolutes. For complex phenomena, such as human health and behavior, it is possible to entertain many different conceptual frameworks for interpreting a given situation. How we choose to resolve the ambiguity of the situation has a bearing on our assessment of probabilities.

In the case of a weather forecast, for example, a probability can only be defined *relative to* a particular conceptualization of current reality. Within this context, we might say that our uncertainty is just like that which we would have about drawing a white ball from an urn containing seven white and three black balls. Then, there are two questions to consider. First, is our conceptualization of the actual situation essentially correct? Second, in such a situation as we have conceptualized, would this analogy to an urn with seven white balls and three black balls be valid?

If the world is such that our conceptualization is essentially correct, we might be able to test the reality of our probability empirically. We might have, or be able to obtain, some data available on the outcomes for a representative sample of similar situations in the past. These data would provide a valid estimate of the real probability. So, in this sense, the forecast of 70% can be said to be objectively right or wrong. From this perspective, observing a single sunny day after this prediction would provide some weak evidence tending to suggest that the probability might be "wrong." Observing ten such mornings, of which only two were rainy, would imply much stronger evidence.

Suppose, however, that the particular situation at hand has been misconceived. Then, the data collected would not necessarily be similar to this situation in all relevant respects. In that case, the prediction could be wrong not because it was a faulty estimate of an unknown probability, but because it was an accurate estimate based on faulty evidence. As Keynes posited, we cannot assess "the probability of a statement on given evidence, by determining its probability in relation to quite different evidence." Laplace believed that people differed in their probability estimates mainly because they possessed varying *information*. He failed to appreciate what troubled Jacob Bernoulli: that they might also disagree because of ambiguity pertaining to the relevant evidence.

CHAPTER 10

THE DECISION FACTORY

It is a beautiful early spring morning on the outskirts of London in 1919.[1] The 29-year-old Ronald Fisher, deep in contemplation, walks briskly along the two-mile route from his home to the local post office. There, he intends to mail a letter that will alter his life for good or ill. A small cloud of smoke emanates from the pipe that has become almost a permanent fixture in his mouth. For the last few weeks, he has suffered an agony of uncertainty, but he is now firmly resolved. The path he has chosen is unconventional, but offers the best chance to accomplish something truly significant.

So far, his working life has been one of utter frustration, despite the great promise of his undergraduate years at Cambridge, and the unquestioned brilliance he displayed there in studies of mathematics, astronomy, and biology. He is especially bitter about being forced to sit out the recently concluded Great War, rejected from military service because of his extreme nearsightedness. Professionally he has tried his hand at teaching mathematics in secondary school and performing statistical analyses for an investment house. He considers himself an abject failure in both of these endeavors.

Willful Ignorance: The Mismeasure of Uncertainty, First Edition. Herbert I. Weisberg.
© 2014 John Wiley & Sons, Inc. Published 2014 by John Wiley & Sons, Inc.

As the post office comes into view, Fisher hesitates slightly and ruminates for the hundredth time on the opportunity he is walking away from. Karl Pearson has offered him the post of chief statistician at the Galton Laboratory. There he would be at the forefront of research in modern statistical methods, especially as applied in biology. However, he would be working in the shadow, and under the thumb, of the autocratic Pearson. Still, the position at the Galton Laboratory would afford him a comfortable income, especially important now that he is married and about to start a family. Until a few weeks ago, he had seen no other viable prospect.

Then, like a *deus ex machina*, this unexpected alternative option had suddenly materialized. Rothamsted! That venerable agricultural experimentation station in Harpenden seemed an unlikely venue for realizing his ambitions. Until, that is, he had met with its director, Sir John Russell. They had chuckled as Russell recounted how Fisher's tutor at Cambridge had written in his letter of recommendation that Fisher "could have been a first class mathematician had he stuck to the ropes, but he would not." Undoubtedly, Pearson felt the same way, but Russell seemed to comprehend that the "ropes" were much too constraining for someone like Fisher. Yes, the decision was clear: Rothamsted it must be!

BEYOND MORAL CERTAINTY

When Fisher began his tenure at Rothamsted in 1919, statistical methods were almost entirely concerned with problems in which large volumes of data were in hand. For example, Galton's original biometric studies involved observations on hundreds, or even thousands, of individuals. While not adequate to provide "moral certainty" to suit Jacob Bernoulli, the resulting statistics, such as a calculated frequency or mean value, were usually good enough for most practical purposes. Consequently, statisticians tended to denigrate the importance of the "small-sample" problem.

Something Brewing

Perhaps the most revolutionary turning point in statistical thinking resulted, oddly enough, from the attempt to brew a better beer. William

Sealy (W. S.) Gosset (1876–1937) graduated from Oxford with a first-class chemistry degree in 1899. Eminently practical, Gosset eschewed an academic career and went to work for the Guinness Brewery in Dublin.[2] He was employed by Guinness until his death in 1937, eventually rising to become its Head Brewmaster. His recruitment in 1899 was part of a progressive campaign by the company to adopt modern scientific and engineering practices. Gosset, it turned out, was ideally suited to lead these efforts. He possessed exceptional managerial and technical talents, was extremely personable, and had a particularly good head for mathematics.

Much of the research being pursued by Guinness concerned the best methods for growing barley and hops, the main ingredients of Guinness's signature "stout porter" beer, now known simply as Guinness stout. Field experiments were being conducted, comparing the yields and quality of various seed types, soils, fertilizers, and so on. However, the results often proved equivocal, because there were many factors that could determine these outcomes. Each combination of treatment conditions required a substantial plot of land on which it could be tested, and the number of available plots was quite limited. So, the variability among the plots in a research study often obscured the "signal" of interest.

Suppose, for example, that a new type of seed was being compared with the current standard in an experiment that involved 20 plots of land. Then, 10 of these plots might be chosen to receive the new seed and 10 would get the standard. After the harvest, the yield of each plot (say, bushels of barley) would be measured. The result would be a set of data consisting of 20 numbers. From these data, it would be natural to calculate the average yield per plot for the two experimental groups. The treatment yielding the higher average would *appear* to be the winner in this competition, but there was a problem.

As a hypothetical, imagine the average yield for the standard treatment was 20.1 bushels per acre, while the new, and presumably improved, seed produced 24.2 bushels. How close was the estimated difference of 4.1 bushels per acre to the true causal effect, and how confident could the scientists be that the new seed was truly superior to the standard? These were very difficult questions to answer for two main reasons.

One reason was that the experimental units assigned to the two different treatments may have been too dissimilar. Various factors besides the

Landmarks of Probability

1600	
1654	Pascal & Fermat
1657	Huygens
1700	
1713	Bernoulli
1718	De Moivre
1764	Bayes & Price
1774	Laplace
1800	
1837	Poisson
1838	De Morgan
1843	Mill
1843	Cournot
1849	Ellis
1854	Boole
1866	Venn
1892	Peirce
1900	
1921	**Keynes**
1921	**Knight**
1922	**Fisher**
1926	**Ramsey**
1926	**Neyman & Pearson**
1928	**Von Mises**
1937	**De Finetti**
1949	**Reichenbach**
1954	**Savage**
1959	**Popper**

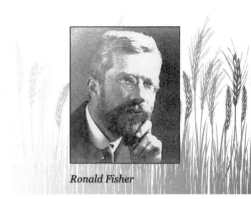

Ronald Fisher

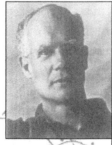

Egon Pearson

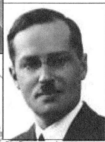

Jerzy Neyman

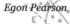

different seed types might have affected the yields. If these factors were not balanced in a way that equalized their overall impact on the outcome, the observed outcome difference would be *biased*.[3] That is, this causal effect would be *confounded* with the effects of the hidden factors.

A common way to deal with possible confounding was to find matched pairs of the plots of land that shared all *known* relevant characteristics. Soil composition, drainage, and insect infestation are examples of possible confounding factors. By assigning the new treatment to one plot and the standard to a matched plot nearby, this variability could, in theory, be controlled. However, in practice, some confounding factors were either not known or difficult to measure. So, matching and similar strategies required much skill to employ and still could not truly guarantee that experimental control was adequate.

Furthermore, even when the experimental control was thought to be virtually perfect, there would be a second difficulty. The estimated causal effect could be influenced by "random" variation. By random, we mean causal factors whose effects were transitory or irregular. Such random factors would on average have a similar impact on the different experimental groups, so no systematic error (bias) would result. However, the "noise" generated by these uncontrolled factors might, by chance, create an apparent treatment effect.

Assume that my hypothetical seed-comparison experiment generated the data shown in Table 10.1. The average apparent difference favoring the new seed was 4.1 bushels per acre, an increase of approximately 20%. But was this difference really meaningful? Could it possibly have resulted entirely from the random variation among the plots of land? That was the question that Gosset was trying to answer. To do so, he needed advice from the greatest statistical guru at the time, Karl Pearson. So, in 1907, he convinced Guinness to send him off for a year of special training in Pearson's department at University College in London.

From this fount of all statistical wisdom, he imbibed the latest knowledge of data-analytic methods. As a result, he wrote two highly original papers related to the probability distributions in small samples of a mean value (average) and of a correlation coefficient. In 1908, these were published in Pearson's house organ, *Biometrika*, the first academic statistical journal.[4] However, Guinness required Gosset to publish under a pseudonym, so the author was identified simply as "Student."

TABLE 10.1   Hypothetical Field Experiment: Comparing Mean
Yield (Bushels)

Pair Number	New Seed Type	Standard Seed Type	Difference
1	16.5	17.2	−0.7
2	22.7	20.1	+2.6
3	30.4	26.2	+4.2
4	19.3	20.2	−0.9
5	28.8	18.1	+10.7
6	26.8	17.5	+9.3
7	21.6	22.5	−1.9
8	28.8	22.2	+6.6
9	21.4	19.3	+2.1
10	25.6	17.7	+7.9
Mean	**24.2**	**20.1**	**+4.1**

A Tale of Two Students

Fisher first became aware of Gosset's two *Biometrika* articles while still a
student at Cambridge in 1912. His advisor, the astrophysicist F. J. M.
Stratton (1881–1960), had introduced him to statistical theory in the
context of astronomical measurement problems. During the nineteenth
century, great progress in astronomical research, as well as geodetic surveys of the earth, had been achieved. This scientific research depended
on imperfect measurement techniques. It was necessary to obtain multiple observations and derive from them the best possible estimate of a
true position or distance. Mathematicians, going back to Carl Friedrich
Gauss (1777–1855) and Laplace, around 1800 had been working out the
mathematical "theory of errors."[5]

By the turn of the twentieth century, the mathematical analysis of measurement problems had become quite refined, but this technology had
spread very little into other areas of research. In particular, problems of
variation in biological and social sciences were not terribly concerned with
"measurement error." The measurements were quite precise, and the variation of interest (e.g., height, weight, wingspan, and petal size) in animal,
plant, and human populations came mainly from real individual differences rather than observational error.

Variations in human populations were sometimes regarded as deviations from an ideal type. The construct of the *homme moyen* (average man),

introduced by Adolphe Quetelet (1796–1874) in 1835, was sometimes interpreted as a racial or national exemplar.[6] However, this so-called average man was an abstraction, not a real person. Moreover, Quetelet and the many social scientists he inspired studied very large groups. So, the small-sample theory of measurement errors was not recognized as relevant to the biological and social sciences during the nineteenth century.

Student's first paper dealt with the question of how much random variability could be expected when a mean (average) was being estimated based on a small number of observations. This issue was central to determining whether an experimental effect could reasonably be attributed to chance variation or not. The critical factor was the ratio between the mean difference observed and a measure of variability called the "probable error."[7] The larger this ratio, the less likely was chance as an explanation.

The catch was that the probable error had to be *known*. For example, in astronomy, where the statistical theory was most highly evolved, the probable errors of various instruments and observational procedures were typically quite well known based on long experience. In agricultural experiments, on the other hand, the "errors" were not attributable to imperfect measurement equipment or technique, but to the unknown causal factors at work. Therefore, the probable error of the underlying distribution was not known. It usually had to be *estimated* from the same data that were being utilized to estimate the mean itself.

In large samples, very little error would be introduced by simply replacing the true (unknown) probable error by the estimated one. Thus, the standard formula could be used, ignoring the slight error introduced by this approximation. However, in small samples, this error could be substantial, and the standard formula would need to be adjusted in some way. So, Gosset asked himself how this adjustment could be accomplished, and derived a solution, which was then published in his first *Biometrika* article.

In the context of his time, Student's paper was an outlier. Student had an answer, but nobody was asking the question. Experimental scientists did not understand his result and statisticians thought it a mathematical curiosity, of little scientific utility. Who would have any use for such small-sample methods? Once again, a major potential development related to probability was ignored, and once again, was rescued from oblivion quite by chance. In this case, it was a precocious Cambridge undergraduate rather than a Dutch nobleman who came to the rescue.

R. A. Fisher was intrigued by Gosset's mathematical results and found a way to prove them rigorously by applying his unique geometrical approach. Stratton, Fisher's tutor, encouraged him to write up his proof and send it to Gosset. A correspondence between Fisher and Gosset ensued, initiating a long-term personal and professional relationship between the two. For nearly a decade, Fisher and Gosset were perhaps the only two people in the world who truly understood Student's formula, let alone appreciated its potential importance.

When Fisher finally landed at Rothamsted in 1919, the creation of modern statistical theory and practice began in earnest. Student's original article had lit the way, and Fisher soon realized that Gosset's ideas could be clarified and extended in many fruitful ways. Within three years, Fisher had laid the foundations for modern statistical analysis based on mathematical probability. His 1922 landmark paper began with his conception of probability, which I discussed in Chapter 9. He went on to propose several original theoretical concepts, and to apply his new ideas to practical problems related to the agricultural research being conducted at Rothamsted.

Shortly thereafter, Fisher set to work on a research methods manual, published in 1925 as *Statistical Methods for Research Workers*.[8] In it, he explained the principles and the methods for the design and analysis of controlled experiments. Recognition of its importance was not immediate:

> The book did not receive a single good review. The reviewers, faced with a volume so new in philosophy, scope, and method, were unimpressed with its virtues. They criticized the predominance in it of Fisher's own work ... And they regarded the whole treatment as of very narrow interest, dealing as it did with small samples ... Fisher was beginning to expect this sort of reception for his original work.[9]

Soon, however, the scientific world began to catch on. Fisher's landmark first book eventually went through 14 editions.

Fisher went on to generate hundreds of articles and reports, wrote several more classic books pertaining to both statistics and genetics, was invited to lecture at universities around the globe, and received many prestigious awards. He was elected to the Royal Society in 1929, receiving its Darwin Medal in 1948, primarily for his contributions to population genetics, and in 1952 was knighted by the newly crowned Queen Elizabeth II.

Contriving Ignorance

I mentioned above the two methodological problems faced by experimentalists: confounding and random variability. By 1923, Fisher had come to realize that both of these could be solved by a kind of statistical aikido. In most practical situations, attempting to exert strict experimental control over all important sources of variability was a fool's errand. Fisher saw that it would rarely be feasible to engineer sufficiently equivalent groups to assure a valid comparison. There was simply not enough information about the relevant characteristics of the individual units. So, rather than tackle this problem by decreasing the uncertainty about the various sources of variation in order to control them better, he took the opposite tack. He proposed to *perfect our ignorance* by assigning treatments completely at random.

Fisher's idea of artificial randomization would become the cornerstone of modern experimental design, but was revolutionary in the 1920s. At that time, even the idea of taking a random sample to estimate a percentage or mean of some parameter in an actual population of people was uncommon. For example, political polling, which had existed for about a century, often relied on a "convenience" sample that happened to be feasible, but which could entail substantial bias. Somewhat more scientific was to design a "purposive" sample that was designed to be as representative of the population as possible. It was not until the 1930s that the unconventional notion of selecting individuals in a random manner started to be widely recognized as the best way to assure representativeness.[10]

The beauty of random sampling was that it converted a situation that was ambiguous into one for which the metaphorical lottery assumption was literally true! The process underlying a purposive sample was intended to yield a representative sample but could have been biased in unknown ways. In Fisher's conception, the method of sampling might unwittingly focus on a relevant subset, thus effectively sampling from a subpopulation that differed from the whole population of interest. By willfully ignoring all individual characteristics rather than trying to balance them explicitly, random sampling avoided potential bias *and* created a situation in which the probability distribution of the sampling error would be precisely known.

To implement a random sampling method required first a list of the entire population of interest, termed the sampling frame. For example, a telephone survey of consumers in a particular geographic area might utilize the appropriate telephone directories in order to specify the frame. Then, a system had to be set up to select individuals as if they were being drawn just like tokens in a lottery, or well-mixed balls in a large urn. When the population of interest comprised thousands, or even millions, of individuals, creating a random sample was not a trivial exercise.

Eventually, statisticians created tables of random numbers. These tables contained a long series of digits in a particular order that had been generated by a mechanical process assumed to be effectively random. For example, such a series might be developed by spinning a well-balanced roulette wheel many times. The resulting tables of random numbers could be used in various ways.

Suppose we desired to choose a 1% random sample from a sampling frame of 10,000 potential voters. Then, we could start at any point in the table and note the subsequent four digits. If the digits were 4519, individual 4519 on our sampling-frame list would be selected. Then we could take the next four digits and continue until we had obtained all 100 individuals for our sample. Of course, duplicates would need to be eliminated. (How well I remember such tedious exercises from personal experience during graduate school.)

The first published table of random numbers appeared in 1927, and the largest table, containing one million digits, was generated by the Rand Corporation in 1955.[11] Soon afterward, these "hard-copy" tabulations began to be replaced by computer-generated "pseudorandom" number sequences. Pseudorandom numbers are created by mathematical algorithms that produce sequences of numbers that display no obvious regularities, although the numbers are fully determined by an underlying formula.

Today, it is easy to generate pseudorandom numbers for many purposes using widely available software packages. However, when Fisher originated the idea of randomized experimentation around 1923, random sampling was not common. No published random-number tables existed. So, Fisher and his colleague Frank Yates (1902–1994) had to develop their own "home-grown" table in order to implement random assignment of treatments.

Given this primitive state of the technology for scientific sampling, even for a simple population estimate, it is remarkable that Fisher perceived clearly the critical importance of randomization for comparative studies. By introducing random assignment of treatments, Fisher took the logic of random sampling one step further. Just as contrived ignorance could assure the validity of a simple mean derived from a sample, so it could also guarantee a valid comparison between two treatment options.

Statisticians at that time were not all immediately persuaded. They understood that randomization provided a means of approximately equalizing the average values of all confounding factors that might exist. In this way, the estimated outcome difference between experimental groups would be unbiased. However, some statisticians were concerned that purely random allocation of the treatments could also result in estimates that were more variable than those derived using purposive allocation. That is, by giving up explicit control when the main determinants of the outcome were in fact known, Fisher may have been reducing the bias at the cost of increasing the random variability.

Fisher understood this trade-off and devised various experimental designs that would allow a few designated factors to be controlled explicitly. Such experimental arrangements were known as *factorial designs*.[12] However, for any remaining uncontrolled or unknown factors, Fisher insisted that random allocation of treatments was absolutely essential. In his mind, not only was randomization a way to eliminate bias, but also the *only* method of rigorously accounting for uncontrolled variability among the experimental units.

It was true, he acknowledged, that the actual variability between experimental groups might sometimes be reduced by a purposive approach. However, we could never really know how large the effect of any remaining variability might be. So, we could not adjust properly for this residual variability. For example, could a difference of 4.1 bushels per acre plausibly be the result of unknown differences between the plots of land that had received the new and old seed types? How could we know? Student's formula was effectively a way to test the hypothesis that *for each plot* the outcome would not depend on which treatment was being administered.

This was, according to Fisher, the "null hypothesis" that was being tested. It was not sufficient, he believed, to apply a test of the weaker hypothesis that the *average* outcome for all plots would be identical. In that case, Student's formula would not necessarily provide a valid test of whether there was a true difference between the treatments. In addition, there would be no way to know *how* misleading the use of the standard test might be.

Fisher was the first to understand the nature of such problems, and therefore to grasp the full importance of randomization. The essential problem, he realized, was to ensure that different experimental groups could (under the null hypothesis) be regarded as random samples drawn from the *same population* of units. That is, the causal process that generated each sample must be identical. Only then could Student's test assure us that an observed average difference was unlikely to have arisen by chance.

How, though, could we be sure that the experimental groups would be formed by identical causal processes? Clearly, the "matrix of causal conditions" that determined the intrinsic variability among the experimental units (e.g., plots of land) could not be controlled. But it would still be feasible to guarantee that the process, *whatever it might be*, would be the same for different experimental groups. This could only be accomplished by introducing an element of randomness at the stage of assigning the units randomly to the different treatment modalities.

Statistical Significance

Before the twentieth century, the notion of a formal statistical test of significance did not exist. The first such procedure was developed by Karl Pearson in the 1890s.[13] Much of Pearson's research was concerned with finding the appropriate mathematical description of a probability distribution. For example, he might be analyzing the weight distribution of a certain species of animals. So, he would need to compare the empirical distribution with a theoretical distribution believed to hold. Alternatively, he might wish to determine whether or not the distributions in two different populations were similar to *each other*, rather than to some specified distribution.

In such situations, the empirical difference of interest was influenced by random variability in addition to the systematic difference. To deal with this issue, Pearson devised the Chi-square (χ^2) test. This test required that the variable of interest (length, weight, coloration, etc.) had first to be sorted into a small number of categories, if not already in that form. Pearson wanted a valid criterion that could be used to test whether the frequencies observed in the various categories conformed to the specified theoretical expectation.

In a paper published in 1900 that introduced his new method, Pearson borrowed some data from his friend and colleague Walter F. R. Weldon (1860–1906). Weldon was a biologist who often collaborated with Pearson on studies of animal populations. Weldon in 1894 had performed a "simulation" study to understand better the effects of random variation.[14] To represent a true unknown characteristic of interest, he artificially generated observations for which the underlying theoretical distribution was known. Weldon was trying to find out how close the observed frequencies of the various outcomes would come to the theoretical probabilities.

For example, suppose he knew that a certain measurement of a particular species of insect might assume any integer value between 0 and 12. Moreover, the *theoretical* probability associated with each value was known. Then, if he obtained measurements on thousands of these insects, how close would the observed frequencies of the various possible values be expected to come to these theoretical values? Conversely, how large would the deviations need to be to indicate that the theoretical values were in fact incorrect? At that time, there was no statistical procedure to answer such questions.

Weldon's experiment involved tossing a set of 12 dice over and over again. Each time a die among the 12 landed as a 5 or 6, he counted that as one "success." So, the theoretical distribution he had in mind was a "binomial distribution" in which there were 12 Bernoulli trials, each with a probability 1/3 of success. On each toss of the 12 dice, the expected number of successes was four, but the actual number could range from 0 to 12. Weldon's total series consisted of 26,306 tosses of the 12 dice, and he recorded the outcome (number of successes) for each toss.

The resulting data are shown in Table 10.2. The empirical frequencies are close to those predicted, but there are some evident deviations. Were these "discrepancies" enough to discredit the theorized distribution? Applying his new Chi-square testing procedure, Pearson concluded that indeed they were. He stated that "the odds are 62,499 to 1 against such a system of deviations on a random selection."

TABLE 10.2   Weldon's Dice Experiment: 26,306 Throws of 12 Dice

A "Success" = 5 or 6		
Hits Among 12 Dice	Observed Throws	Expected If $P = 1/3$
0	185	203
1	1149	1216
2	3265	3345
3	5475	5576
4	6114	6273
5	5194	5018
6	3067	2927
7	1331	1255
8+	526	493
Total	**26,306**	**26,306**

Pearson's innovation represented a major breakthrough. However, it was only an approximate test that would not work well for the much smaller samples that Gosset had in mind. Moreover, dividing numerical outcomes, such as yields of barley, into a small number of categories would be arbitrary and inefficient. So, Gosset adapted Pearson's idea of significance testing to fit the context of agricultural or industrial experimentation.

At the time, there was no standard way to express the results of a significance test. Suppose the observed value of the test statistic, such as Pearson's Chi-square, was very large. Then, the probability that such a large value could arise "by chance" would be very small. In Pearson's original example, the probability of a value as large as the one actually observed was extremely small. However, Pearson did not suggest how large a value was needed to rule out the null hypothesis being tested? Could a criterion be established to decide when the evidence was sufficient to "reject" the null hypothesis?

In the early 1900s, it seems that certain rough guidelines were established, but no hard-and-fast criteria. Gosset in his 1908 paper had suggested a rule of thumb that was equivalent to approximately 0.05 that "for most purposes, would be considered significant." Fisher, in his highly influential 1925 book appeared to endorse the 0.05 criterion as well. However, he regarded the choice of cutoff as a prerogative of the researcher, who would apply his professional judgment within the particular scientific context.

From his perspective, reaching a 0.05 level of statistical significance indicated that the effect (such as an estimated mean difference between two seed types) might be worthy of being taken seriously. Anything with a P-value above 0.05 would not be very surprising. A result with a P-value of 0.01 or less would imply strong evidence that the result was not a statistical fluke. Fisher offered this advice not as an attempt to promulgate a strict rule, but rather as a guideline and personal preference that he believed other researchers might find useful.

For him, statistical design and analysis was an integral component of the ongoing *process* of scientific research. Fisher seemed to regard scientific research as a high calling undertaken in the service of bettering the world. His early enchantment with the eugenics movement now seems misguided, but is an example of a youthful idealism that was never fully extinguished. The darker side of his idealism was a kind of intransigence that left him virtually isolated on some issues. For instance, he never accepted the mounting evidence implicating tobacco smoking as the main cause of lung cancer.

Fisher has often been characterized as irascible and intolerant. There is ample evidence that he was not an easy man to deal with. However, his attitude stemmed in part from his frustration about what he saw as the corruption of scientific practice. Science, he felt, was not about solving specific technical problems, narrowly defined. Rather, its mission was to facilitate rational thought by expanding and refining the store of valid knowledge on which such thought could draw:

> If, however, scientific findings are communicated for the enlightenment of other free minds, they may be put sooner or later to the service of a number of purposes, of which we can know nothing. The contribution to the Improvement of Natural Knowledge, which research may accomplish, is disseminated in the hope and faith that, as more becomes known, or more surely known, a great variety of purposes by a great variety of men, and groups of men, will be facilitated.[15]

In this light, the idea of slavishly applying a strict cutoff for statistical significance would have been anathema to Fisher. He treated the P-value as simply a piece, albeit an important piece, of the total evidence to be taken into consideration by the scientist. In the abstract, the *P*-value did not answer a scientific question. So, it is ironic that Fisher is often blamed today for the mindlessly ritualistic obeisance to statistical significance that later developed.

DECISIONS, DECISIONS

Fisher conceived of the research enterprise as primarily intended to generate potentially useful knowledge. The specific manner in which this information could be applied to reach conclusions, he preferred to leave somewhat ambiguous. Attempting to state a "decision problem" too narrowly or explicitly, he believed, would run counter to the ideal of scientific exploration. However, soon after he had laid out some basic principles for statistical analysis, a pair of his early admirers tried to resolve the ambiguity, much to Fisher's chagrin.

An Odd Couple

When Fisher was starting out at Rothamsted in 1919, his primary future *bête noire* was launching his academic career as a lecturer in mathematics at Kharkov University in Poland. Like Fisher, Jerzy Neyman (1894–1981) was a mathematical prodigy whose early life was somewhat rocky.[16] The Russian Revolution and related political crises affecting Eastern Europe had caused major disruptions to his education and career, including health problems and several weeks' imprisonment. Somehow, Neyman managed to survive relatively unscathed.

During his student days, Neyman was introduced to Karl Pearson's writings, which shaped his philosophical outlook and stimulated his interest in probability and statistics. In 1921, Neyman moved to Warsaw, in anticipation of a promised academic post. To support himself while waiting for this appointment to materialize, he became involved in statistical research at a local Agricultural Institute and at the State Meteorological Institute. Finally, in the fall of 1923, he joined the faculty of the University of Warsaw. By 1924, he had published several papers related to agricultural research. However, opportunities in Poland were quite limited, so he sought and received a year-long fellowship to study with Karl

Pearson in London, which was followed by another fellowship to pursue advanced mathematics in Paris.

During his year in Paris, Neyman was visited by Karl Pearson's son, Egon (E. S.) Pearson (1895–1980). Egon was attempting to follow in his father's large statistical footsteps, but also to carve out his own niche. During Neyman's time in London, he and E. S. Pearson had become friendly. Just before Neyman had left for Paris in late 1926, the younger Pearson suggested some new theories that he and Neyman might be able to develop by working together. When the two met in Paris, they discussed Pearson's ideas, leading to a long-distance collaboration that began when Neyman returned to Warsaw in May, 1927.

Neyman and Pearson were quite different in many ways, but complemented each other well. Pearson was reserved, patrician, and intuitive, but somewhat insecure regarding his mathematical talent. Neyman was a survivor; he was ambitious, perhaps somewhat cocky, and adept at rigorous mathematical analysis. Their joint effort proceeded sporadically until 1933, when Pearson "inherited" his father's position as Chairman of the Department of Statistics at Cambridge. He was then able to arrange for Neyman to join his faculty, where their collaboration flourished until 1938, when Neyman received an unexpected offer. Would he be interested in coming to teach at the University of California at Berkeley? Neyman accepted, and over the next 50 years established what was generally considered the premier center of mathematical statistics in the world.

From Knowledge to Decisions

When E. S. Pearson first wrote to Neyman in late 1926, he had been inspired by a comment in a letter from W.S. Gosset.[17] Pearson had been casting around for some general principle or criterion "beyond that of practical expediency" that could be used to compare alternative possible statistical testing procedures. He admired Fisher's brilliance, but was not comfortable with Fisher's intuitive justifications for why he favored certain particular testing procedures over other possibilities in various situations. Gosset's comment supplied what seemed to Pearson an important missing element.

Gosset had suggested that a significance level (*P*-value) weighing against a null hypothesis could not *by itself* be meaningfully interpreted. Suppose, wrote he, that Student's test resulted in a *P*-value of 0.00001 under a null hypothesis of no true difference between two treatments. Would this *necessarily* imply that the null hypothesis was highly unlikely to hold? Not so fast, argued Gosset.[18] Logically, it would depend on whether or not there was an *alternative* hypothesis under which the evidence would have arisen with "a more reasonable probability."

Perhaps Gosset was an admirer of Sherlock Holmes, who famously admonished his friend Dr. Watson: "How often have I said to you that when you have eliminated the impossible, whatever remains, however improbable, must be the truth?"[19] In other words, it is not the absolute degree of probability that matters, only its relative probability compared with other possible alternatives. In the statistical context, when the evidence suggests a (null) hypothesis is very improbable, we ought to be sure there is some *more* probable explanation before counting it out.

Gosset's remark gave Pearson his first inkling of where he and Neyman might be able to make their mark:

> Gosset's reply had a tremendous influence on the direction of my subsequent work, for the first paragraph contains the germ of an idea which has formed the basis of all the later joint researches of Neyman and myself. It is the simple suggestion that the only valid reason for rejecting a statistical hypothesis is that some alternative explains the observed events with a greater degree of probability.[20]

For example, consider a test statistic to distinguish between a single null hypothesis H_0 and a single alternative hypothesis A. Suppose, however, that this test statistic would have the same probability distribution under A as under H_0. Then, no matter what *P*-value would occur, no discrimination *between* the two hypotheses would be provided.

In order to discriminate, the test statistic's probability distribution must *differ* depending on which of the two possible hypotheses is operative. Moreover, the more sensitive this distribution is to which hypothesis is true, the more confidently can we "reject" the null hypothesis. Put simply, we ought to *choose* (decide upon) the explanation that is most consistent with (i.e., least placed in doubt by) the data. Starting with this seemingly plausible premise, Pearson and Neyman went on between 1926 and 1938 to lay the foundations of an elaborate theoretical framework.

This Neyman–Pearson decision theory aimed to place the derivation and comparison of possible statistical tests on a rigorous logical and mathematical footing. Eventually, several innovations were developed that proved especially useful in the context of industrial product development and quality control. Most notable were the concepts of a *confidence interval* and the *power* of a statistical test. The confidence interval is essentially a range of values for the parameter of interest (e.g., a probability or mean) that is consistent with the data in a specific mathematical sense. The power is a measure of the sensitivity of the statistical test to detect a true effect when it exists.

Neyman and Pearson initially saw themselves as refining and extending Fisher's groundbreaking ideas. Indeed, Fisher was at first cautiously supportive of their efforts. It was an exciting time for the field, with rapid adoption and expansion of small-sample statistical methods. By the 1940s, the modern statistical paradigm had fully emerged. It was based mainly on Fisher's basic approach to statistical estimation and testing, amended by the Neyman–Pearson innovations.

The core concept of Neyman–Pearson theory was to evaluate any particular procedure for making statistical inferences in terms of its long-run properties as a *decision-rule*. Each application of a particular procedure, such as a test or confidence interval, was regarded as a random occurrence in a hypothetical sequence of decisions. A statistical test, for example, was judged by its long-run performance. Specifically, was the frequency of errors sufficiently low? A primary preoccupation of mathematical statisticians in the 1950s and 1960s became the derivation of tests and confidence intervals that could be proved optimal in the sense of committing the fewest errors.

In effect, the principle of willful ignorance was expanded by Neyman and Pearson to encompass *testing occasions*. A statistical procedure was effectively being patterned after an industrial machine. The main "product" of such a mathematical device was a *decision* to accept or reject the null hypothesis. In this light, the level of statistical significance was recast as the probability of making an error of Type I, pronounced as "type one." A Type I error meant that the test would *reject* the null hypothesis when it was actually true. Fisher's 0.05 significance level became the usual default "setting" for operating the statistical machinery.

Once the Type I error probability, or "alpha level," had been set (usually at 0.05), the second "operating characteristic" of the machine could be considered. This was the probability of accepting the null hypothesis when it was false, or Type II error. Conversely, the probability of avoiding a Type II error (by correctly rejecting the null hypothesis when it was false) was termed the power of the statistical test. So, the usual objective in designing a test was to obtain the maximum power possible at the 0.05 (or other stipulated) alpha level. However, the power would depend on the particular alternative hypothesis and was therefore somewhat arbitrary. This led to the idea of determining a gold standard procedure that would have maximum power regardless of the particular alternative hypothesis.

This brief overview only scratches the surface of the many technical issues raised by the Neyman–Pearson decision-theoretic approach. These issues required advanced mathematical methods to unravel. As a result, the field of statistics became increasingly viewed as a branch of applied mathematics. Statistics departments in academia became dominated by mathematicians rather than applied researchers. The highly technical problems of interest to the professors of mathematical statistics became increasingly divorced from the practical concerns of applied statisticians, let alone clinicians.

Rage Against the Machine

By the mid-1930s, several disputes over various methodological issues had begun to separate Fisher from Neyman and Pearson. Fisher grew increasingly disenchanted with the wrong turn that he perceived the field of statistics to be taking, spearheaded by his erstwhile disciples. When E. S. Pearson had been appointed Chairman of the Department of Statistics at Cambridge in 1933, Fisher had become the Galton Professor in the Department of Eugenics. When Neyman subsequently joined Pearson's group the following year, the level of tension soon grew palpable. Given this untenable situation, Neyman's departure was inevitable.

The source of their irreconcilable disagreements was a deep difference of philosophical perspectives, exacerbated by a clash of strong personalities. At the risk of greatly oversimplifying, I would boil the philosophical differences down to two main issues. First, Fisher regarded statistical design and analysis as inseparable from broader issues of scientific research and inductive inference. So, he was reluctant to regard the scientist's task as entirely reducible to an abstract problem of mathematical analysis. Second, Neyman viewed statistical methods through the narrow lens of frequentist probability. Fisher's more nuanced concept of probability I have previously tried to describe.

In Fisher's view, statistical methods ought to facilitate the growth of *scientific knowledge* by sharpening the process of *inductive reasoning*. Inductive reasoning, he thought, could not be reduced to pure logic:

> In inductive reasoning, we are forming part of the process by which new knowledge is created. ... inductive reasoning is the study of the embryology of knowledge, of the process by means of which truth is extracted from its native ore in which it is fused with much error.[21]

This kind of metaphorical rhetoric was lost on Neyman, the hard-headed mathematician and positivist. Neyman appreciated Fisher's seminal methodological contributions, but wanted to replace what seemed to him Fisher's woolly-headed intuitions with rigorous mathematical logic.

To accomplish this program, he required some new principle upon which a mathematical superstructure could be constructed. That principle was the idea of choice between alternatives that Pearson had initially derived from Gosset's letter. In his discussion of Fisher's 1935 paper, Neyman clearly stated this principle:

> Now what could be considered as a sufficiently simple and unquestionable principle in statistical work? I think the basic conception here is the conception of frequency of errors in judgment.

This was to be the rock upon which he and Pearson would erect their new statistical edifice. They had redefined the fundamental problem confronting the statistician. No longer was the summarization of data and production of general knowledge the primary focus. The hazy notion of "inductive reasoning" would be supplanted by the precise and operationally defined concept of "inductive behavior." Inductive behavior was predicated on the idea that the probability distribution of a test statistic was interpretable in terms of actual frequencies. Setting a *P*-value of 0.05 as the criterion for rejection meant that the test would incorrectly reject a true null hypothesis 5% of the time in the long run. But, nothing could be said about the probability of being right or wrong on any specific testing occasion.

Fisher argued that this imaginary series of indistinguishable testing occasions was meaningless. He interpreted the 0.05 in relation to the particular test at hand; a value of the test statistic that reached a P-value of 0.05 would be rather surprising if the null hypothesis were true. The strength of this surprise would be similar to what we would experience upon drawing a black ball out of an urn that contained 19 white balls and a single black one. The P-value, according to Fisher, was a piece of evidence meant to be considered by the scientist in the context of all other knowledge and information available.

Fisher rejected the idea of implicitly extending willful ignorance to a sequence of future testing occasions. Recall his remark about probability, if properly understood, applying to events or statements that were "singular and unique." Thus, the evidence provided by a significance test pertained to that individual testing occasion. Knowing that a particular testing procedure was correct 95% of the time would not tell you how likely it was to be correct on *this* occasion.

After 25 years of feuding, Fisher and Neyman had come no closer to understanding each others' perspectives. In a paper entitled "Silver Jubilee of my Dispute with Fisher" in 1961 (the year before Fisher's death), Neyman wrote:

> The subject of the dispute may be symbolized by the opposing terms 'inductive reasoning' and 'inductive behavior.' Professor Fisher is a known proponent of inductive reasoning. After a conscientious effort ... I came to the conclusion that, at least in the sense of Fisher, the term is empty.[22]

For his part, Fisher acknowledged grudgingly that inductive behavior had some validity in certain areas such as game theory and industrial quality control. But he regarded its employment in scientific research as a dangerous perversion:

> The Natural Sciences can only be successfully conducted by responsible and independent thinkers applying their minds and their imaginations to the detailed interpretation of verifiable observations. The idea that this responsibility can be delegated to a giant computer programmed with Decision Functions belongs to the phantasy of circles rather remote from scientific research.[23]

When Fisher penned these words in the mid-1950s his battle against the "giant computer" was already lost. By the time I was studying statistics as a graduate student in the late 1960s, the Neyman–Pearson version of statistics had come to predominate. Here is how the subject of statistics was introduced in a popular text published in 1959:

> Years ago a statistician might have claimed that statistics deals with the processing of data. As a result of relatively recent formulations of statistical theory, today's statistician will be more likely to say that statistics is concerned with decision making in the face of uncertainty.[24]

Fisher's nightmare of a computer programmed with decision functions has become an everyday reality. Rather than informing a "responsible and independent thinker" who can use her "mind and imagination," the computer has effectively taken over the primary responsibility for making inferences.

The Bayesian Revival

Neyman and Pearson had succeeded in resolving the ambiguities of Fisher's more intuitive approach to testing and estimation. Their solution was to recast the problem of statistical inference in operational terms, as a matter of making decisions. Furthermore, by focusing on behavior over the long run, their approach remained squarely within the objectivistic frequentist framework. This had the advantage, from their viewpoint, of taking subjective judgment out of the equation. The statistician or researcher did not have to interpret the results of a statistical procedure, but simply to make sure that the procedure was implemented correctly. Then, the conclusion to be reached would be made automatically.

The emphasis on decisions was (and still is) either explicitly or tacitly accepted by most practicing statisticians. However, there have always remained some who are uncomfortable with the frequentist underpinnings of Neyman–Pearson doctrine. In Chapter 8, I explained how the use of Bayes's Theorem to obtain inverse probabilities had fallen out of favor around 1840. Then in the 1920s, Frank Ramsey and Bruno de Finetti tried to breathe new life into this long-discredited idea. Their ideas stimulated a brilliant mathematical statistician, Jimmie Savage, to lead a revolt against the Neyman–Pearson dominance.

For Savage and his followers, the statistician's primary task was to calculate the posterior probability distribution of the parameter of interest (e.g., probability or mean value):

> The difficulty in the objectivistic position is this. In any objectivistic view, the probabilities can apply fruitfully only to repetitive events, that is, to certain processes; … Thus, the existence of evidence for any proposition can never, on an objectivistic view, be expressed by saying that the proposition is true with a certain probability. Again, if one must choose among certain courses of action in the light of experimental evidence, it is not meaningful, in terms of objective probability, to compute which of these actions is most promising.[25]

These latter-day Bayesians accepted wholeheartedly the idea that statistical inference was really about decision-making under uncertainty. However, in their view, all probabilities were inherently subjective, or as Savage preferred, *personal*. So, there was no philosophical or ideological problem in expressing uncertainty as the probability that a proposition (hypothesis) was true. Indeed, following Ramsey and de Finetti, Savage defined probability in terms of personal betting behavior. A person's probability was simply a useful measure of the odds at which she would be willing to wager.

From this perspective, a statistical test had a different interpretation. Rather than a behavioral long-run strategy, it was a guide to action in the present instance. Take the simplest case of a choice between a null hypothesis H_0 (say, zero difference in yield of barley) and an alternative A (say, at least 5 bushels greater using a new fertilizer). Let us denote the statistical evidence by E. Then, the Bayesian would like to obtain the two probabilities: $P(H_0|E)$ and $P(A|E)$. This seems completely straightforward and relevant to the problem at hand. Yet, this appealing Bayesian methodology remains controversial. Why?

Part of the resistance is attributable to the sheer mathematical difficulty in many situations of calculating the posterior probability distributions. However, the main reasons are philosophical. In general, the idea of relying on subjective probabilities in matters as serious as scientific research leaves most statisticians feeling somewhat queasy. There seems to be an inherent contradiction between the presumed objectivity and authority of science and the injection of personal beliefs.

Savage was well aware of this objection and addressed himself to those who "consider probability an objective property of certain physical systems" and who thus "look on any personal view of probability as, at best, an attempt to predict some of the behavior of abnormal, or at any rate unscientific, people." To such critics, he responded cogently that science cannot and should not be devoid of personal judgment:

> I would reply that the personalistic view incorporates all of the universally acceptable criteria for reasonableness in judgment known to me, and that, when any criteria that may have been overlooked are brought forward, they will be welcomed into the personalistic view. The criteria incorporated in the personalistic view do not guarantee agreement on all questions among honest and freely communicating people, even in principle. That incompleteness, if one will call it that, does not distress me, ...[26]

Savage rejected in principle the platonic ideal of true probabilities upon which all reasonable scientists could, or necessarily should, ultimately agree.

The adoption of subjectivism opened the door for using Bayes's Theorem to generate posterior probabilities of hypotheses. In theory at least, this method can be applied in any situation. However, there is one not-so-small difficulty. As I have explained previously, to start up the Bayesian engine, you need to plug it into a prior probability distribution. This is the real sticking point. Where does this prior distribution come from? There are two main approaches to this delicate problem.

One approach relies on Laplace's venerable principle of insufficient reason. When we are completely ignorant about the operative source (cause, hypothesis, distribution), we simply assume that all such sources are equally likely. This was also Bayes's postulate, which he hoped might solve the problem of induction. In effect, we regard the value of the unknown hypothesis as a random draw from a metaphorical lottery. As I have discussed, this superficially appealing idea can run into serious problems of ambiguity.

Remember, for example, Keynes's troublesome urn with the two different plausible ways that the unknown distribution of the proportion of white balls could be specified. In short, there is no unique way to translate pure ignorance into a prior distribution. Some Bayesians have adopted a pragmatic attitude toward this dilemma.[27] They regard the prior distribution as an approximate representation of our ignorance and rely on the fact that a substantial amount of data will eventually swamp the impact of the prior.

From this perspective, it may be possible to define a prior that is somewhat vague or "uninformative." Using such an uninformative prior, the precise form of the prior will often not matter much. However, an element of arbitrariness still enters the picture to some degree. Moreover, the impact of this arbitrariness might not be trivial, especially when we deal with a complex statistical model.

A second approach is to take the bull by the horns and select a prior distribution intended to reflect the existing state of knowledge. This knowledge might be entirely personal, or it might represent some consensus of scientific opinion. Consider the problem of medical diagnosis. The prior distribution that the patient has Condition X is often called the *base rate* of this condition in some relevant population. This base rate has a major effect on the posterior probability of Condition X after the patient's results on diagnostic testing are obtained. If the base rate is known, even approximately, then to determine the posterior probability using Bayes's Theorem is straightforward and uncontroversial. If, on the other hand, we have only a vague sense of the true base rate, or no idea at all, the posterior probability will be ill-defined.

Now imagine a much more ambiguous problem—analyzing the result of a pivotal clinical trial to evaluate the efficacy of a new drug. Assume that we have some information, based on previous small-scale studies, to suggest that the new treatment is somewhat better than a placebo. We also have some relevant data from animal studies and basic biochemistry. Should this prior knowledge be taken into account somehow? Is our knowledge sufficient to allow us to formulate a prior probability distribution of the improvement in response rate compared with a placebo? Such questions are very difficult to answer. As a result, although Bayesian analysis has made inroads in certain domains, it remains somewhat outside the mainstream of scientific research.

MACHINE-MADE KNOWLEDGE

Scientific research entails a set of activities and procedures that are not readily reducible to a simple formula. The process of generating new scientific knowledge depends on the interplay between

- hypothesis generation within a context of accepted *theory*;
- techniques to exert experimental *control*;
- methods for obtaining relevant *data*;
- analyses for hypothesis *testing*; and
- additional studies for refinement and *replication*.

The validity and credibility of a scientific finding is a product of the researcher's skill in carrying out these tasks.

During the past 50 years, however, one criterion has come to assume undue importance—statistical significance. More than any other factor, attaining statistical significance at the conventional 0.05 level has become a passport to presumed validity. A significant result is often interpreted to mean that the hypothesis being tested is in some sense true, or real. In this way, the less objective criteria that used to enter consideration tend to be discounted. In effect, study interpretation has to a large extent become automated, or algorithmic.

This situation, which is now so predominant, did not come about all at once. Initially, as I explained, the basic idea of testing for statistical significance was invented by Karl Pearson. In the 1920s, Fisher formalized and developed this idea much more extensively in the context of randomized agricultural experiments. In such a randomized study, the significance level (*P*-value) provided evidence that an observed effect might be *causal*. If an average difference between two seed types, for example, was highly significant, the only plausible explanation was that one treatment *caused* more grain to grow than the other.

As the use of randomized experimentation expanded into various industrial applications, reliance on statistical significance as a criterion for causality became more firmly established. So, when randomized experimentation penetrated the field of medical research in the 1950s, the *P*-value assumed a prominent role. Initially, this was not problematic in light of the kinds of medical interventions being studied. For the most part these were various types of antibiotics or vaccines for which the effects were quite uniform and context-independent.

However, by the 1970s, medical research had become focused primarily on complex chronic conditions such as cancer, heart disease, diabetes, and arthritis. In addition, applications of statistical methods had expanded widely to include epidemiology, economics, and various social sciences. These fields rely mainly on *observational* studies, in which randomization is not feasible. Statisticians were careful not to refer to the correlations they uncovered in these studies as causal, but the connotation of statistical significance as warranting an effect as "real" had become almost universal.

The transition of statistical significance from one valuable *aspect* of the research process to a virtual seal of approval has had profound consequences. Even for randomized studies, the importance of statistical significance has been oversold. In the various applications in biomedical and social science today, the relevant theory and degree of experimental control are often relatively weak. Moreover, there are many practical challenges involved in implementing studies without introducing bias. For example, there may be problems of (nonrandom) missing data or patient dropout that can undermine the intended research design. Therefore, the presumed link between statistical significance and causality cannot be taken for granted.

In *observational* studies, the situation is even worse; the advantages that would be conferred by randomization do not exist, even in theory. So, a result can be highly significant, but not necessarily causal. For example, a significant correlation between two variables can be the result of some uncontrolled third variable. Such *confounding* can complicate the interpretation of study results in many ways, as discussed extensively in the methodological literature.

Ideally, science advances by discovering causal relationships that are stable; these relationships can be expected to *persist*. Those relationships that endure not only over time, but also under a broad range of conditions are of most value. In many studies, however, certain of the causal conditions responsible may be transitory or local. Consequently, even a truly causal effect may not hold up over time. Statistical significance cannot by itself establish persistence and generality. To do that, it is necessary to *replicate* the results at different times and under different conditions.

There is no doubt that statistical significance remains a valuable tool in the scientist's arsenal, especially under the tightly controlled conditions of a well-implemented randomized experiment. However, the degree of corroboration it provides should not be construed as *absolute*; rather, this evidence must be evaluated in the context of the overall design, conduct, and analysis of the study. To the extent that mechanical interpretations based solely on statistical criteria are mindlessly cranked off the assembly line of research, science is being impoverished.

CHAPTER 11

THE LOTTERY IN SCIENCE

The core idea underlying mathematical probability is that it is often useful to regard a particular aspect of the world as a metaphorical lottery. This expedient of regarding observed variability *as if* it has resulted from a lottery has provided many practical benefits. However, it can be a serious mistake to forget that this metaphor is not *real*. In reality, there exist actual generating processes that exhibit varying degrees of regularity. At one extreme, there are processes that are for all practical and completely deterministic purposes, such as Newton's laws of motion. At the other extreme are the subatomic phenomena described by quantum mechanics, which appear to be completely random.

Most of applied science deals with processes situated somewhere between these extremes. So, strictly speaking, the lottery model does not apply. In general, something akin to Peirce's "would-be" or Popper's propensities might be a more valid conception. However, the lottery model implicit in additive mathematical probability has come to dominate our thinking. We attempt to separate neatly the presumed regular causes from the presumed random "error." Beginning with Galton and Pearson, our statistical theory has been built upon the idea that all "unexplained" variability must be treated as essentially random.

Willful Ignorance: The Mismeasure of Uncertainty, First Edition. Herbert I. Weisberg.
© 2014 John Wiley & Sons, Inc. Published 2014 by John Wiley & Sons, Inc.

This assumption may seem innocuous, but in fact has had profound consequences. It has led us in many contexts to conceive (and treat) individuals as indistinguishable. This reductionism has proved particularly useful as a means of "managing" populations *en masse*. From a corporate or government viewpoint, it is highly efficient to categorize millions of individuals into broad classes. Willfully ignoring all other factors is necessary for their purposes. Thus, probability and statistics may serve as an essential component of a technology for dealing with large groups.

This technological function is not in itself either good or bad, but it is susceptible to a variety of abuses. So, it is critical not to overlook the potential implications for dehumanization that can be facilitated by this technology. The Lottery in Babylon, a short story by Jorge Luis Borges, presents an eerie portrayal of a mythical world that is *truly* ruled by randomness.[1] Over time, every aspect of life has gradually come to be governed by an all-powerful Lottery, presumed to be operated by a shadowy Corporation. The intentions of this mythical organization, if indeed it exists at all or ever did, become subject to wild speculations. In the end, everything meaningful in "Babylon" has been totally obliterated, even a sense of one's personal identity. Nothing any longer is certain. Nothing is under anyone's control, and no one is personally responsible.

There is something deeply haunting and sinister about this tyranny of chance, a sense of something gone terribly wrong. In more pessimistic moments, I experience a similar feeling about our current research enterprise. For me, the joys of science have always revolved around the excitement of new and often unexpected discoveries. Research is ideally a quest for deeper knowledge and insight. Extracting truth from its native ore, as Fisher described this process, can be a source of great satisfaction. Indeed, I was originally drawn to statistics as a field of study primarily for this reason. Sadly, much of what passes for biomedical and social science today lacks these attractive qualities, as the line between science and technology has been blurred.

SCIENTIFIC PROGRESS

Technology is a two-edged sword.[2] It is the great facilitator of advancement toward predefined ends. Statistical methodology has become merely a special kind of technology that is geared toward making decisions. Much of science also entails decision-making. Indeed, the need to make good decisions is a prime motivation for much analytic effort. However, by attempting to optimize a specific decision that happens to be currently in view, we may be sacrificing broader or longer-term objectives.

Fifty years ago, John Tukey suggested that we are often better served by fashioning informational building blocks whose future utility remains somewhat ambiguous. Tukey drew an important distinction between decisions and conclusions. Like Fisher, Tukey argued that scientific progress results from the establishment of a body of knowledge that has broad potential relevance:

> This body grows by the reaching of conclusions- by acts whose essential characteristics differ widely from the making of decisions. Conclusions are established with careful regard to evidence, but without regard to consequences of specific actions in specific circumstances.... Conclusions are withheld until adequate evidence has accumulated.[3]

Tukey, himself a consummate mathematical statistician, decried the increasing emphasis on complex technical solutions designed to achieve optimality for narrowly defined decision problems. He advocated paying increased attention to "exploratory" analysis aimed at detecting "indications" that might cumulatively and incrementally lead to solutions of complex problems.

Tukey and a handful of colleagues regarded *exploratory* analysis as akin to detective work, which is needed to provide a broad and deep evidentiary base for subsequent *confirmatory* analyses. They appreciated that, unlike confirmatory analysis, data exploration required other tools besides probability theory. In fact, Tukey wrote an entire book on *Exploratory Data Analysis* that never even mentioned the word probability![4] His intent was to turn the attention of statisticians in another direction:

> The processes of criminal justice are clearly divided between the search for the evidence ... and the evaluation of the evidence's strength ... In data analysis a similar distinction is helpful. Exploratory data analysis is detective in character. Confirmatory data analysis is judicial or quasi-judicial in character.... As all detective stories remind us, many of the circumstances surrounding a crime are accidental or misleading. Equally, many of the indications to be discerned in bodies of data are accidental or misleading.... *To fail to collect all appearances because some—or even most—are only accidents would, however, be gross misfeasance* ...[5]

Tukey hoped to restore a balance between open-ended discovery of potentially important context-dependent information and mathematical techniques for sorting the signal from the noise. The ultimate decisions, he believed, were mainly in the province of those with substantive knowledge. The role of data analysis was to provide quantitative evidence and to assist, but not to replace, the substantive expert to sift through and interpret the evidence. By focusing exclusively on decision-making, the researcher was effectively cutting the clinician out of the "judicial" process of evaluation.

Tukey's division of responsibility between the exploratory (investigative) and confirmatory (judicial) functions roughly parallels the two dimensions, ambiguity and doubt, that can contribute to uncertainty. Investigation is more open-ended and inclusive, attempting to clarify the relevant circumstances surrounding the crime. Before sufficient evidence has been amassed, it may be impossible to frame the issue in terms of the probability of guilt for a particular suspect. In science, resolving ambiguity by acquiring relevant evidence and refining hypotheses generally must precede the decision-making stage. Progress in science, just as in crime-solving, requires a balance between exploration and confirmation.

Tukey was far ahead of his time. In the 1960s, sources of data and powerful computational tools to explore data were very limited. But as these constraints are being lifted, his message is becoming timely. Consider, for example, the two areas of research I mentioned in Chapter 2: the benefits of early childhood educational programs and the efficacy of aspirin for prevention of heart attacks. Each of these is usually framed simplistically as a policy decision problem. Should early educational intervention be widely implemented? Should aspirin be prescribed routinely? In each case, a simple yea or nay is expected. Not surprisingly, the answers to such poorly posed questions have largely failed to expand the boundaries of our useful knowledge.

Early Childhood Education

Evaluations of early childhood programs, especially Head Start, *have* yielded some important general conclusions. We have learned that such interventions cannot by themselves produce substantial improvements in long-term academic performance. It is also likely, though less certain, that some particular types of "high-quality" programs have the potential to provide a variety of benefits to particular categories of children and their families. These general conclusions were evident by the 1970s, but research activity for over 40 years has largely persisted in ignoring them.

Instead, the vague hypothesis that preschool programs *in general* can exert a strong and lasting impact on academic performance has been examined again and again, with essentially the same negative results. As an unfortunate consequence, real opportunities to identify specific factors that *might* make a real difference for *some* children have been squandered. There is no doubt that enriched early education is a good thing, but also no doubt that it is expensive and variable in its implementation and effects.

Creative research designed to identify *which* subgroups (if any) of children can receive the most long-term benefit from *which* types of initiatives might help to inform judgments about how best to allocate finite resources. In other words, research must seek to identify specific characteristics of children and families coupled with specific attributes of educational programs that could yield the most leverage for positive change. Put in Fisherian terms, we must attempt to *recognize* certain *relevant* variables that distinguish individuals in meaningful ways. The kinds of knowledge we are capable of acquiring might be less certain than that provided by a "rigorous" experiment aimed at reaching a definitive answer. But, the "indications" accumulated might contribute to solutions in the future in ways that we cannot yet envision.

At huge expense and opportunity-cost, we continue to search for simplistic, context-independent, causal factors. Statisticians call the presumed impact of such factors the "main effects." The main effects are *assumed* to be of primary importance. Focusing on potential interactions is largely forbidden, at least until the main effects have been established. I have called this prevailing attitude the *main-effect fallacy*. If Peirce and Popper were right, this approach is upside-down. I interpret Peirce's notion of a "would-be" to be a property of something that determines its behavior *in combination with* the relevant existing circumstances. This propensity exists but can rarely if ever be isolated, because there is no "occasion that would bring out the full consequence" of the would-be. So, if the relevant causal processes are indeed something like propensities, then virtually everything is highly context-dependent.

If so, the main effects may be no more real than Quetelet's "average man," and hunting for these unicorns an exercise in futility. Worse, by committing the main-effect fallacy, we fail to notice any real interactive effects that may be hiding in the underbrush. Perhaps worse still, our research contributes almost no real insight to move us forward. A true *science* of education would develop general principles along the lines of Tukey's *conclusions*. These would form the foundation for technologies to implement these principles. To focus directly on identifying improved technologies before establishing a firm scientific underpinning is a recipe for failure.

Aspirin for Prevention

In a similar way, clinical studies of aspirin for cardiovascular prevention have yielded some important conclusions. We know that the risk of a myocardial infarction (MI) can be reduced for some individuals. Moreover, we know that a remarkably low dose of aspirin is necessary to achieve this benefit. We also know that a major potential effect of aspirin is to increase the risk of bleeding events, which in rare cases can be very serious. The biological mechanisms that cause these effects are understood in some detail. Basically, aspirin reduces platelet aggregation, the tendency for blood to clot. This effect is beneficial for preventing an MI, but can occasionally cause harmful bleeding. Finally, evidence is emerging that indicates low-dose aspirin may reduce the risks of several types of cancer, although the extent and mechanisms of these protective effects are not yet well understood.

What is clear from over 40 years of research is that aspirin can be highly effective in reducing mortality and morbidity for certain individuals. What remains unclear is exactly *for whom* the benefits outweigh the risks, and by how much. In part, the failure to obtain this knowledge stems from our lack of necessary biological theory. For instance, relevant genetic information has only recently begun to be available. However, a major obstacle is the statistical paradigm itself.

Early studies focused on a very high-risk population, men who had previously experienced an MI. These "secondary prevention" studies indicated that a low dose (less than 100 mg) of aspirin per day could reduce the probability of a second MI by about 30%. Moreover, the increase in bleeding events was very small. Subsequent research has mainly attempted to learn whether these benefits would extend to a much broader "primary prevention" population, men and women without a previous MI.

The results have been disappointing. Aspirin does provide some protection, but the effect is less dramatic than for those at very high risk. In addition, the risk of bleeding-related side effects is somewhat greater, though still quite low. These results are not very surprising, because aspirin's anti-clotting ability causes much of both its beneficial (reducing MIs) and deleterious (increasing bleeds) clinical effects. Thus, the consequences of a reduced clotting tendency will differ across individuals and be most favorable for those with a high predisposition for clotting, as evidenced by a prior cardiovascular event.

In this light, attempting to make a simple yes/no determination about aspirin use for a broad population seems misguided. There is no "average person" when it comes to such a complex medical recommendation. The probability of suffering an MI depends on many factors (genetic predispositions, other concomitant medications, age, gender, etc.). Aspirin will have an impact on this probability, but its effect may depend on a variety of individual characteristics, circumstances, and future eventualities.[6]

Physicians know all this, but the evidence-based recommendations they receive relate to broad reference classes, not to specific individuals. So, the physician is urged to ignore most of the individual factors she might deem pertinent. If she does attempt to adjust for them judgmentally, she may do so hesitantly and apologetically. But imagine that research during the past 40 years had focused more on reaching some conclusions about who might reap the benefits of aspirin therapy and why.

There are two possible ways such an alternative universe would have turned out. In one scenario, we would have garnered some useful knowledge to refine our evidence-based recommendations for individual doctors and patients. In another, we would reluctantly have concluded that our knowledge base was insufficient to identify meaningful individual variation. Even in this disappointing situation, there might be a silver lining. We might have discovered some promising statistical "indications" that suggested new avenues of research. Perhaps one of these new directions would now become interpretable in light of progress in relevant areas of basic science. For example, an unfolding understanding of human genetics to an extent that was unimaginable circa 1980 might hold the key to why and how aspirin might be highly beneficial for some but inadvisable for others.

FOOLED BY CAUSALITY

The indisputable success of probability theory and statistical thinking has engendered a great irony. On the one hand, we are being bombarded with advice to anticipate ubiquitous unpredictability and randomness. The main message seems to be that most of our causal explanations of reality are fantasies we make up to achieve a false sense of security. Our tendency to concoct unsubstantiated theories is termed the *narrative fallacy*. We can supposedly do better by relying more on hard data and less on our intuitions. We are advised to accept the vagaries of chance and attain a more sophisticated understanding of probability and statistics.

The irony here is that we are entering an era in which these valuable lessons, while often helpful, are becoming oversold. Like the proverbial generals who always fight the last war, we fail to grasp some important changes that are transpiring. Yes, we are often "fooled by randomness," and susceptible to a variety of "cognitive biases," and oversimplifications. Our analytical weaknesses are not difficult to document. But to dwell almost exclusively on these flaws opens us to another type of error.

In the conduct of scientific research, we have the choice of a half-empty or half-full perspective. We must judge whether we really do understand what is going on to some useful extent, or must defer to quantitative empirical evidence. Statistical reasoning seems completely objective, but can blind us to nuances and subtleties. In the past, the problem was to teach people, especially scientists and clinicians, to apply critical skepticism to their intuitions and judgments. Thinking statistically has been an essential corrective to widespread naiveté and quackery. However, in many fields of endeavor, the volumes of potentially relevant data are growing exponentially.[7] Therefore, willful ignorance must become more strategic, allowing us to move beyond main effects and discern fruitful avenues for more refined analyses. Unfortunately, the capacities for critical judgment and deep insight we need may be starting to atrophy, just as opportunities to apply them more productively are increasing.

Heuristics and Biases

In 1854, George Boole published *The Laws of Thought*.[8] Of central importance, according to Boole, was the calculus of probability. However, Boole would have been stunned at the extent to which mathematical probability has become the very touchstone for rational thinking. Exactly 100 years later, another influential treatise revealed how far things had come. In *Clinical vs. Statistical Prediction*, psychologist Paul Meehl propounded a radical thesis: for guiding clinical decisions, at least in the context of psychology, "actuarial" predictions based on statistical frequencies were nearly always more reliable than those based on subjective clinical judgment.

In 138 pages of elegant and thoughtful prose, Meehl laid out the arguments for and against using an actuarial, or as we might say today an *algorithmic*, approach to prediction. While acknowledging the importance of clinical insight for therapeutic intervention, he produced empirical evidence that clearly supported the actuarial approach for making diagnostic predictions:

> In spite of the defects and ambiguities present, let me emphasize the brute fact that we have here ... some 16 to 20 studies involving a comparison of clinical and actuarial methods, *in all but one of which the predictions made actuarially were either approximately equal or superior to those made by clinicians*.[9]

Meehl's little monograph ruffled many feathers and has spawned a huge literature. His basic finding has been quite consistently replicated and extended to many other areas of decision-making. In the 1970s, Meehl's seminal work stimulated what has come to be known as the "heuristics and biases" (HB) theory of cognition. The main founders of this approach were two Israeli-born psychologists, Daniel Kahneman and Amos Tversky (1937–1996). Along with many of their followers, these pioneers developed the field of behavioral economics, for which Kahnemen received the Nobel Prize in Economics in 2002.[10]

Kahneman and Tversky perceived that judgments, and the decisions that flow from them, are often less than optimal. Their criterion of optimality was based on classical economic theory for decision-making under uncertainty. Theoretically, a rational decision-maker takes into account a range of possible future outcomes. For each possible alternative option under consideration, he then assesses the probabilities associated with the possible outcomes and the value (utility) of each. Ideally, he compares the resulting expected utility of each available option and selects the one that yields the highest expected utility. Their research has done much to disabuse academic economists of the idea that economic actors are rational decision-makers in this sense.

In his recent popular exposition, *Thinking, Fast and Slow*, Kahneman explains the genesis of the HB theory he and Tversky originated:

> Social scientists in the 1970's broadly accepted two ideas about human nature. First people are generally rational, and their thinking is generally sound. Second, emotions such as fear, affection, and hatred explain most of the occasions in which people depart from rationality. Our article challenged both assumptions without discussing them directly. We documented systematic errors in the thinking of normal people, and we traced these errors to the machinery of cognition rather than to the corruption of thought by emotion.[11]

The HB research program has generated thousands of studies about the simplifying shortcuts (heuristics) we commonly apply, and the mistakes (biases) that result. A major aspect of this research concerns probability and statistics, which are regarded as gold standards for logical thinking. In numerous experimental settings, HB research has attempted to test whether we correctly apply rational (probabilistic) decision-making as assumed by economic theory. These studies have repeatedly shown that we appear to be very poor practical statisticians.

Kahneman alludes to two distinct systems of thinking. "System 1 operates automatically and quickly, with little or no effort and no sense of conscious control."[12] *System 1* thinking is generally easy and *fast*. (When driving to pick my wife up at work, I am mostly operating with System 1.) "*System 2* allocates attention to the effortful mental activities that demand it, including complex calculations." System 2 thinking is hard and *slow*. (While attempting to write this paragraph, I am making heavy use of System 2.)

Theoretically, System 1 is said to be intimately connected to our innate intuition (or illusion) of causality. It has evolved to make us aware of important factors in our environment that we perceive, rightly or wrongly, as causal agents. We can then respond unconsciously in a reasonably appropriate manner when these factors are encountered. In a stable environment, System 1 can be highly adaptive and efficient. But, it is not very useful for dealing with novel situations or complex problem-solving.

That is where System 2 comes in: "Statistical thinking derives conclusions about individual cases from properties of categories and ensembles. Unfortunately, System 1 does not have the capability for this mode of reasoning; System 2 can learn to think statistically, but few people receive the necessary training." So, our inability to apply correctly the logic of probability and to analyze statistics is alleged to be a main source of irrational behavior. We rely on System 1, because it is easier and provides the familiar and comforting illusions of causality. Probability and statistics are inherently difficult for us and can be challenging to employ correctly, even for those with specialized training.

The message that we cannot, in general, trust our intuition and judgment is disheartening. But at least, we are told, we can be a little *less* biased by studying statistical theory, and fighting gamely against our naturally irrational inclinations. However, even that path may often be foreclosed if Nassim Taleb is right. He correctly emphasizes that the world is far more unpredictable than implied by standard probability theory.[13] So, there may be no recourse but to expect the unexpected, and attempt to adopt strategies that are resistant to large unanticipated shocks, or even profit from them.

To make matters worse, even purported subject matter experts in many areas are quite poor prognosticators. For example, most financial analysts and stockbrokers are generally no more (or less) successful than market averages, except occasionally by chance. Those who emphasize our weak predictive abilities often cite the research of Philip Tetlock, author of *Expert Political Judgment*. Tetlock has documented the fallibility of experts when it comes to predictions of future political and military developments. Tetlock adduces evidence that "foxes," who are flexible and pragmatic, are somewhat better than "hedgehogs," who are wedded to grand theories and less open to alternative viewpoints. But, even the foxes lose out to statistical models, just as in Meehl's studies of psychological diagnoses:

> Quantitative and qualitative methods converge on a common conclusion: foxes have better judgment than hedgehogs. Better judgment does not mean great judgment. Foxes are not awe-inspiring forecasters: most of them should be happy to tie

simple extrapolation models, and none of them can hold a candle to formal statistical models. But foxes do avoid many of the big mistakes that drive down the probability scores of hedgehogs to approximate parity with dart-throwing chimps.[14]

Ouch!

Are We Really So Dumb?

There are doubtless many ways in which the "average person" and even the statistically sophisticated professional can easily become confused about probabilities. So, if mathematical probability is truly such a critical aspect of logical thinking, we are all in serious trouble. Before reaching this pessimistic conclusion, however, let us critically consider the basic assumption that underlies much of the heuristic-and-biases program. Is mathematical probability really the proper yardstick for measuring rationality?

Recall that mathematical probability is a very recent invention. Moreover, as Keynes and Knight explicitly recognized, rational thinking about uncertainty cannot be confined to this special form of probability. The more qualitative sense of probability that was familiar to Jacob Bernoulli had important aspects that are not captured by the laws of mathematical probability. Recognition of these lost aspects has partially motivated innovative work on the theory of *belief functions*, pioneered by Dempster and Shafer in the 1970s and Zadeh's *possibility theory*.[15]

These and some other proposals explicitly regard the usual laws of probability as inadequate to handle fully the nature of our uncertainty. The proposed solutions are developed within a mathematical framework capable of expressing a broader conception of uncertainty. These efforts aim to quantify the total evidence by combining the sources of relevant information, especially empirical data. A variety of mathematical rules for combining such evidence have been proposed and their implications elaborated. Perhaps because of their complexity, however, practical applications so far have been quite limited.

Another critique of the HB perspective has been offered by psychologist Gary Klein. Klein rejects the notion that optimal decisions and actions depend on optimization of some "objective function" based on probability theory and statistics.[16] In *Sources of Power*, he summarizes a research program that has been termed "naturalistic decision-making" (NDM). This approach was inspired by studies of master chess players undertaken in the 1970s. Klein and his colleagues have attempted to determine how true experts in fields such as firefighting, emergency medicine, and military strategy use intuitive insight to inform their decisions. These researchers generally view the heuristics that guide such master practitioners in a positive light.

At a high level, proponents of NDM have identified the recognition-primed decision (RPD) strategy as the main source of expert proficiency. The core idea behind RPD was first articulated by the multifaceted genius Herbert Simon (1916–2001) in 1992:

> The situation has provided a cue: This cue has given the expert access to information stored in memory, and the information provides the answer. Intuition is nothing more and nothing less than recognition.[17]

In this view, expertise consists largely in having a relevant store of remembered occasions that are similar to the present one, and the ability to recall an appropriate instance. The expert does not need to consider multiple options and find the best; rather, he immediately grasps the essence of a problem and "recalls" a *satisfactory* solution, although not necessarily the absolute *best* one.

Both Klein and Kahneman assert that in order for real predictive skill to develop, the expert must be trained in a "high-validity" environment:

> First, the environment must provide adequately valid cues to the nature of the situation. Second, people must have an opportunity to learn the relevant cues.... Skilled intuitions will only develop in an environment of sufficient regularity, which provides valid cues to the situation.[18]

Their disagreement is mostly a matter of emphasis. Thinking more about situations like political analysis and psychological evaluations (low-validity), Kahneman and company are persuaded that true expertise is rare. Focusing more on situations like chess playing and emergency medicine (high-validity), Klein and his colleagues emphasize that real expertise can and often does develop.

Attempting to delineate the requisite *conditions* for validity of clinical insight is an important step forward. Furthermore, recognizing relevant "cues" based on an environment with "sufficient regularity" does seem important. However, the RPD formulation cannot be the whole story. Both sides in the Kahneman–Klein discussion regard *statistical regularities* as the main source of potentially relevant information. The environment is seen as providing a regular series of relevant cues, and the budding expert's job is to observe and assimilate this externally generated data.

This seems much too passive, however, almost Pavlovian. Where do these cues come from, and how are they recognized? Surely, acquiring expertise entails a more active and complex engagement with the flux of experience. To categorize a situation mentally must require more than simply observing it and filing it away. A refined conceptual framework must be formed in tandem with, and helping to shape, the process of observation. Without such an evolving conceptual framework, the *meaning* of the situation will be unclear. Consequently, the motivation for noticing and remembering it will be weak or nonexistent.

Another prominent critic of the heuristics and biases assumptions is psychologist Gerd Gigerenzer. He has spearheaded a program of research to uncover the "ecological rationality" underlying many of our judgments and decisions. Gigerenzer has written cogently (in my opinion) about the positive value of many "fast and frugal" heuristics.[19] A fast and frugal heuristic is "a strategy, conscious or unconscious, that searches for minimal information and consists of building blocks that exploit evolved capacities and environmental structures." Gigerenzer argues that such "ecological" strategies, grounded in our evolutionary development (and presumably calling mainly on System 1) can often be far more reliable and efficient than the "optimizing" analytical solutions attributed to System 2.

One of his favorite examples is the manner in which an athlete is able to catch an object projected into the air from a great distance (think baseball, football, frisbee, etc.). A System 2 solution might entail a complex calculation based upon the equations of physics. In contrast, a baseball outfielder reacts to a fly ball hit in his general direction by unconsciously employing a simple rule of thumb: "When a ball comes in high, a player fixates his gaze on the ball, starts running, and adjusts the speed so that the angle of gaze remains constant."[20] According to Gigerenzer, such a heuristic should not be seen as merely a poor substitute for the more complex mathematical analysis, but is often superior.

Gigerenzer's heuristics can be regarded as the procedures employed by the navigator in the submarine metaphor. Having evolved to be strongly coupled with the external environment, these heuristics function well in most circumstances. Most important, they help reduce uncertainty by efficiently resolving ambiguity. In contrast, statistical technology lodged in System 2 depends on the absence of ambiguity and can be misleading when substantial ambiguity is present.

Gigerenzer suggests that our standards of rationality, especially pertaining to probability and statistics, are flawed. We may *seem* to be "irrational" because we cannot perform abstract mathematical and logical operations easily. But this "content-blind norm" is the wrong criterion to use. In its place, he proposes an ideal that is more appropriate for actual human circumstances:

> We can easily agree how experiment participants have or have not violated the truth-table logic or some other logical law in an experimental task. But proponents of the heuristics-and-biases program count the first as human irrationality and the second as rationality. I do not. I believe that we need a better understanding of human rationality than that relative to content-blind norms. These were of little relevance for *Homo sapiens*, who had to adapt to a social and physical world, not to systems with artificial syntax, such as the laws of logic.
>
> The concept of ecological rationality is my answer to the question of the nature of *Homo sapiens*. It defines the rationality of heuristics independently of optimization and content-blind norms, by the degree to which they are adapted to environments ... *Homo sapiens* has been characterized as a tool user. There is some deeper wisdom in that phrase. The tools that make us smart are not bones and stones, but the heuristics in the adaptive toolbox.[21]

There is no doubt that mathematics, in general, and probability theory in particular, are among the most adaptive "tools" ever invented. Mathematical probability is an instrument for dealing with uncertainty and variability. It was first conceived and refined by a few great thinkers, whose contributions I have described in previous chapters. However, it is a mistake to imagine that this wonderful tool is *all* that we need in order to think effectively about uncertainty and variability.

As a recent addition to our adaptive toolbox, it resides in System 2, which greatly limits its utility. Statistical thinking has not had a chance to become integrated into any unconscious heuristics, but instead must be laboriously learned and applied. Assessing a probability certainly requires consideration of any *recognized* empirical frequencies. But it may also involve *insight*, an intuitive perception of underlying causal dynamics.

Insight can play a role in part by helping to define an appropriate reference class and to identify particular variables on which to condition. Insight undergirds judgments of *recognizability*, in Fisher's sense. Thus, it is the basis for exercising willful ignorance intelligently.

Beyond this technical function, however, insight is central to expert decision-making.[22] In particular, it is needed to identify the cues that are central to the RPD theory. At their worst, such intuitions can represent wishful thinking, but at their best, they are flashes of brilliance like those described by Malcolm Gladwell in *Blink*. Klein's program of respecting intuitive power and seeking to understand its sources has been extremely valuable. However, the RPD formula for explanation is inevitably limited. The art of framing probabilities depends ultimately on metaphysical considerations that cannot be linked *directly* to observed frequencies alone.

The cues do not come ready-made, but must be selected or constructed within some theoretical framework. *This* situation is reminiscent of some other one I can recall in certain particular respects that are salient to me. From this fabric of previous experiences, I somehow fashion my expectations of what may happen now or in the future. Klein explains how the expert can mentally play out various hypothetical implications based on manipulating a sophisticated conceptual model. In this way, probabilities can sometimes be assessed when the environment is relatively low-validity.

Note that the metaphorical-lottery perspective does not necessarily imply that there is an actual, potentially observable, series of events that is analogous to selections from a lottery. In fact, it may often be the case that the heavy analytical lifting is actually performed by System 1 rather than System 2. Framing a numerical probability would then be secondary, merely an attempt to translate a vague intuitive sense of uncertainty into a manageable form. The *Blink*-like insights described by Gladwell seem to work this way. So, too, do the epiphanies that are sometimes experienced immediately upon waking up, the morning after an evening spent wrestling with a difficult dilemma.

Frank Knight pondered the conundrum of how such judgments of probability are possible:

> It is manifestly meaningless to speak of either calculating such a probability *a priori* or of determining it empirically by studying a large number of instances. The essential and outstanding fact is that the 'instance' in question is so entirely unique

that there are no others or not a sufficient number to make it possible to tabulate enough like it to form a basis of any inference of value about any real probability in the case we are interested in. The same obviously applies to most of conduct, and not to business decisions alone. Yet it is true, and the fact can hardly be over-emphasized, that a judgment of probability is actually made in such cases.[23]

Where does this probability come from? That is a profound mystery. It cannot be just a matter of recognition, because the situation has unique and novel aspects.

Knight's answer appears to prefigure Gigerenzer's concept of ecological rationality:

> The ultimate logic, or psychology, of these deliberations is obscure, a part of the scientifically unfathomable mystery of life and mind. We must simply fall back upon a 'capacity' in the intelligent animal to form more or less correct judgments about things, an intuitive sense of values. We are so built that what seems to us reasonable is likely to be confirmed by experience, or we could not live in the world at all.[24]

This statement regards the ultimate source of intuition as ineffable but expresses optimism that expert intuition can sometimes penetrate the web of confusion about causal processes to some useful degree.

The expertise of the successful entrepreneur, according to Knight, lies in her ability to see more deeply and accurately what is happening, and likely to happen. So, here is the essential paradox. The entrepreneur, or any creative individual, can formulate probabilities and make decisions by an "act of ultimate responsibility," and will enjoy or suffer the consequences. But in the particular instance, she will never really know whether her judgments were good ones, regardless of the outcomes.

Knight may well be correct to say that the psychological wellspring of our probability judgments is unfathomable. However, neuroscientist Antonio Damasio has offered some clues. He draws on recent brain science to suggest that the HB view of rationality commits "Descartes' error" by sharply separating thought and feeling.[25] Damasio advances a *somatic-marker hypothesis* that posits a close link between imagining something and simultaneously reacting emotionally. A somatic marker is a positive or negative emotion or bodily feeling that has been "connected, by learning, to predicted future outcomes of certain scenarios."

Damasio's somatic markers may help to explain Gary Klein's examples of effective intuitive decision-making. For instance, in situations involving complex human interactions, a person must implicitly make assessments of probabilities. According to standard economic theory, he should employ a complex cost-benefit evaluation for a possible action being contemplated. This analysis would consider both the probability of each possible outcome and its utility. The theoretical index of the action's worth would then be calculated as the mathematical expectation.

This artificial idealization places the locus of decision-making, including probability estimation, entirely within the realm of conscious intellect. In reality, our brains and nervous systems deal with uncertainty in an elegant symphony of conscious and unconscious processes, in which thought and feeling are intertwined. In Damasio's theory, somatic markers play a pivotal role:

> Somatic markers do not deliberate for us. They assist the deliberation by highlighting some options (either dangerous or favorable), and eliminating them rapidly from subsequent consideration. You may think of it as a system for automated qualification of predictions, which acts, whether you want it or not, to evaluate the extremely diverse scenarios of the anticipated future before you. Think of it as a biasing device.[26]

So, the somatic-marker machinery generates "biases" that are critical to efficient functioning. However, these are *useful* biases.

According to Damasio's schema, somatic markers incline us toward decisions that seem preferable by virtue of both high value *and* low risk. Interestingly, this simultaneous accounting for both utility and probability is consistent with the old pre-mathematical concept of "expectation." Perhaps these deep neurobiological roots explain why expectation long preceded our modern ideas of utility and probability. This perspective turns our usual understanding of rationality on its head.

We generally regard feeling and emotion as obstructions to the operation of "cool reason." So, the ability to manipulate the abstract mathematics of probability becomes paramount, and the possibly value-laden context is secondary. But in complex circumstances, it would be highly inefficient to proceed by "rational" cost-benefit analysis. So, for example, the business executive or political leader may be faced with a fluid and highly ambiguous reality, and the necessity to react continually in real time. Like the baseball player chasing a long fly ball, he lacks the luxury of careful calculation to evaluate alternatives:

> Intellectuals analyze the operations of international systems; statesmen build them. And there is a vast difference between the perspective of an analyst and that of a statesman. The analyst can choose which problem he wishes to study, whereas the statesman's problems are imposed on him. The analyst can allot whatever time is necessary to come to a clear conclusion; the overwhelming challenge to the statesman is the pressure of time. The analyst runs no risk. If his conclusions prove wrong, he can write another treatise. The statesman is permitted only one guess; his mistakes are irretrievable. The analyst has available to him all the facts; he will be judged on his intellectual power. The statesman must act on assessments that cannot be proved at the time he is making them.[27]

Somatic markers are fast and frugal; they attend to ambiguity as well as doubt by rapidly filtering our complex perceptions. In this way, the "blooming, buzzing confusion" of experience is transformed into useful information.[28] Of course, these biases may turn out to be biased in the HB sense as well. They can only function well if our implicit causal "theories" of what is going on are well coupled with reality.

Kathryn Schulz, in *Being Wrong*, her fascinating meditation on uncertainty illustrates in many ways how the ability to rapidly resolve ambiguity is an essential human strength. Consider the way we perform the task of reading. I suspect that reading entails a continual process of subliminally anticipating what is likely to come next. Our expectations depend on the words we have just read, as well as the context that has been evoked by earlier reading. Schulz offers the example of how we respond when asked to complete a sentence that begins: "The giraffe had a very long ... ." The word "neck" involuntarily springs to mind. In a particular context, we may predict what the general character of the next sentence or paragraph might be.

Our intuitions will often prove misguided and are always subject to correction as we read on, but the efficiency of our interpretive process is generally facilitated by this dynamic speculative engagement with the unfolding text. Indeed, whether and how we learn new information may be mediated by our emotional reaction when our implicit predictions are not fulfilled. In this respect, we would have a significant edge over a computer program that has been trained to "read" and to "understand" text.

The computer might have the benefit of access to an enormous database of statistical information about word frequencies and usage. However, it would be at a huge disadvantage when it comes to disambiguation. So, completing a sentence about a giraffe may literally be "child's play" for us, while it may be quite complicated, or even virtually impossible, for the computer:

> We care about what is *probable*. We determine what is probable based on our prior experience of the world, which is where evidence comes in: we choose the most likely answer to any given question based on the kinds of things we have (and haven't) experienced in comparable situations. Over the course of our lifetimes, we've observed some things about giraffes, sentences, and sentences about giraffes, and based on those observations, we make an educated guess about this particular sentence concerning this particular giraffe. Significantly, it doesn't matter how *much* we've observed about sentences and giraffes. Unlike Descartes, we aren't interested in whether we have ample evidence to support a given conclusion—which is just as well, since, as the computer's conundrum shows, we almost certainly do not. All we're interested in is whether whatever evidence we *do* have supports one conclusion better than another. That's why four-year-olds can answer this question, despite their comparatively limited experience with sentences and (one assumes) even more limited experience with giraffes.[29]

By *probable*, Schulz clearly does not mean mathematical probability, and by *evidence* she does not mean only observed frequencies of similar situations. Her concept of probability assessment encompasses the capacity to resolve ambiguity via some high-order mental processing for which we humans seem especially well wired. It is perhaps reminiscent of Jacob Bernoulli's probability.

Paradoxically, the highly touted "successes" of computers in besting human champions at chess and in the TV game of Jeopardy highlight the limitations of "artificial intelligence."[30] These victories represent impressive technological achievements. Yet, each was only possible within a highly structured and unambiguous realm of knowledge. Even a minor perturbation of the structure would require a major new investment of effort to accommodate. For instance, suppose that the rules of chess were modified in some way, say by allowing one piece to move twice consecutively one time in a game. Presumably, a human expert would possess the flexibility to adapt much more easily and quickly to such a change.

STATISTICS FOR HUMANS: BIAS OR AMBIGUITY?

It cannot be denied that we often err in our assessments and actions far more than we realize. In particular, we tend to over-interpret statistical patterns by reading more into them than is warranted. In this regard, many HB studies are insightful and illuminating. However, I believe that HB researchers can exhibit a subtle bias of their own; let us call it *willful ignorance bias*. It is a tendency to interpret events as random draws from easily specified general populations, thus favoring statistics over insight. Consequently, the rich context that *may* be relevant is willfully ignored. Because of this bias, many problems that are actually quite ambiguous may appear to be amenable to statistical analysis.

I believe that many of the statistical "errors" commonly observed in HB experiments are attributable to ambiguity rather than to defects in the "machinery of cognition." The questions posed to experimental subjects are *abstracted* from a realistic context. Consequently, the respondent is confronted with an ambiguous situation in which the pertinent cues are minimal. The situation faced by the subject is similar to that which I discussed in connection with the Monty Hall and Two Envelope games. Without clearly specifying a protocol to indicate exactly how the metaphorical-lottery analogy applies, the problem has no definitive answer.

Because the questions are divorced from a real context, a respondent may try to fill in the blanks with intuition or judgment. This behavior would be adaptive in many actual situations, but is arguably "incorrect" in the artificially restricted laboratory environment. In a real-life situation, a person generally has both a cognitive interest and an emotional investment of some kind. A problem that arises within a complex or ambiguous situation may trigger numerous potential responses, including a sense of uncertainty about the meaning of the question and a desire for more information to reduce the ambiguity. As Jacob Bernoulli noted, if a decision is not mandatory, then "we should suspend our actions until we learn more."

The Representativeness Fallacy

One of the hallmark "proofs" of our cognitive limitations involves our tendency to confuse probability with typicality, or *representativeness*.[31] We tend to associate higher probabilities with events that seem to represent our stereotypical expectations. This is deemed a fallacy because evidence of representativeness does not necessarily increase the mathematical probability. Here is an example of the kind of problem posed in the heuristics-and-biases experimental research:

> Roger W is 42 years old. He is married and the father of three young children. After studying engineering in college, he enlisted in the air force, and served in the first Gulf War. He rose to the rank of major and was honored for his performance in several combat missions. Roger is a natural leader who commands respect, and thrives on taking responsibility in difficult situations.

Of the following, which is the most probable?
Roger is an airline pilot.
Roger is a teacher.
Roger is a chef.

Your first instinct might be to opt for the first choice. If so, you have supposedly committed the fallacy of predicting by *representativeness*. Roger's profile is most consistent with our stereotype of an airline pilot. However, there are vastly more teachers than airline pilots. According to the HB theorists, this "base rate" should be weighed strongly. Based on this objective statistical evidence, the probability Roger is a teacher is much greater than the probability he is an airline pilot. But is reliance on representativeness truly a reflection of irrational bias?

Roger's profile is so definite that it tends to swamp any perceived relevance of frequencies in the general population. These statistics would not necessarily be based on an appropriate reference class. Perhaps if we could obtain more information about Roger's background, we might decide whether or not the general population would be a reasonable referent. For instance, suppose we knew that both of his parents were teachers and that Roger enjoyed coaching his children's soccer teams. Knowing such facts might affect our judgment.

Of course, this artificial problem lacks any broader context to help resolve the ambiguity. In the abstract, there can be no definitive answer. That said, I would not dispute that most of us have a tendency toward overreliance on representativeness. We really do prefer causal insight to dry statistics. However, in real situations, this is not always wrong.

The Conjunction Fallacy

Perhaps the most controversial and perplexing of the HB studies begins with a brief description of a fictitious woman by the name of Linda[32]:

> Linda is 31 years old, single, outspoken, and very bright. She majored in philosophy. As a student, she was deeply concerned with issues of discrimination and social justice, and also participated in antinuclear demonstrations.

Which alternative is more probable?
Linda is a bank teller.
Linda is a bank teller and is active in the feminist movement.

Please give this one a little thought before reading on.

If you are like most people, you chose the second statement. If so, according to probability theory, you were wrong (and irrational). Why? The set of bank tellers who are also feminists is a subset of the set of bank tellers in general. The mathematical probability of event A (being a bank teller) *and* event B (being a feminist) must therefore be less than the probability of just being a teller. In general, the probability of the conjunction of two events, say A and B, can be no greater than the probability of either individually. Failure to recognize this basic law of mathematical probability is called the *conjunction fallacy* by the HB researchers.

Now suppose that Linda's best girlfriend Lorna has virtually identical characteristics. Consider the following two possibilities:

Lorna has blonde hair.
Lorna has blonde hair and blue eyes.

Again, which is more probable? This one is obvious; possessing both characteristics is less probable than having only one.

Why do so many of us get the probability "right" in the Lorna Problem, but "wrong" in the Linda Problem? According to HB theorists, the answer is the lack of a plausible causal back-story for Lorna, compared with a compelling one for Linda. So, Linda's case (but not Lorna's) evokes our instinct to imagine possible causal explanations. This *narrative bias* may be at work to some degree, but is only part of the story here.

Notice that hair and eye color are completely irrelevant to Lorna's political or occupational activities. Thus, the Lorna problem invites us to ignore her personal characteristics. It is easy to regard her as a generic member of the class of young women, and to frame our probability judgments accordingly. In the case of Linda, however, there is ambiguity about our interpretation of what it means to be a bank teller. For instance, has Linda chosen this occupation in the context of her career aspirations, or only as a temporary expedient? Perhaps she is a graduate student in sociology who is supporting herself until she can launch her academic career.

The ghost in the probability machine here is the real *context* of Linda's work experience. When asked simply about her likelihood of being a teller, we naturally assume this refers to her chosen profession. In this light, being a teller seems quite improbable given her background. On the other hand, considering whether she might be a bank teller *and* an active feminist suggests other possibilities. Perhaps we are being asked to consider her broader lifestyle, not just her occupation. Thus, the (presumed) evidence underlying our judgments may *differ* for these two questions. As Keynes explained, the probabilities in such a case cannot be compared directly; they lie on different conceptual paths.

Of course, in this laboratory exercise, we have no grounds for deciding *which* interpretation is appropriate to each of the questions, respectively. But in the real world, we might attempt to resolve the ambiguity by asking for clarification of the question, or by seeking more information about Linda's actual situation. Moreover, if the problem were modified to eliminate the ambiguity, I suspect that the "bias" would largely evaporate. For example, suppose we were told:

> Linda is 31 years old, single, outspoken, and very bright. She majored in philosophy. As a student, she was deeply concerned with issues of discrimination and social justice, and also participated in antinuclear demonstrations. Recently, Linda decided to take a part-time job temporarily in order to make ends meet.

Now, select which of the following statements is more probable:
Linda is a bank teller.
Linda is a bank teller and is active in the feminist movement.

Explaining that her current job is merely a temporary expedient makes Linda's choices seem less contradictory. So, the relevant evidence supporting each of the possible statements is much more aligned. It now becomes more reasonable to compare the two by applying the laws of mathematical probability. In this light, the second statement may be deemed less probable than the first.

Finally, it is worth considering why, in the standard version of the Linda problem, we experience such a strong gut feeling that being a bank teller and feminist is more "probable." I believe that our connotation of probability is something like that which Jacob Bernoulli, or for that matter Kathryn Schulz, would clearly understand. This is a wider and arguably more natural sense of probability that in some fashion recognizes ambiguity as well as doubt. From this perspective, representativeness bias is not necessarily a defect in the "machinery of cognition." Rather it is a fast and frugal heuristic that often serves us well, especially when System 2 thinking is ineffective because we lack sufficient time or data.

The Allure of Causality

Here is another problem that is purported to demonstrate our biases regarding probability judgments[33]:

> A cab was involved in a hit-and-run accident at night.
>
> Two cab companies, the Green and the Blue, operate in the city.
>
> You are given the following data:
>
> - 85% of the cabs in the city are Green and 15% are Blue.
> - A witness identified the cab as Blue. The court tested the reliability of the witness under the circumstances that existed on the night of the accident and concluded that the witness correctly identified each one of the two colors 80% of the time and failed 20% of the time.

What is the probability that the cab involved in the accident was Blue rather than Green?

Most people seem to be influenced by the assumed reliability rate much more than the frequencies of the two types of taxis. Therefore, their answers are close to 80%. According the HB theorists, this is a flagrant error, since this is obviously "a standard problem of Bayesian inference." In other words, a logical response would, at least intuitively, balance the

TABLE 11.1 Simple Statistics for the Runaway Taxicab Problem

	ID = Green	ID = Blue	
Cab was Green	68	17	85
Cab was Blue	3	12	15

P(Cab was Blue | Identified as Blue) = $^{12}/_{29}$ = 0.41

base rate of 85% against the reliability rate of 80%. So, they ought to choose a probability a bit less than 50%. The mathematically "correct" result, obtained by applying Bayes's Theorem, would be 41%.

Even for many professional statisticians, performing the Bayesian calculation is not trivial and may require a paper-and-pencil computation. The simplest way to obtain this result is to reduce the data to four frequencies, as Gigerenzer has suggested (see Table 11.1).[34] We can imagine that out of 100 accidents, 85 would involve Green cabs, of which 68 (80%) would be correctly identified by the witness, and 17 (20%) would not. Blue cabs would be involved in 15 accidents, in 12 (80%) of which the witness would correctly identify the cab's color and three (20%) would not. So, only 12 of the 29 cabs that the witness would have seen as Blue would actually have been Blue.

The HB researchers assert that we generally err by tending to lean much more on causal stories than on statistical facts. To demonstrate this phenomenon, they tested an alternative version of the runaway taxi problem. The first part of the problem statement was modified to read:

- The two companies operate the same number of cabs, but Green cabs are involved in 85% of accidents.

With this alternative specification, the probabilities reported by respondents in the HB research are fairly consistent with the 41% dictated by the Bayesian analysis.

Kahneman interprets this result as confirmation of the "causes trump statistics" theory. He argues that in the first version, there are dry statistics (percentage of cabs Green) to consider along with a causal story (witness testimony).[35] So, the causal narrative wins out. In the second version, there are two balancing causal stories. In place of the bare statistical frequency, there is the idea of a "hit-and-run, which naturally evokes the idea that a reckless Green driver was responsible." This account certainly has some plausibility. The salience of causal information is undoubtedly one element that influences the subjects' responses. However, Kahneman overlooks another important aspect of the information given. In its original formulation, the problem is highly ambiguous.

What does it mean that 85% of the cabs in the city are Green? This raises a host of questions. For example, do the cabs service the same neighborhoods? Do they operate during exactly the same hours? Are their drivers equally well selected and trained? Are their drivers equally accident-prone? Are company disciplinary policies equivalent for driving infractions? It is a long stretch from having 85% of the cabs in Boston, for instance, to being responsible for 85% of the accidents, let alone the hit-and-run accidents, that occur in the Allston neighborhood at night.

There is ample evidence that decision-makers tend to discount ambiguous information in making decisions under uncertainty. They can, of course, be *forced* to decide, as in this artificial exercise. However, their normal impulse is to give less weight to more ambiguous data, even to the extent of violating the axioms of mathematical probability. Ellsberg's Paradox, which I discussed in Chapter 9, discusses an experiment demonstrating just this point.[36] As Knight and Keynes theorized, confidence in an assessment of probability plays a role, along with the value of the probability itself. Ellsberg argued eloquently that those who exhibit such behavior should not necessarily be construed as irrational: "Indeed, it seems out of the question summarily to judge their behavior as irrational: I am included among them." And obviously so am I!

The second version of the runaway taxicab problem is much less ambiguous than the first. The fact that 85% of the *accidents* involve Green cabs does imply that the rate of accidents for Green cabs is much higher than that for Blue cabs. However, this can be attributed to a variety of factors besides the recklessness of individual drivers. For example, the Green cabs might operate mainly in areas of higher traffic density. Nonetheless, data related to accidents are much more relevant than data about the number of cabs. So, it is not surprising that subjects tend to give somewhat more weight to this information than to the general statistics about the numbers of cabs.

Put differently, the set of accidents occurring seems much closer to the real reference class of interest than the set of cabs operated. The best reference class would be something like "hit-and-run accidents under conditions similar to those that actually occurred." Presumably, if we altered the problem statement a bit more as follows, the results would be quite different:

- The two companies operate the same number of cabs, but Green cabs are involved in 85% of hit-and-run accidents similar to that which actually occurred.

This is much less ambiguous; accordingly, the presumed relevance of the base-rate data becomes more evident.

Finally, the runaway taxicab problem illustrates the general difficulty posed by Bayesian statistical analysis in general. The fundamental tenet of Bayesian theory is that a prior distribution can be specified. From the classical perspective, prior probabilities are essentially personal representations of uncertainty *in the form of a metaphorical lottery*. However, there is no guarantee that our perceptions of the situation are structured in such a way as to justify such a formulation. Knowing that 85% of cabs in the city are Green in a real situation would not automatically translate into a prior probability estimate of 85% that any particular hit-and-run cab was Green.

In many cases, our level of relevant knowledge is much weaker, or even virtually nonexistent. The disagreement between Bayesians and frequentists arises from a clash between two extreme positions. Bayesians assume that our prior uncertainty should *always* be framed in terms of mathematical probabilities; frequentists assume it should play no role in our deliberations. Very little serious attention has been paid recently to approaches that attempt to reconcile or transcend these dogmatic extremes.

REGRESSION TOWARD THE MEAN

Perhaps the most widespread and misunderstood kind of error related to probability is the phenomenon of *regression to the mean*. I mentioned in Chapter 2 the invention of correlation and regression by Sir Francis

Galton. These closely related and enormously important concepts were devised originally to explain data about heredity. Galton had found that on almost any characteristic, the offspring of humans, animals, or plants tended to be less extreme than the parents.

The phenomenon of regression to the mean can appear in many different guises and is often a source of great confusion. Although essentially a mathematical truism, it can appear to imply the existence of some invisible force, like gravity, pulling each individual back toward mediocrity. As the heuristics-and-biases studies suggest, we are prone to invent causal explanations. To avoid this misconception, it is critical to understand that regression is fundamentally a property of populations, not of individuals. A group of extreme individuals on a certain variable are *on average* less extreme on some other correlated variable. To jump from this fact to the conclusion that any particular individual will be less extreme is not justified.

Explaining Regression Effects

The most common situations in which regression causes practical difficulties are those in which repeated observations of the same individual occur. For example, suppose that a professional athlete achieves the best performance of his career during his tenth season. Based on this successful year, he may negotiate a lucrative long-term contract for future years. All too often, however, his performance level during the following year will drop off significantly. Does this necessarily indicate that his skills have begun to decline, as often supposed?

For concreteness, let us consider a hypothetical example in a business context. Suppose I tell you that Joe's income for the past year was $300,000. What might be a reasonable prediction of his income for the current year? In the absence of any additional information, you might say $300,000. Now, imagine that you are the president of Acme Realty, and Joe is one of your star brokers. You have just learned that this year he will be making $180,000. Should you be surprised? Worried?

You might be concerned that Joe has lost some of his mojo, and search for a plausible explanation of this precipitous decline. On the other hand, you might simply chalk the change up to the regression effect. After all, the average income of all brokers in his region is only around $60,000.

So, perhaps last year was a "chance" aberration. If so, you would have expected this year's income to regress back toward the overall mean to some extent.

We can think of last year's income as a *predictor* of this year's.[37] How well it predicts depends on the correlation between the values for two different years. If the correlation is high, then we expect this year's income to be quite close to last year's income. If the correlation is low, then it should be close to the population mean. As a result, if the correlation is high, then this year's value will be a good predictor of next year's. If it is low, then the best prediction for next year's value would be somewhere between this year's value and the overall population mean. At the extremes, the best prediction if the correlation is 1.0 would be this year's value; the best prediction if the correlation is 0.0 would be the overall population mean.

Predictions for Individuals

The magnitude and direction of a regression effect depends on reference population that is assumed. In our example, if you conceive of Joe as having been selected from your total employee population, you may expect his income this year to regress toward the overall average of $60,000. On the other hand, why should it not instead regress toward the mean of Joe's own incomes in recent years? This might be much higher, say $150,000. Or, perhaps, it would regress toward some other hypothetical subpopulation of brokers, such as those in Joe's region or office.

How can we know which is the "right" population on which to perform a regression analysis? Actually, this is a meaningless question. It assumes that the regression effect is a phenomenon that pertains to an actual individual; strictly speaking, it does not. It can be considered relevant to a specific person only to the extent that we regard that person as indistinguishable from others with that same predictive value in the specified population.

In its original applications, the human population of interest was generally well specified. Galton was typically studying some attribute, such as height, of British children in relation to the same attribute in their parents. He observed that the son of a tall father would tend to be somewhat shorter (i.e., closer to the mean of British men) than his father. There was no ambiguity about which particular population was appropriate to consider. So, the mathematical formulas he and later Pearson developed were ideal for this situation. However, Galton's epiphany that correlation and regression might be applicable quite generally was somewhat naive. The mathematical formulas were certainly general, but the appropriate reference population might be unclear, as in the example of Joe, the real estate broker. It is this ambiguity that often results in confusion when the concept of regression to the mean is invoked in practical applications.

The Regression of Science

In 2005, a research methodologist named John Ioannidis unleashed an intellectual firestorm. He published an article that purported to prove what some of us have come to believe, or at least suspect.[38] The article was provocatively titled: "Why Most Published Research Findings are False." This article touched a raw nerve, resulting in over 1500 published responses as of this writing, weighing in for and against Ioannidis's controversial position. The technical details of his argument are not especially noteworthy, but the conceptual issues raised are vitally important.

One illuminating way to think about these issues is through the lens of regression to the mean. Ioannidis essentially took a page out of the heuristics-and-biases book to shine a light on the entire research process. Daniel Kahneman emphasizes the prevalence of an *optimistic bias* among entrepreneurs. They may be intellectually aware that about two-thirds of all new businesses fail in their first few years of operation. However, most believe that *their* ventures are the exceptions. Displaying such *overconfidence* is a serious cognitive bias, according to the HB theory.

Regression to the mean plays a large role in what is happening. The entrepreneur is typically encouraged by some early successes, perhaps in the context of a small-scale start-up scenario. On this basis, she may forecast even greater success as her firm's operations are refined and expanded. However, much of the initial good fortune may have been attributable to conditions that can be considered random. Moreover, her business decisions may, to some extent, be geared to these conditions, since she does not perceive their transitory nature. As a result, the subsequent performance of new companies that seem exceptionally promising is often much worse than anticipated, and closer to the average of all new ventures.

In the realm of science, something quite similar occurs. Most researchers are optimistic about their ability to obtain a positive result that confirms a certain theory or hypothesis. In practice, this usually means achieving an effect that is statistically significant, with a P-value less than 0.05. In many fields, studies that are published in widely read journals are virtually *required* to achieve statistical significance. Thus, researchers have a strong incentive to attain this coveted benchmark.

Like the entrepreneur, the scientist whose results are statistically significant may feel confident that his findings are valid. After all, the small P-value is widely accepted as the standard for deciding that the hypothesis has been confirmed. So, he might be very confident that another study designed to *replicate* this research would continue to support his hypothesis. Moreover, an academic journal is likely to take a similar position.

Suppose, however, that we consider the entire process of research and publication within a scientific field. The P-value produced by any particular study can be regarded as a random draw from an unknown population of P-values. The nature of this population is extremely complex. It can be influenced by a variety of scientific issues, and also by the motivation, competence, and ethics of individual researchers. As a result, the subset of studies that obtain significant P-values may contain many "false-positives."

Suppose we were to replicate all of these apparently significant studies. A substantial proportion of these studies would not turn out significant upon replication. Moreover, the average P-value for the replicated studies might be much higher (i.e., less significant) than the corresponding average P-value obtained in these studies originally. This replication average would have regressed toward the average P-value in some relevant population of studies, whatever that population might be.

Ioannidis argues that if all the published studies were actually replicated, the majority would fail to achieve the conventional 0.05 level of significance. But here is the rub: almost no such replication is ever performed. So, it is only occasionally, and in special circumstances, that this regression effect is actually observed. In those rare cases, the mysterious evaporation of a previously accepted finding is typically viewed as an actual loss in potency of the effect, rather than as evidence that there was never a true effect at all. Reasons for this alleged "decline effect" are then vainly sought.

Does the prevalence of the apparent decline effect imply that we should be highly skeptical of all published research findings? That depends. As I explained above, regression effects are relative to a specific population. In this case, a relevant population might be all of the studies in a particular scientific discipline, or subdiscipline. However, adopting such a general reference population means that we *ignore* any specific information that might suggest a relevant subset to which the study belongs.

There are obviously many factors that might be considered in this regard. For example, the reputation of the scientist or the source of study funding might affect the chances of obtaining statistical significance. So, although the concept of regression to the mean is theoretically applicable in some fashion, the ambiguity pertaining to the research process makes it impossible to quantify the magnitude of the regression effect. In the end, we must face up to an inconvenient truth: our system for generating scientific knowledge no longer operates as advertised.

By establishing the level of statistical significance as the "score" for judging research, we have set ourselves up for a massive regression effect. Those findings that are based on studies that achieve the most extreme outcomes, as judged by the P-value criterion, are virtually guaranteed to regress toward mediocrity to some degree. Moreover, as Ioannidis points out, the enormous incentive to achieve significance encourages researchers to engage, often unconsciously, in practices that lead to biased design, analysis and reporting. These practices can thus exacerbate the extent of such regression.

Is there a way to avoid the regression of science? The answer is surprisingly simple, *in principle*. We must recognize that probability theory *alone* is insufficient to establish scientific validity. There is only one foolproof way to learn whether an observed finding, however statistically significant it may appear, might actually hold up in practice. We must dust off the time-honored principle of *replication* as the touchstone of validity. Ideally, each study should be validated by collecting new data and performing a new analysis. Only when the system demands and rewards independent replications of study findings can and should public confidence in the integrity of the scientific enterprise be restored.[39]

The importance of replication is already recognized to some extent in commercial applications of statistical modeling. Practitioners of business analytics understand that independent replication is a *sine qua non* before a predictive algorithm can be deployed for routine use. Furthermore, since circumstances can change, repeated testing and possible adjustment of the predictive model may be needed. Surprisingly, in scientific research, there has been very little serious discussion of the idea that validation based on replication ought to become required.

Somewhat encouragingly, a number of recent articles have called attention to this critical lacuna in the process of scientific research and publication. Various potentially helpful methodological suggestions have been offered, albeit so far largely ignored. To understand the reasons for this resistance, we must turn not to methodology, but to sociology. A whole generation of researchers has become acclimated to the norm that statistical significance is by itself an imprimatur of validity. The belief systems and reward structures are so skewed toward a focus on P-values, that Fisher's original, more limited, function of this criterion has been forgotten.

To reform this situation, we must begin to ask basic questions. What are the legitimate purposes and the limitations of statistical testing? What kinds of independent replication are needed in various types of situations? How can research be organized and communicated to facilitate widespread routine validation? How can the *systems* of research evolve to offer incentives for the kinds of cooperation that are necessary to encourage routine validation? What institutions and professional roles may be needed to implement high-quality validations? Because of the myth that statistical significance somehow guarantees validity by itself, such important questions are rarely raised, let alone seriously addressed.

CHAPTER 12

TRUST, BUT VERIFY

It is 3 P.M. on a depressingly cloudy Thursday afternoon in early March of 1969.[1] I am a graduate student in the Harvard Statistics Department, somewhat bored as I listen to a distinguished invited speaker. Jerome (Jerry) Cornfield is a world-renowned leader in the development of statistical methods for epidemiology and medical research.[2] Today, he is discussing recent clinical trials being conducted by the National Cancer Institute, where he is currently a leading biostatistician. It is a subject unrelated to my thesis topic, so my mind wanders.

At some point, though, I am struck by a troubling thought. It occurs to me that randomized clinical trials of new treatments are really very crude. Given the inevitable improvement of biological knowledge, especially with respect to genetics, won't we soon have the ability to predict individual outcomes of medical treatments very precisely? Can't we expect that our categorization of disease states will become increasingly sophisticated? We will then be able to define subsets of individuals who are quite homogeneous; the probability of a cure, for example, within each such subset will be close to one or zero.

What I find disturbing is the possibility that statistical methods, based on probability theory, might become obsolete. Here I am about to embark

Willful Ignorance: The Mismeasure of Uncertainty, First Edition. Herbert I. Weisberg.
© 2014 John Wiley & Sons, Inc. Published 2014 by John Wiley & Sons, Inc.

on a career that might become irrelevant to the highly advanced science of the twenty-first century that I imagine will exist. At the end of the talk, we students are encouraged to ask questions. I tentatively raise my hand, am called upon, and haltingly struggle to articulate my concerns. Cornfield summarily dismisses my exaggerated expectations for science as unrealistic fiction, not to be taken seriously. Abashed, I sink back into my seat, hoping that my ill-conceived question will be quickly forgotten.

Nearing a half-century down the road, Jerry Cornfield's skepticism has proved completely justified, *so far*. There is little "danger" that statisticians will be going out of business any time soon. Statistical analyses aimed at determining general effects applicable to broad populations remain the norm. Statistical significance remains the main criterion for deciding whether or not an observed effect or correlation is scientifically valid. In the previous chapter, I suggested that this approach is becoming obsolete, as evidenced by the decline effect highlighted most notably by John Ioannidis.

A NEW PROBLEM

The modern statistical paradigm evolved under conditions quite remote from those prevailing today. In the 1920s, applied scientific research was still conducted mainly by a very small intellectual elite. The men (almost all were) of science were educated at a handful of exclusive universities and resided primarily in a few cosmopolitan centers. Their research programs were typically unique and isolated efforts. Communication between scientists occurred at a slow pace, and was limited to written letters and occasional publications in the few academic journals then existing in any particular field. The subject matter of the research was primarily related to areas in which the basic theoretical framework was fairly well-established, such as physics, chemistry, geology, and biology. Analysis of social and economic issues was still mainly philosophical, and to some extent religious, in nature.

Modern statistics was invented in large part to solve one particular pressing problem of the time: *small samples*. With data in short supply, a little had to go a long way. However, each experimental observation could be affected by a wide variety of uncontrolled factors. Separating the signal of interest from this complex of extraneous sources of "chance" variation was challenging. Fisher and his followers realized that by treating the uncontrolled variation as essentially random, mathematical probability theory could be brought to bear. Within this well-developed mathematical framework, a very difficult problem could be reduced to one that was manageable. Statistical tests of significance, and the subsequent development of statistical decision theory, addressed the critical question of whether random chance could be a plausible explanation for an observed effect or correlation.

Fisher was aware that mathematical probability depended on what I have called willful ignorance. Like Laplace, he perceived that probability has an "as-if" character that is relative to our limited knowledge. However, methods based on this useful expedient soon took on a life of their own. Statistical methodology transitioned from a helpful technology to aid scientific reasoning into a central aspect of scientific practice. Statistical significance in particular came to play a dominant role.

In many respects, this new perspective was quite fruitful. During the industrial expansion of the mid-twentieth century, probability-based statistical techniques yielded handsome dividends. However, soon these successful practices started to become a model for research in the *human* sciences, such as medicine, psychology, sociology, education, and economics. Why shouldn't these statistical methods be applied to studies of human populations and activities? Couldn't we apply such rigorous techniques as regression analysis and randomized experiments in the "softer" sciences to generate new knowledge?

Alas, the past 50 years have demonstrated just how naive such well-meaning proposals really were. There is a fundamental difference between the human sciences and the "harder" sciences. This difference pertains to the degree of ambiguity about the causal processes at work. In the physical and biological sciences, the "occasions" being observed can be described relatively simply, and the particular properties being analyzed are quite limited in scope. Moreover, the relevant scientific theory regarding these properties is widely understood and almost universally accepted. Furthermore, the boundaries of this accepted theory, or paradigm, are also clearly delineated. Thus, what lies *outside* these boundaries can be reasonably regarded as purely random.

For example, suppose that a material scientist is studying the response of a new metal alloy to various kinds of stress. He is performing an experiment in which measurements are obtained using sophisticated instruments. Under each specified set of conditions, multiple measurements are made. The outcomes of the measurements can vary slightly because of subtle unknown factors. However, this variability is essentially random; the individual observations are like indistinguishable draws from a metaphorical lottery.

Studying *people* and making predictions about their behavior, individually or in groups, is quite another matter. When the units of analysis are different human beings under varying particular conditions, the *context* of each observation is much more ambiguous. This context may include relevant characteristics of the person and of the circumstances in which the observation is occurring. For example, suppose we are studying the effect of a new drug on some disease and are estimating the probability of a cure. The effect of the drug may depend to some degree on the particular person, the exact nature of the condition, and various external factors.

When efficacy is highly context-dependent, an overall probability in some general population of patients is not very meaningful. There is simply too much *ambiguity* about the context. Only if such ambiguity can be resolved satisfactorily for our purposes can we move into the realm of *doubt*. Then, we may be able to conceive of a metaphorical lottery in which some fraction of "chances" favor the event of interest. With respect to a particular reference class, the degree of evidence for the occurrence of an event could be represented on a scale between zero (impossible) and one (certain).

Furthermore, we might be able to identify historical occasions that we deem similar to the hypothetical chances in our metaphorical lottery. Then, statistical data can come into play. For example, we can find the percentage of patients who recover after receiving the new drug and compare this with the recovery rate after being treated by conventional means. The fraction of actual observed occasions on which an event occurs provides an estimate of a probability. However, it is not in any sense *the* probability. Rather, it is a probability that is appropriate to chances *as we have chosen to conceive them*.

In the case of a new drug, it is usual to describe the patient population for which the drug is suitable. However, this specification may be quite general. We know the drug's benefits and the risks might vary according to individual characteristics, but lack a theory or sufficient data to determine any "recognizable subsets" of the general population. So, we default to the main effect in the hope that it provides the best guidance for the clinician until and unless we can determine otherwise.

The fundamental flaw in this logic is the implicit assumption that the context is only weakly relevant. In the case of a metal's tensile strength, this willful ignorance of the context is entirely appropriate. In some studies on humans, the event of interest *may* be quite independent of the context as well. For instance, the effect of an antibiotic on an acute infection may be unrelated to any measurable characteristic of the individual or her circumstances. However, for most of the events or properties studied today in the biomedical or social sciences, the causal processes involve complex interactions between the individual and the environment.

For instance, a new medication to control the progression of diabetes or heart disease can hardly be expected to have the same impact on all individuals. When it comes to effects of psychological and social interventions, or political policies, the potential for such complexity grows exponentially. In this light, the main effect may not necessarily be a first-order conclusion subject to possible further refinement; it may be virtually meaningless! Moreover, if the main effect happens to be weak or nonexistent, potentially fruitful research to identify individual differences may be abandoned prematurely.

The conventional wisdom at the moment is to focus primarily on main effects because that is the best we can do, at least for now. Even those who recognize the drawbacks of average effects are resigned to this pessimistic conclusion:

> How should clinicians proceed? First, they should recognize that even compromised knowledge is better than complete ignorance.... reliance on average effects as measured in good clinical studies is likely to produce better outcomes than is intuition or habit.[3]

The fallacy here is that clinicians rarely if ever operate on the basis of "complete ignorance." Rather, they must routinely draw upon their professional intuition to some extent in dealing with individual cases. How can they do otherwise? Their expertise in doing so is a major aspect of their perceived value.

Are such deviations from evidence-based generalities truly just "stories," as the heuristics-and-biases school would have it? The fact is we have not the foggiest idea how much better (or worse) in any concrete situation the clinician performs by attempting to think for himself. The apparent superiority of actuarial decision-making discovered by Meehl is certainly a warning to be heeded.[4] When the contextual information is limited or weakly relevant, statistical information is indeed very difficult to beat. But it is a mistake to assume that there *are* no relevant subsets just because we cannot recognize them at present.

Digging deeper into data to uncover such relevant subsets is apt to become increasingly feasible in coming decades. Fisher and Neyman were attempting to solve the problem of small samples in an environment of scarce data, limited communication technologies, and fairly strong scientific theory. Statistical models based on mathematical probability represented a major step forward. In contrast, we stand at the doorstep of a future that will be radically different. Already we are beginning to amass an enormous and permanent repository of "data" in various forms. Our emerging challenge is not how to make do with limited data, but rather how to exploit the *potential* of this virtually unlimited resource.

I believe that framing our options as a choice between the "compromised knowledge" of statistical main effects and the "complete ignorance" of pure clinical intuition will soon come to seem ridiculously simplistic. Instead, both scientists and clinicians will recognize that the dimensions of uncertainty can be explored from a number of different angles. The primary task for data analysts will be to resolve the ever-present ambiguity in productive ways. We can regard ambiguity resolution as the foundation upon which probability assessments (in Keynes's broad sense) can be constructed. *Mathematical* probability will sometimes, but not always, be the final form in which to express our conclusions.

Appreciating ambiguity may be perceived by some as a step backward in terms of scientific method. I disagree. I regard it as an infusion of intellectual honesty. Thanks to new technologies, a much more fine-grained differentiation among individuals is becoming practical. Understanding meaningful statistical patterns will be increasingly important, but will require a radically new mindset. The necessary attitude seems to me encapsulated in a phrase made famous by President Ronald Reagan in the context of nuclear arms reduction negotiations: *Trust, but verify!*[5]

The rift between clinical and statistical viewpoints cannot be bridged by a compromise between these incommensurable approaches. Rather it will require researchers to maintain a *dynamic tension* in which, paradoxically, both approaches are simultaneously exercised to the fullest. What I have in mind for scientific researchers is the attitude of a chess master facing a difficult opponent. Here is a summary by Paul Tough, who interviewed Elizabeth Spiegel, herself a chess expert and teacher, regarding a recent study conducted in Ireland:

> Unsurprisingly, the expert players analyzed their positions more accurately than the novices. What was surprising was *how* they were better. In a word, they were more pessimistic. When the novices found a move they liked, they tended to fall prey to confirmation bias, to see only the ways that it could lead to success; ignoring possible pitfalls; the Eeyore-like experts, by contrast, were more likely to see terrible outcomes lurking around every corner. They were able to falsify their hypotheses and thus avoid deadly traps.
>
> When I asked Spiegel about the Dublin study, she said she agreed it was a good idea for a chess player to be a bit pessimistic about the outcome of any particular move. But when it comes to a person's chess ability as a whole, she said, it was better to be *optimistic*. It's like public speaking, she explained: if you're not a bit overconfident when you step up to the microphone, you're in trouble. Chess is inherently painful, she said. 'No matter how good you get,' she told me, 'you never stop making stupid, stupid mistakes that you want to kill yourself for.' And so, part of getting good at chess is feeling confident you have within yourself the power to win.[6]

Sounds a lot like research.

Maintaining precisely this delicate (and often painful) balancing act of trusting your instincts in general, while doubting your every move, is what I mean by the dynamic tension necessary for research excellence. Both theory and data are important, but each must be tempered by the other. The analogy to chess is instructive. In chess, the machine must ultimately prevail because of its superhuman memory and blazing computational speed. Within the tightly constrained structure of the chessboard and rules of the game, these "technical" capabilities reign supreme. In such a situation, expertise truly is merely a matter of recall and calculation, and insight is just a poor substitute for our relatively limited competence in these skills.

In chess, the analysis of a position is completely unambiguous. There is really only one way to interpret what is going on, and the computer is much better at discovering what is relevant than we are. Flashes of insight provide pleasing explanations for us mere mortals, but are "really" completely superfluous. Where we humans *could* shine, however would be if resolving some ambiguous aspect of uncertainty were required. Change the rules even slightly and the computer's massive database of past games becomes irrelevant.

In scientific research, what Kahneman calls System 1 and System 2 ways of thinking are *both* involved, interacting in complex ways. Analysis of historical data and complex calculation (System 2) are essential to test hypotheses, but imagination and insight (System 1) are needed to generate productive theories. To solve the problems and seize the opportunities of Big Data will require a new kind of interplay between formulating causal theories and determining their validity. Out of the dynamic tension between these "opposing" activities may emerge a closer and more respectful relationship between scientific research and clinical practice.

The dynamic tension between trust and verification was explained eloquently by the pioneering physiologist Claude Bernard (1813–1878), one of the greatest scientists of the nineteenth century:

> Feeling gives rise to the experimental idea or hypothesis.... The whole experimental enterprise comes from the idea, for this it is which induces experiment. Reason or reasoning serves only to deduce the consequences of this idea and to submit them to experiment.
>
> An anticipative idea or an hypothesis is, then the starting point for all experimental reasoning. Without it, we could not make any investigation at all nor learn anything; we could only pile up sterile observations.[7]

So, we must start out with a theory or conceptual framework within which to frame our hypotheses. We must have faith in our ideas, but always be prepared to abandon them if necessary in light of evolving empirical evidence:

> If we are thoroughly steeped in the principles of the experimental method, we have nothing to fear; for, as long as the idea is correct, we go on developing it; when it is wrong, experimentation is there to set it right. We must be able, then, to attack questions even at the risk of going wrong. We do science better service, as has been said, by mistakes than by confusion, which means that we must *fearlessly push ideas to their full development, provided that we regulate them and are always careful to judge them by experiment.* The idea, in a word, is the motive of all reasoning, in

science as elsewhere. But everywhere the idea must be submitted to a criterion. In science the criterion is the experimental method (emphasis added).[8]

When our understanding is confused, we cannot make progress. Attempting to resolve ambiguity is thus a necessary precondition for research. By trusting our theories *provisionally*, we can avoid piling up sterile observations. But we must, simultaneously subject our ideas to the sternest forms of critical examination. Only in this way can we:

> ... avoid setting up a sort of opposition or exclusion between practice, which requires knowledge of particulars, and generalizations which mingle all in all.
>
> A physician, in fact, is by no means physician to living beings in general, not even to the human race, but rather, physician to a human individual ... Only after delving, then, as deeply as possible into the secrets of vital phenomena in the normal and pathological states can physiologists and physicians attain illuminating and fertile generalizations.[9]

TRUST, ...

By emphasizing the centrality of statistical methodology, scientific research today displays a fundamental *lack* of trust in the validity of insight and intuition. From a historical perspective, we have come full circle. Before the seventeenth century, the opinions of presumed experts were trusted as the main source of authoritative evidence. This seems strange to us, and naive, because we have so much more factual information about the world at our disposal. By the end of the twentieth century, the "hard facts" represented by statistics had become the touchstone of scientific truth.

As I have explained, probability and statistics are predicated on a narrow view of uncertainty. In order to frame a probability, our uncertainty must be expressed as a degree of doubt. There must be little ambiguity about the nature of the facts that are being analyzed, and the frequencies being calculated. In science, the desire to avoid ambiguity has resulted in a generally positivistic outlook. Only statements pertaining to properties or behaviors that can be directly observed and measured are licensed as truly *scientific*. Theories based on more abstract metaphysical conceptualizations generally fail to receive this imprimatur.

The shortcomings of positivism have long been recognized by many philosophers of science. Whitehead emphasized the intellectual poverty of limiting our gaze to past statistical regularities:

> The speculative extensions of laws, baseless on the Positivist theory, are the obvious issue of speculative metaphysical *trust* ... The point is, that speculative extension beyond direct observation spells some *trust* in metaphysics, however vaguely these metaphysical notions may be entertained in explicit thought. Our metaphysical knowledge is slight, superficial, incomplete. Thus errors creep in. But, such as it is, metaphysical understanding guides imagination and justifies purpose (emphasis added).[10]

Whitehead was pointing out how all scientific thought is premised on some implicit metaphysical substrate. Trust in this conceptual foundation emboldens and enables the scientist to move forward with confidence and motivation. Like the chess master, the scientist expects to succeed ultimately, because she trusts in her deep theoretical knowledge and educated intuition.

Whether such trust is warranted for any individual researcher can depend on many factors. Ironically, we have very little *scientific* knowledge about the qualities that give rise to superlative research. There is today a broad presumption that the quality of scientific research depends much more on methodology than on personal expertise. So, our emphasis tends to be on training scientists in *technique*, rather than in, say, logic or creativity. This primarily methodological conception of science has in some areas led to a plethora of technically sophisticated but uninspired or trivial studies.

By confusing science with technology, we misconstrue its true nature. The scientist must be an adventurer in the realm of new ideas, not simply an assembler of "sterile observations." It is one thing to notice that causal explanations are often misleading or based on wishful thinking, quite another to conclude that statistical summaries should always trump intuitive judgment. It is true that sound theories are not easy to discover and establish, but their value often far outweighs that of straightforward statistical information. A theory, in Whitehead's words, allows "speculative extension beyond direct observation."

Part of the current skepticism about the importance, or even the existence, of true insight, derives from a basic misconception about probability. An expert is commonly defined as someone who is capable of making accurate *predictions*. So, expertise is often judged by comparing predictions about specific events with observed frequencies of occurrence. In those situations in which relevant statistics are available, such comparisons are possible and may indeed provide an important indication of expertise. By this criterion, as Meehl suggested, human intuition seems no better than statistical algorithms, and sometimes worse.

Suppose, however, that we are dealing with a situation that is fraught with ambiguity. Is predictive skill a valid standard for assessing expertise? In such a context, it may be difficult or impossible to represent our uncertainty as a mathematical probability. Forcing the expert to frame his uncertainty so precisely may be artificial. Before this uncertainty can be placed on a numerical scale, it would be necessary to substantially resolve the ambiguity. The ability to resolve ambiguity productively is as much a hallmark of expertise as the ability to analyze preexisting data.

Consider the kinds of uncertainty dealt with in Philip Tetlock's research on predictions made by political scientists.[11] Imagine attempting to predict whether at least one nation will secede from the European Union within the next 10 years. Such an event is extremely vague because there are so many complex scenarios under which the future might unfold. Most of us could not begin to hazard a guess. What about an expert political scientist?

I would argue that the political expert might possess some real *insight*. By this, I mean that his mental "model" of the relevant reality would be much more refined than mine. It could draw upon a much richer reservoir of learning and experience. Of course, this does not necessarily mean that the expert's assessment would be correct; here we have the problem of the submarine navigator again. The expert's opinion might plausibly describe what is going on in the world, but still run aground on some overlooked factor. The point is that the expert's perspective is more likely than the layperson's to be useful for dealing with the situation. Much as I may have disliked many of Henry Kissinger's policy recommendations, if I were President I would certainly listen carefully to his opinions.[12]

All that may be true, you may be thinking, but what good is such expertise if it cannot generate accurate predictions? My answer is that in a real-world context, the problem is usually not simply a matter of passive prediction, but of taking effective *action*. The real question of interest might, for example, be not whether a country will exit the EU, but what are the relevant economic and political forces at work? Answers to that question might suggest additional questions related to the possible course of future events and how it might be influenced. Responding to such questions could suggest a number of subsidiary issues and possible strategies. Ideally, the insightful political scientist could contribute useful ideas to policy discussions. Equally important, she may suggest some fruitful means to obtain additional data to clarify the causal dynamics at play.

In a context that is so ambiguous, expertise can ideally help to navigate successfully through a series of challenges, even when the obstacles are not well understood. Indeed, an important aspect of expertise may be the wisdom to avoid prematurely offering firm numerical probability estimates. Rather, the expert in such a situation might be wise enough to refrain until the ambiguity has been sufficiently reduced. As Bernoulli counseled, we must try to withhold judgment until it becomes absolutely necessary to act or decide. By reducing all problems to matters of prediction, we are willfully ignoring ambiguity. Consequently, we tend to devalue the expert's role in resolving ambiguity because it cannot be measured objectively.

We have become accustomed to thinking that the sole function of science is to provide *answers*. However, science progresses as well by refining our *questions*. Often the key to a great discovery lies in reformulating the question. The Indian philosopher Jiddu Krishnamurti noted that "if we can really understand the problem, the answer will come out of it, because the answer is not separate from the problem."[13] In my experience, a hallmark of the true expert researcher or clinician is the ability to pose a fruitful question.

... BUT VERIFY

The great virtue of trusting one's gut is the increased possibility of discovering something important. Asking insightful questions and making educated guesses can lead to new opportunities. The thrill of making an important new discovery is a critical driver of research effort, but entails a considerable chance of being wrong. Without a healthy measure of self-confidence, who would assume this risk? On the other hand, unbridled optimism must be tempered by constant testing of our speculations against empirical data.

From a historical perspective, the "invention" and proliferation of *data* is a remarkable and quite recent development. Like the air we breathe, quantitative information now constitutes a ubiquitous backdrop that is simply always "there." We have forgotten that a few centuries ago, there *were* no data in our modern sense! Recall that around 1660, John Graunt hit upon the novel idea of compiling crude records of births and deaths into tables that could be analyzed for meaningful patterns. A quarter-century later, Jacob Bernoulli conceived the notion of quantifying uncertainty mathematically by analyzing large collections of similar previous occurrences. These geniuses were anomalies, in part because their world lacked all but the most minimal and rudimentary sources of data.

Gradually, as technology advanced, the volume of scientific, commercial, and administrative data grew steadily. Statistical methods, in tandem with mathematical probability, became the primary means of summarizing the data. However, the amount and scope of the data remained quite limited, because data storage was restricted to hand-written tabulations and printed copies. Moreover, until the mid-twentieth century, computation was almost exclusively by paper-and-pencil methods. In this pre-digital environment, statistical methods were severely limited because databases were small, difficult to obtain, and time-consuming to analyze.

The computations necessary for data analyses can be performed much faster today, but the basic methods have changed little. The main concern of the statistician remains the assessment of whether an observed pattern in data can plausibly be attributed to random variability. If the "null hypothesis" can be rejected, then the pattern can prima facie be regarded as something *real*. The primary criterion for making this determination is the test of statistical significance, based purely on probability theory. With few exceptions, the observed significance level (P-value) for each study is based on its data alone. The test ignores the broader context of many other studies and tests that are also being performed, and the various forces, including biases, that may affect the true probability of finding a statistically significant result.

In the early days of significance testing, there were very few tests actually being conducted in any research area. So, there was little danger that a multiplicity of studies would increase the true probability of achieving significance well above its nominal value (usually taken to be 0.05). Moreover, statistical significance was originally interpreted as merely *suggestive* of something worth considering seriously. A single study with a P-value less than 0.05 was evidence, but still far from proof. Real validation entailed replication in additional studies as well as plausibility in light of other relevant scientific theory and evidence.

Today, however, the situation is quite different. There are many studies going on in any given field, and multiple tests may be conducted within any study. This situation has resulted in the problems highlighted by John Ioannidis, which can only be expected to worsen unless our research methodology can adapt to a new reality.[14] The technological watershed occurring today promises to be at least as momentous as the advent of recorded data in the seventeenth century. That remarkable and unexpected breakthrough had enormous unforeseen consequences. We stand now at the threshold of a similar breakthrough: virtually unlimited data storage and manipulation capabilities made possible by computer technology. The ramifications of this staggering development are barely beginning to be felt, but will certainly include dramatic changes in how we do research.

The massive increase in captured data will present great *opportunities* for new scientific discoveries on an unprecedented scale. However, these opportunities will be accompanied by novel challenges. Some of these relate to the ambiguity of the available data. Rather than well-organized tables of numbers describing the values of a few pre-defined variables, the raw data may take a variety of new forms. Sources of potentially analyzable data already include text, conversation, music, photography, and video, all recorded in various media and formats. So, one set of challenges/ opportunities will be to transform this abundance of potentially useful information into more structured forms that can be productively analyzed.

How mathematical probability will be applied for analyzing the resulting databases is not clear. With huge volumes of data, we will uncover many more correlations that can pass muster according to conventional tests of significance. However, the nominal P-values will no longer provide a valid indication of whether or not such empirical relationships are *persistent* in the sense of reflecting causes likely to continue operating in the future. In a sense, statistical significance functions only as an imperfect proxy for the causal persistence that is aimed at by scientific research.

In a world of very limited data, there was not much opportunity to repeat experiments in order to provide direct evidence of an effect's persistence. Statistical testing effectively served as a substitute for replication, and it was usually adequate in the context of agricultural and industrial research. It became tacitly accepted that if random variability could effectively be eliminated as an explanation, the effect must be real, and therefore likely to continue. However, for the reasons I have discussed in the previous two chapters, this rationale is becoming less and less compelling. Statistical significance simply does not mean what it used to.

If conventional statistical methods based on mathematical probability are becoming unreliable as a proxy for actual replication, what may replace them? Fortunately, the huge increase in data has the potential not only to yield insights derived from statistical patterns, but also to test their validity through true replication. I say *potential* because existing methodology for replication is not yet very sophisticated. For the most part, research methodologists have not focused extensively on the complex issues that can arise in performing validation through replication.

One reason for this failure is that the problem cannot be reduced entirely to a mathematical form. For instance, a fundamental problem is to determine whether an apparent causal relationship will *generalize* to other situations of practical interest. Will an educational program proven effective under limited conditions continue to be effective when much more widely adopted? Will a drug that appeared safe in clinical trials turn out to have adverse effects when prescribed in general practice? Such questions of generalizability or "external validity" require some combination of technology and clinical expertise to address.

A second important dilemma related to validation arises from the astronomical numbers of potential predictive variables that exist in certain contexts. Research on genomics is a prime example. In this research, it is obvious that some kind of replication is *de rigueur*, because "false discovery rates" are extremely high when testing many thousands of genes for a causal effect on some outcome of interest. A number of different approaches have been suggested to deal with this problem. However, statisticians have tended to concentrate almost exclusively on complex modeling techniques that are based on probability theory. For example, when testing hundreds of thousands of genes to identify the few that cause a certain disease, the threshold P-value may be lowered from 0.05 to 0.0000001.

In this way, the probability of falsely detecting a gene (or set of several genes) that achieves significance by chance is greatly reduced. However, the catch-22 is that the probability of discovering a truly causative gene is *also* greatly reduced. This dilemma is especially problematic when there are multiple genes, possibly working together in some manner, each of which contributes only modestly to the outcome. The probability that such genes will emerge from a very stringent screening process is low. Finding a balance between the conflicting demands of discovery and validation is recognized as a critical challenge. Much less understood, however, is that the solutions do not lie exclusively within the realm of probability theory.

There are two main avenues for improving the discovery process in these "high-dimensional" situations. First, theoretical knowledge and insight can often be helpful in focusing attention on a promising subset of variables. Understanding causal processes will often improve the chances of success, and of identifying factors that are interpretable by clinicians. Clinical insight applied to individual cases will depend on understanding causal mechanisms, not just blind acceptance of black-box statistical models.

Second, validation of statistical associations culled from massive databases *must* depend primarily on repeated testing on data that were not used to suggest the association. The basic reason is that any procedure for "fitting" a predictive model attempts to obtain the best predictive accuracy within the data used for the analysis. Ironically, however, such a procedure is guaranteed to "over-fit" by responding to some random variation (noise) as well as to the true predictive relationship (signal). Therefore, the *apparent* accuracy within the original sample is bound to be exaggerated to some extent. Developing sophisticated new techniques to minimize overfitting will become increasingly important as part of the solution to this conundrum. However, the only way to obtain a true (unbiased) measure of the model's accuracy is to try it out on a new sample of observations.

To date, the critical importance of independent replication has been recognized more by practitioners of *predictive analytics* and developers of *machine learning* techniques than by statisticians and scientists. Much of this work occurs in the context of business problems, especially those related to market research. Best practice in this area includes at least two levels of validation. One level involves only the study's own data; the other requires independent data from at least one additional study.

Using only the study's own data, the total dataset is divided randomly into an *analytic* or *training* sample for model derivation and a *hold-out* subset that is put aside for validation. For each individual in this hold-out sample, the outcome is predicted based on the model derived from the analytic data. The predictions are then compared against the actual outcomes for the individuals in the hold-out sample. This independent validation on a hold-out sample provides an unbiased estimate of the model's predictive accuracy. More sophisticated versions of the hold-out principle may also be utilized.[15]

Performing well on a hold-out subset should be viewed as a minimum requirement. At the next level, the model can be tested on a completely independent sample. For example, data on a different region or time-period may be used. Making accurate predictions for this independent sample provides solid evidence that the model *may* work well in general. However, ongoing feedback on its performance "in the field" is necessary to determine if conditions may have changed, requiring an update or revision of the model.

I have argued that statistical significance will become a much less useful criterion in the new world of large and more complex databases. This will be especially true for the process of *discovering* potentially meaningful relationships. Generating promising indications of such relationships requires the kind of open-ended exploration that John Tukey advocated 50 years ago, for which he understood that mathematical probability would be largely irrelevant. On the other hand, Tukey saw correctly that probability-based methods would continue to play an important *confirmatory* role.

If we encourage more creativity in generating and exploring hypotheses, we will inevitably increase the chances of over-fitting, resulting in many false discoveries. Suppose, for example, that we are testing 10,000 genes to determine if any of them can increase the risk of colon cancer. Assume that one of these, Gene X, actually does have a substantial effect. If we perform 10,000 statistical tests using a significance level of 0.01, we would expect

Gene X to appear significant. But, in addition, we might find 100 of the other tests statistically significant as well. Of all the 101 genes flagged, we would not know which would truly be related to colon cancer.

Suppose, however, that one of these genes happens to have a plausible biological rationale. We could then decide to test it again in a new sample of people, perhaps a hold-out subset of those in the original study. If this test yields a significance level of 0.01 or less, we would have fairly strong evidence that Gene X is indeed a real risk factor. This simple hypothetical illustrates how statistical significance can be valuable as a tool for validation of indications that are discovered by a more open-ended exploratory methodology. Analyzing an independent sample essentially restores the conditions under which the significance test is valid. Regardless of how the predictive model has been derived, and how much over-fitting may have occurred, the resulting model is subjected to a fair test on a new playing field.

THE FUTURE

Creating a culture of science in which independent validation becomes a primary criterion for scientific acceptance will help to regain public trust. Knowing that their findings will be subjected to independent scrutiny will impose a higher standard of proof on investigators. At the same time, however, it will free them up to follow promising leads and refine hypotheses. Requiring real validation will blunt the inhibitions that result from the pressure to achieve statistical significance or bust. Because both data exploration and independent validation require substantial skill and effort, the quantity of research being generated may well decrease as a result. However, the quality should improve greatly.

One particularly important improvement can result from much less emphasis on *main effects*. Under the present reward system, statistical significance is the most important criterion. Average effects on broad populations are favored in part because they have the best chance to produce a P-value of 0.05 or less. More subtle effects that pertain to particular subgroups have less statistical *power* to attain significance. These realities play strongly into the inertia currently preventing a move away from these main effects. In contrast, a strong emphasis on replication would shift the incentive structure toward finding effects that could stand up to the rigors of trial by independent data and analysis.

At present, even requiring researchers to provide access to their data to enable simple *reproduction* of a study's findings is not feasible.[16] Investigators generally regard the data as their private preserve, to be jealously guarded from prying eyes. As a result, even blatant errors in the analyses underlying findings published in respected journals rarely come to light. There is almost no systematic effort to discover such defects, which we must assume to be grossly underreported. There are simply no incentives for the original authors to solicit, or for other investigators to conduct, even basic reproduction of results. More meaningful replication of study findings by analyzing independent data faces even more daunting obstacles. Obtaining the necessary data and performing the analysis are costly and time-consuming, if even made possible at all, and offer little ultimate payoff.

Going forward, this situation must and can change. In a world of cheap and plentiful data, it should become feasible to institutionalize some forms of routine independent validation.[17] Eventually, methods and standards for replication of study results will evolve. Proper validation will become an essential component of research activity. Statistical significance testing in some form will remain important, but will be returned to its rightful place as a piece of evidence, not the main criterion for decisions regarding publication. Journal editors and reviewers will insist on some form of *real* validation before accepting papers for publication.

Our current methodological orthodoxy plays a major role in deepening the division between scientific researchers and clinical practitioners. Prior to the Industrial Age, research and practice were more closely tied together. Scientific investigation was generally motivated more directly by practical problems and conducted by individuals involved in solving them. As scientific research became more specialized and professionalized, the perspectives of researchers and clinicians began to diverge. In particular, their respective relationships to data and knowledge have become quite different.

The research scientist became regarded primarily as a *producer* of new knowledge, while the practitioner became a *consumer*. Science in the twentieth century became increasingly seen as a product, to be manufactured and shipped out to customers in the form of lectures, books, and journal articles. As this knowledge industry has developed, the sheer volume of scientific information has grown enormously. Whether the value of this information has increased commensurately is highly questionable.

Scientists and practitioners inhabit quite different professional worlds. Researchers are immersed in a world of sophisticated technology and quantitative analysis. In many fields, the techniques of probability and statistics are central. Data are the stock in trade that researchers collect, organize, and analyze. In studying human beings, the subjects are reduced to sets of numerical values that purport to capture their relevant characteristics. Individuality is submerged, so probabilities and correlations can emerge.

The world of quantitative research has become divorced from the world of the clinician. When involved in complex statistical modeling, researchers must necessarily lose sight of the individual human beings whose pale reflections are encapsulated in the data being manipulated by their computer programs. Their ultimate goal may be to help real people, but their immediate focus is on the technical challenge. Concentrating on this immediate objective, a scientist can easily forget the flesh-and-blood people behind the numbers.

Practitioners, on the other hand, typically deal with concrete problems faced by individual human beings. The situations they face are often so ambiguous that the relevance of general statistical conclusions may be unclear. The neatly packaged main effects that are offered by researchers ignore too much of what they observe about each particular individual in front of them. However, they are powerless to adapt or adjust the evidence-based general recommendations to fit their specific situation. They must *either* accept blindly the statistical "product" or choose to override it with clinical intuition. Neither solution seems quite right.

Both practitioners and statisticians are locked into a feedback loop that strongly reinforces the status quo.[18] Practitioners (and many applied researchers) are intimidated by the authority of statistical methodology. Their limited training in these methods, focused on main effects and significance testing, leaves them with the impression that there are no alternatives. Therefore, they do not demand more nuanced and relevant kinds of information. Conversely, statisticians (and many theoretical research methodologists) do not perceive a demand for new approaches, since their current methods are so widely accepted and used. So, they are not motivated to rock the boat. I am hopeful that in the near future this unsatisfactory stasis can change, as our relationships to data continue to evolve.

I suspect that the absolute separation between the production and consumption of knowledge will come to seem rather artificial. The model for the research process in the twentieth century was something like industrial manufacturing; the emerging model of the future seems to be more like a social network. Everyone involved in generating and using scientific research will become increasingly interconnected; a range of new roles for dealing with data will develop. A variety of new enterprises, both public and private, may spring up to mediate between databases and those who can potentially make use of their contents.

How this sort of transformation will occur is truly *uncertain*, in the broadest sense of the word. However, we are already beginning to witness a rapid evolution of information-related industries such as software development, entertainment, education, marketing, and publishing. Scientific research will inevitably evolve as well to become more relevant and effective within a more networked and computationally unlimited future. Statistical methods must adapt to this evolution by focusing on the real challenges and opportunities that will arise. This may require methodologists to move out of the comfort zone of main effects and prespecified tests of hypotheses:

> A major challenge of tomorrow will be to extract valid causal information from complex databases in a way that takes much fuller account of personal characteristics. Increasingly, there will be a demand for solutions that are tailored to smaller and smaller subgroups, and even to individuals. To develop methods of analysis that can meet this challenge, statisticians will need to question many of the assumptions on which traditional approaches have been constructed. This will not be easy or comfortable, but is essential if real progress is to be made.[19]

Unlike the past, the future will present an embarrassment of data riches. The problem will be to transmute various sources of raw data into a form that is analyzable. The sheer volume of data will require new approaches for organizing and summarizing the raw data. Already, some medical researchers envision a "digital revolution" in healthcare, facilitated by emerging technology.[20] Before too long we may start to accumulate a full database of biological readings taken continually throughout a person's entire life, perhaps via tiny subcutaneous implants. The data could be transmitted to a personal storage server where it will remain permanently on file.

Data analysts of the future will develop software and methods for deriving valuable information that is potentially useful for research. The overwhelming amount and variety of raw information about personal health and behavior will call for judicious application of willful ignorance in creating standardized databases. In addition to collecting and analyzing the digital exhaust from normal activity, it will become possible to conduct some kinds of experiments much more efficiently. No longer will a sample of experimental subjects need to be present in one physical location. The subjects could in many cases participate remotely, with study data sets contructed automatically by querying their personal databases.

For those situated more toward the consumption end of the data processing spectrum, the emphasis will be on ways to access and interpret the data. Perhaps the clinician, or even the patient in some cases, will have the capability of performing various "on-demand" customized studies. Sources of data could be acquired from providers at a nominal cost instantaneously and assembled for analysis. The data analysis might be performed using the products and services offered by a wide range of data intermediaries.

Imagine, for instance, that a patient in the year 2050 is deciding whether to begin taking aspirin to ward off heart disease and cancer. In conjunction with his medical advisors, he must choose a precise dose, timing, and method of ingestion, tailored to his complete medical history and individual needs. The volume of data and complexity of the analysis are far beyond anything we can imagine today. The software allows many simulations to be easily carried out to determine probabilities of various outcomes under different treatment choices. These probabilities apply to the individual patient, although they are derived in part by analyzing the data from many previous patients.

The specific ways in which such possibilities may be realized are impossible to spell out. I cannot begin to imagine how "statistical" software might look a few decades from now. Perhaps it will be something like the "data garden" envisioned by popular science fiction writer Tad Williams:

> Technologists had their own names for such things, ... but whether it was called an interface, a data display, or a dream library, what had begun a century before as an attempt to conceptualize information in ways that people other than engineers could understand, starting with crude images of the most mundane business objects—file folders, in-boxes, wastebaskets—had expanded along with the power of technology, until the ways in which information could be ordered and acted upon were as individual, even peculiar, as the people who used it.... It had the look of a jungle, a place where things grew and fought, altered, adapted, where strategies blossomed spectacularly then failed, or bloomed and survived, or simply absorbed the moisture of informational existence and waited.... The virtual flora altered with the information they symbolized, changing shape and habit as the database relations shifted.[21]

Of course, there will be many ethical as well as technical problems raised by the potential of knowing so much more about everyone. Can we minimize exploitation for economic or political ends, while reaping the benefits for human health and well-being? Certainly, our historical record on this score is quite mixed.

MINDFUL IGNORANCE

Prior to 1654, the concepts of chance and uncertainty were quantified only in the most nebulous way. Chance was associated with the arbitrariness and capriciousness of mythical forces that were utterly inscrutable. Our modern idea of randomness was unknown. Uncertainty was a function of our limited human understanding about the true underlying causes. This primal uncertainty encompassed both ambiguity and doubt, which were not clearly differentiated. The interchange between Pascal and Fermat represented a watershed moment: it ushered in a series of somewhat fortuitous further developments that led to mathematical probability.

A century later, uncertainty was starting to be widely regarded as subject to mathematical laws. This momentous step was made possible by implicitly reframing probability as a degree of doubt within the well-defined context of games of chance. Ambiguity pertaining to the conceptual framework within which this measure could be applied was effectively ignored. As a result, chance became "tamed" and was no longer completely unfathomable and attributed to the whims of the gods. The lottery became the model for the operation of chance more generally.

By the early nineteenth century, this metaphorical-lottery conception had spread into many other domains. Randomness, similar to that which exists in an idealized lottery, was regarded as an inherent aspect of natural and social phenomena. The laws of chance were deemed responsible for the ubiquitous statistical regularities that were being discovered. Empirical frequencies of a diverse collection of important events, such as births, deaths, marriages, thefts, and suicides were found to be remarkably constant over time and often across geographical areas. Laplace famously observed that even the number of undeliverable letters winding up in the dead letter office of the Paris postal system varied little from year to year.

These apparently law-like patterns raised questions about their meaning. Did they represent evidence that human free will was an illusion?[22] Were there real social forces that produced a "budget" of events, regardless of individual actions and decisions? Such questions were intimately bound up with debates about the nature of probability, as I discussed in Chapter 8. In popular literature, social critics including Twain, Dickens, and Balzac satirized the pretensions of those like Quetelet who perceived in these apparent statistical constancies the hand of natural law, or even divinity.

Eventually, the angst felt by many intellectuals of the nineteenth century regarding probability and statistics gave way to agnosticism by the early twentieth. Probability became simply accepted as the logic of uncertainty, without worrying about what precisely the word really meant. As a result, few moderns recognize that statistical "reality" applies to populations, but not necessarily to the individuals within those populations.

Mathematical probabilities and the statistics used to estimate them depend on willful ignorance. It is only by ignoring certain specific considerations pertaining to the event or statement in question that a mathematical probability becomes possible. This mathematical probability applies to individuals *en masse*, but must overlook some of what Keynes called the "vague though more important" individual circumstances. The vagueness of what must be ignored may preclude formulation of uncertainty as a numerical probability.

Finally, and most relevant to the problems and opportunities we face today, probability is not destiny. To accept passively that the world is essentially a *lottery*, as in Borges's parable, represents a kind of fatalism. The scientist (like the entrepreneur or chess master) must believe in his ability to succeed, despite the long odds that may exist in general. Research is an unfolding process that continually evolves as evidence is obtained and theory is refined. Chance certainly plays a role in this process, but so do personal qualities like intellect, creativity, perseverance, and courage.

Statistics can often provide useful evidence, but the relationship between statistical frequencies and judgmental probabilities is indirect. The scientist must decide which pieces of contextual information are relevant and which to ignore. This is an essential aspect of the scientist's responsibility that, as Fisher emphasized, cannot be ceded to the data analyst, or worse, to the computer. Evading this responsibility by assuming that a level of statistical significance, or any other purely probabilistic measure, can by itself determine scientific validity is a dangerous delusion.

Mathematical probability is a tool for quantifying uncertainty by drawing an analogy with an idealized lottery. As such, it can only measure the degree of uncertainty as a degree of *doubt*, ranging from 0 (complete doubt) to 1 (no doubt). Probability is a tremendously useful tool, but deals with only a part of uncertainty. Statistical methods based completely on probability theory apply to classes and categories of individuals that must be *given*. Statistical theory glosses over ambiguity about the appropriate categories to choose or create. This ambiguity is either ignored entirely or regarded as a nuisance that gets in the way of rigorous research.

Practitioners are focused to a large extent on ambiguity. They are in the business of resolving ambiguity in productive ways and are often uncomfortable with statistical analyses. Researchers, on the contrary, generally regard their empirical data and mathematical models as imperfect but objective representations of reality. They are in the business of generating inferences in the form of probability statements and are often uncomfortable with qualitative insight. Each of these alternative perspectives is of limited scope. The path toward some kind of fruitful reconciliation must be based on a conception of uncertainty that is more integrative.

Probability entails a delicate balancing act. On the one hand, we must recognize the infinite complexity of the individual case. On the other, we must simplify to achieve useful generalizations by ignoring much of the individual detail. To selectively view only the subset of information we deem relevant, out of all potential information, is to maintain a posture of willful ignorance. This is absolutely necessary in order to generate a mathematical probability statement, but is usually done implicitly and unconsciously. The challenges and opportunities of the future demand that it be done more explicitly and mindfully.

APPENDIX: THE PASCAL–FERMAT CORRESPONDENCE OF 1654

The first extant letter in the exchange contains a response by Fermat to some apparent confusion evidenced in Pascal's previous letter.[1] Fermat attempts to clarify a possible misunderstanding regarding a variation on the problem of determining the fair odds for attempting to obtain a 6 with eight potential throws of a fair die. Suppose that "after the stakes have been made," the players subsequently agree to change the terms.

Instead of winning if a 6 occurs on or before the eighth throw, the player will win only if a 6 occurs for the first time *after* a specified throw, such as the fourth throw. In other words, the player will win if the first point is made between the fifth and eighth throws, but will lose if the 6 comes up in one of the preceding throws (or not at all). What portion of the total amount staked should be given back to the player in compensation for agreeing to this more stringent condition?

It is important to understand that Fermat was not asking how the player's future expectation would change *after* four unsuccessful throws *had actually occurred*. It can be shown that the fair odds in favor of making the point in the remaining four trials would be about 13:12. However, this reduction of the expectation would not be the result of a decision on the player's part but simply to bad luck. So, although his odds against

Willful Ignorance: The Mismeasure of Uncertainty, First Edition. Herbert I. Weisberg.
© 2014 John Wiley & Sons, Inc. Published 2014 by John Wiley & Sons, Inc.

making the point in the four remaining throws would be diminished, the player would deserve no compensation.

Fermat's logic is impeccable but rather confusing to follow:

> If I try to make a certain score with a single die in eight throws, and if, after the stakes have been made, we agree that I will not make the first throw; then according to my theory I must take in compensation 1/6th of the total sum, because of that first throw.
>
> Whilst if we agree further that I will not make the second throw, I must, for compensation, get a sixth of the remainder which comes to 5/36th of the total sum.
>
> If, after this, we agree I will not make the third throw, I must have, for my indemnity, a sixth of the remaining sum which is 25/216th of the total.
>
> And if after that we agree again that I will not make the fourth throw, I must have a sixth of what is left, which is 125/1296th of the total, and I agree with you that this is the value of the fourth throw, assuming that one has already settled for the previous throws.

For concreteness, suppose that I wager $77 that I can make my point in eight throws, and you bet $23 against me. As I explained in Chapter 3, this is approximately a fair bet. Then, suppose I agree (in advance of throwing the die) to lose if my point is made on the first try, but otherwise to continue with all subsequent rolls. Fermat's logic is that (in advance of throwing) I should receive a partial share consisting of 1/6th of the total $100 wagered, or $16.67, as a rebate. He reasoned that staking this amount in hopes of gaining the $100 on the first throw would be a fair wager.

At this point (still prior to any actual throws), suppose I agree to forego as well the potential win on the second throw. Then, by the same reasoning, my rebate should be $13.88 in addition (5/36 × $100), because that is the expectation for winning on exactly the second throw. My total compensation for agreeing to sacrifice both throws should be the sum of these values, or $30.55. Similarly, if I agree to forego the payoffs for the first three throws, my total recompense would be $42.12, and for four throws it would be $51.77.

In modern terms, we would say that the probability is approximately 0.52 that a 6 would occur on one of the first four throws (or on one of any four throws, for that matter). Since the total probability of winning within all eight throws is 0.77, the probability at the outset (a priori) that a 6 will appear *first* within throws five through eight must be 0.25

(= 0.77 − 0.52). As I mentioned, this does not mean that the player's probability of winning after four losing tosses have actually taken place would be 0.25. That probability would be 0.52, which is the same as the a priori probability of winning in four throws.

The difference between 0.52 and 0.25 can be explained by the fact that throwing the first 6 in throws five through eight entails two events: *not winning* in trials one through four and *winning* in one of trials five through eight. The probability of this "compound event" is the product of the respective probabilities of the two component events, which is 0.25 (= 0.52 × 0.48).

This distinction is fairly easy to understand with modern probability theory, but Fermat only had very rudimentary tools at his disposal. So, his explanation appears somewhat ambiguous and must have confused Pascal, who thought Fermat referred to the situation after the first dice had already been cast. In reply, Fermat took pains to clarify his meaning:

> But in the last example of your letter (I quote your own words) you suggest that if I undertake to get the six in eight throws and having thrown three times without getting it, and if my opponent wants me to abandon my fourth throw and is willing to compensate me because I might still be able to get the six, then 125/1296th of our total stakes would be due to me.

> This, however, is incorrect according to my theory. For, in this case, since the one who is throwing has gained nothing in the first three throws, the total sum remains in play, and the one who holds the die and who agrees not to make the fourth throw should take 1/6th of the total stakes as his reward.

In other words, the situation (and the corresponding expectation) regarding the fourth trial would be different, because the "competing" possibility of an earlier 6 would no longer be relevant to the current situation. The fraction 125/1296 would of course represent the probability that the player would win exactly on the fourth trial but not before. Fermat was essentially distinguishing between what we would today call a *conditional probability* of 1/6 (relevant after some other event has already occurred) and an *unconditional probability* of 125/1296 (relevant without reference to any other event).

A real breakthrough here is Fermat's insight that the total stake (expectation) for a player can be subdivided into separate components corresponding to different *ways* (outcomes) in which the event can be achieved.

In this case, the player might win on any of the eight trials. Prior to playing, each of these possibilities can be accorded a certain portion of the total expectation. This share corresponds to the odds of betting on that specific throw. Thus, for example, if we were to bet that the fourth throw would be the winner (i.e., the first on which a 6 turns up), the correct odds would be 1171:125. Calculating the odds that the winner will occur within the first four throws involves summing the incremental shares of the four throws, to obtain the overall fair share, and then converting this share into odds.

Fermat has shifted the focus of attention away from the odds directly and toward the *fraction* of the total stakes. In this way, he reaps certain mathematical advantages that derive from dealing with a fraction rather than with odds. These technical benefits come mainly from the *additive* nature of the calculations. It is much easier to assemble a total fair share in a complex problem by *adding up* the shares of the constituent parts than to work directly with the odds.

In dealing with fractions, Fermat seemed to be on the verge of defining mathematical probability as we now know it, in place of the odds. Indeed, his exposition quoted above refers to fractions (1/6, 5/36, 25/216, 125/1296) that we would naturally interpret as *probabilities*. Indeed, it is hard for us *not* to regard these fractions as probabilities, but Fermat never made this leap. We can only wonder how differently the subsequent history of probability would have turned out if Fermat had, like Cardano, evinced more interest in trying his luck in the gaming salons.

From this point, the correspondence turned mainly to the problem of the points. In his response dated July 29, 1654, Pascal described his general method with some examples. We know that Pascal had been composing a book that would contain the most extensive treatment of combinatorial mathematics to date. While it may have been completed around the time of the correspondence, it was not published until 1665, 3 years after Pascal's death. The complete presentation of his solution to the problem of the points is contained in this *Treatise on the Arithmetical Triangle*.[2]

In the letter to Fermat, Pascal first considers the case in which Player A needs one more point to win, and Player B still needs two more points. We can represent this situation as (A1, B2). Suppose, writes Pascal, that each of the players has wagered 32 pistoles, so that the total pot contains

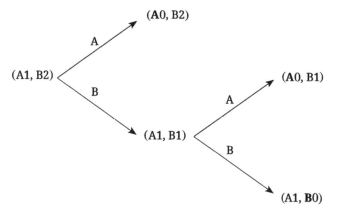

FIGURE A.1   Schematic of the problem of the points: player A lacks 1 point to win and player B lacks 2.

64 pistoles. How should the 64 pistoles be divided? The future progress of the game can be represented by an event tree, as in Figure A.1.

If A wins the first game the match is over because he now lacks zero points, while his opponent still lacks two (A0, B2), so he is the victor, taking all 64 pistoles. If B wins the first game, the match continues (A1, B1). At that point A's expectation would be 32, since the players would then have equal chances of winning the pot. In effect, they would be play-ing a symmetrical game in which the amount wagered by each one was 32 pistoles. Therefore, this sub-game must have a value of 32 pistoles. Hence, the total game can be evaluated as shown in Figure A.2. A's total expectation is the same as if he were playing only a single game, with an

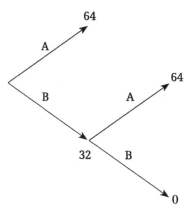

FIGURE A.2   Schematic of the problem of the points showing all possible outcomes when player A lacks 1 point to win and player B lacks 2.

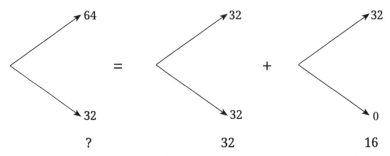

FIGURE A.3   Pascal's evaluation of the unknown expectation in the problem of the points when player A lacks 1 point to win and player B lacks 2.

equal chance of obtaining either 64 pistoles or 32 pistoles, as illustrated in Figure A.2. But how are we to evaluate the expectation of such a gamble?

To us, the answer might seem obvious, but in Pascal's day there was no principle upon which to evaluate such a gamble. So, Pascal's ingenious solution breaks new ground. He analyzes the single gamble with an equal chance of obtaining 64 or 32 as being worth the same as receiving 32 *for certain*, plus an equal chance of winning an *additional* 32. But the equal chance at winning 32 versus 0 is equivalent to a bet in which each player has staked 16 and has an equal chance of winning the pot. The value of this equivalent bet would therefore be 16 for each player. Thus, A has an expectation of 16 pistoles, which together with the 32 he has "for certain" yields 48 in total.

Pascal's resulting complete breakdown of the total gamble is illustrated in Figure A.3. Note that when Pascal states that the player has 32 for certain, he is equating the value of an even gamble that is *worth X* with the value of receiving *X* for certain. So, he really means that the value is at least 32, not that he will actually win at least 32. In fact, he was well aware that the only possible outcomes of the game were 0 and 64.

Next Pascal considers the case when B lacks 3 points and A lacks just one (A1, B3), as represented in Figure A.4. Again, each player wagers 32 pistoles. If A wins the first game, then the match is over (A0, B3) and A collects all 64 pistoles, as in the previous example. However, if B wins the first game, then the players will find themselves in position (A1, B2).

But Pascal has already determined that in this position, A's share would be 48 and B's would be 16. Thus, at the outset (A1, B3), the match would be equivalent to a single game in which A had an equal chance of obtaining

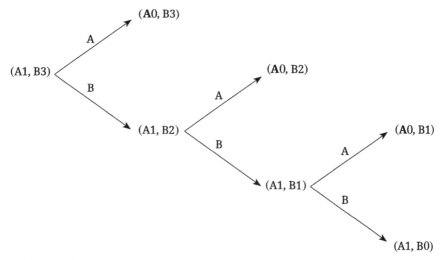

FIGURE A.4   Schematic of the problem of the points when player A lacks 1 point to win and player B lacks 3.

either 64 pistoles or 48 pistoles. This simple gamble would be worth 56 pistoles (see Figure A.5).

If you find this all somewhat confusing on an initial reading, do not feel too bad. It was a struggle for the two most gifted mathematicians in France. Referring to the event-tree diagram in the Figure A.5, you can see that Pascal works back from the tips of the tree to the base. At each

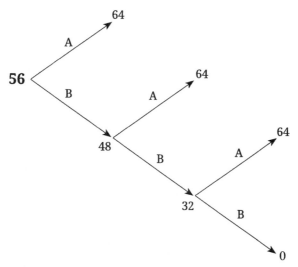

FIGURE A.5   Schematic of the problem of the points showing all possible outcomes when player A lacks 1 point to win and player B lacks 3.

stage, he evaluates the expectation of a gamble in which the player has an equal chance of obtaining either a higher or lower amount. He accomplishes this by taking the average of the two amounts and substituting this fixed value for an uncertain one. Pascal has in effect invented the idea of a *mathematical expectation* in its simplest form. Pascal uses this new idea to obtain what would today be called a *recursive* solution.

In principle, this recursive method can be extended to solve the problem of points for any numbers of points that are lacked by A and B. Indeed, a similar approach can solve much more general problems, such as when there are three players and when the players have unequal skill. However, the combinatorial mathematics involved becomes much more formidable. Indeed, it is astounding that Pascal could develop this approach without the algebraic notation we now take for granted, let alone modern probability theory. Fortunately, Pascal had recently written his *Treatise* and was well equipped for this challenge.

Pascal, in effect, had found a new principle for calculating the expectation that did not depend on enumerating a set of equally likely outcomes. Fermat, as we shall see, devised two solutions. One was rather similar in spirit to Pascal's approach, but the other followed the strategy of finding a clever way to apply the established principle of counting favorable and unfavorable cases, or chances. As we mentioned previously, Fermat's favorite ploy was to divide and conquer. He would attempt to divide the total outcome into component parts. The expectation corresponding to each of these parts could be calculated separately based on the traditional principle of counting favorable and unfavorable cases. Applying this approach to the problem of points, Fermat could move *forward* through the tree instead of backward.

Consider the problem of points just discussed, which begins in position (A1, B3), and refer now to Figure A.6. Fermat observed that player A could win in one of three different ways, and player B in one way. He noted first that A had an even chance of winning the first game and that his share for this chance alone should be half the pot (32 pistoles). However, if he failed in the first game, he could win in the second, which would be worth half of the remaining 32, or 16 pistoles. Here Fermat is applying the same logic he had employed in the simpler problem of making a 6 in eight throws of a die. Finally, if he failed on rounds 1 and 2, his chance of winning in round 3 would be worth 8 pistoles. Adding these, he arrived

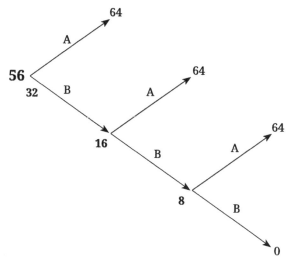

FIGURE A.6   Fermat's evaluation of the problem of the points when player A lacks 1 point to win and player B lacks 3.

at 56 pistoles in total. Once again, he has divided the total expectation into component parts and added them together.

As neat as this solution seems, it was not the one presented initially by Fermat to Pascal. As I mentioned earlier, Fermat was famous for teasing other mathematicians with strokes of brilliance accompanied by precious little explanation. In this case, the wizard of Toulouse may have been doing exactly this, by at first proposing a simple method that worked perfectly, but whose rationale was mystifying. Fermat accomplished his trick by transforming the problem of points into a straightforward enumeration of favorable and unfavorable outcomes.

Fermat suggested that we imagine a hypothetical extension of the match to the *maximum number* of possible games, regardless of the results at any earlier stage. Then, all possible sequences of outcomes could be listed. Each of these sequences could be considered equally likely *prior to the match*. For example, the 16 possible sequences for a match when A needs two points and B lacks three (A2, B3) are shown in Table A.1. Each line in this table corresponds to one possible "path" through the event tree. However, as indicated by shading in Table A.1, some of these paths could never actually occur if the match ended as soon as the outcome was no longer in doubt.

TABLE A.1   Unfinished Game with Starting Position = (A2, B3)

Game 1	Game 2	Game 3	Game 4	Winner
A	A	A	A	**A**
A	A	A	B	**A**
A	A	B	A	**A**
A	A	B	B	**A**
A	B	A	A	**A**
A	B	A	B	**A**
A	B	B	A	**A**
A	B	B	B	**B**
B	A	A	A	**A**
B	A	A	B	**A**
B	A	B	A	**A**
B	A	B	B	**B**
B	B	A	A	**A**
B	B	A	B	**B**
B	B	B	A	**B**
B	B	B	B	**B**

Nonetheless, Fermat argued that we ought to count the number of paths in which each player would win. So, in this particular example, the odds in favor of A are immediately seen to be 11:5. One drawback of this method noted by Pascal was that the "labor of the combination is excessive." For instance, suppose we attempted to solve the problem (A10, B7) by Fermat's approach. Then the maximum number of games would be 16, and there would be 65,556 possible paths to evaluate.

Fermat, the theoretician, was untroubled by such practical difficulties. In principle, his approach provided a general solution to the problem of points. Moreover, Fermat claimed that it would work for the three-player version as well! Pascal was at first quite skeptical of this claim. In his letter, he concedes that this "pretense" of imaginary additional rounds happens to work with two players, and even develops a rationale for why it should. However, he relates that he and Roberval have found a flaw, because (they believe) Fermat's approach leads to problems in the three-player version. Poor Roberval seems especially befuddled by Fermat's thinking. Why, he wonders, should we base our calculation on the maximum number of possible games when the match could end in fewer?

Pascal has a better handle on Fermat's logic, but it turns out he too is a bit confused.

To express his misgivings, Pascal proposes to consider a match among three players, each with an equal chance to win any round. He assumes that player A needs only one point, while each of B and C need two more points to win. We can represent this as (A1, B2, C2). This contest will be completed by the third game at most (see Table A.2). Pascal then gets tangled up in his analysis of what he understands to be Fermat's technique. Since there are three possibilities for each game, there are 27 paths in total (3 × 3 × 3). He observes that in some of the paths, two players *both* seem

TABLE A.2   Unfinished Game with Starting Position = (A1, B2, C2)

Game 1	Game 2	Game 3	Winner
A	A	A	**A**
A	A	B	**A**
A	A	C	**A**
A	B	A	**A**
A	B	B	**A**
A	B	C	**A**
A	C	A	**A**
A	C	B	**A**
A	C	C	**A**
B	A	A	**A**
B	A	B	**A**
B	A	C	**A**
B	B	A	**B**
B	B	B	**B**
B	B	C	**B**
B	C	A	**A**
B	C	B	**B**
B	C	C	**C**
C	A	A	**A**
C	A	B	**A**
C	A	C	**A**
C	B	A	**A**
C	B	B	**B**
C	B	C	**C**
C	C	A	**C**
C	C	B	**C**
C	C	C	**C**

to win. For example, if A would win the first round, but B the next two, wouldn't they both achieve the goal? How then should the division be made?

Pascal was missing the point that Fermat's 27 equally likely cases were really convenient metaphysical devices, not actual outcomes that could all be carried out in reality. Upon receiving this letter, Fermat apparently realized (or did he slyly know all along?) that his reasoning was not so transparent. In his reply, Fermat pulls back the curtain to reveal how his magic has been performed:

> The consequence, as you so well remarked, of this fiction of lengthening the match to a particular number of games is that it serves only to simplify the rules and (in my opinion) to make all the chances equal, or, to state it more intelligibly, to reduce all the fractions to a common denominator.

> So that you will have no more doubts, if instead of *three* games in the same case, you lengthen the pretended match to *four*, there would be not just 27 combinations but 81, and we have to see how many combinations would give one game to the first man before either of the others would get two games, and how many would give two games to each of the other men before the first man gets one. You will find that there are 51 combinations favorable to the first man, and 15 favorable to each of the other two, which comes to the same thing as before.

Fermat then goes on (for Roberval's benefit, ostensibly) to produce a "solution without artifice," namely his method of moving forward through the event tree. Whether or not he had started with this more straightforward approach is unclear, but keeping it hidden would not have been out of character. Fermat goes on:

> And this rule is sound and applicable to all cases, so that without recourse to any artifice, the actual combinations in each number of games give the solution and show what I said in the first place, that the extension to a particular number of games is nothing but a reduction of the several fractions to a common denominator. There in a few words is the whole mystery, which puts us on good terms again since we both seek only accuracy and truth.

Fermat's reduction of several fractions to a common denominator was literally a stroke of genius. He knew that the match could end after one, two, or three games. For each game, the relative proportion of chances would determine the expectations. For instance, the first game could be conceived equally well as entailing three chances (of which A would win in one of these) or nine chances (of which A would win in three). By conceiving the total number of chances as 27 or more for all the individual games, the mathematics was greatly simplified, since all of these chances would be equally possible. In other words, each actual outcome could be expressed as some number of symmetrical outcomes, what we would call today "elementary events."

NOTES

INTRODUCTORY QUOTATIONS

1. Jorge Luis Borges (1941). La Loteria en Babilonia (The Lottery in Babylon) in Ficciones (1944). Buenos Aires: Editorial Sur; Translated by Anthony Bonner and published as Ficciones (1962). New York: Grove Press.
2. Ronald A. Fisher (1959b). Statistical Methods and Scientific Inference, 2nd ed. Edinburgh: Oliver and Boyd, p. 33.
3. Keynes, John Maynard (1921). A Treatise on Probability. London: Macmillan, p. 71.

PREFACE

1. R. A. Fisher's introduction, written in 1955, to Gregor Mendel's papers in Bennett, J. H. (ed.) (1965). Experiments in Plant Hybridisation: Gregor Mendel. Edinburgh: Oliver & Boyd, p. 6.

CHAPTER 1: THE OPPOSITE OF CERTAINTY

1. John P. A. Ioannidis (2005). Why most published research findings are false. *PloS Medicine*, 2: 696–701.

Willful Ignorance: The Mismeasure of Uncertainty, First Edition. Herbert I. Weisberg.
© 2014 John Wiley & Sons, Inc. Published 2014 by John Wiley & Sons, Inc.

2. Jonah Lehrer (2010). The truth wears off: is there something wrong with the scientific method? *The New Yorker*; Samuel Arbesman (2012). *The Half-Life of Facts: Why Everything We Know Has an Expiration Date*. New York: Penguin, p. 155.

3. Gary King (1995). Replication, replication. *Political Science and Politics*, 28: 443–499.

4. John W. Tukey (1962). The future of data analysis. *Annals of Mathematical Statistics*, 1: 1–67.

5. Adolphe Quetelet (1835). *Sur l'homme et le développement de ses facultés, ou Essai de physique sociale*. Paris: Bachelier. Translated as *A Treatise on Man and the Development of his Faculties* (Edinburgh: Chambers, 1842).

6. Siméon Denis Poisson (1837). *Recherche sur la probabilité des jugements en matière criminelle et en matière civile, precédé des règles générale du calcul des probabilities* [Research on the probability of judgments in criminal and civil matters, preceded by general rules for the calculation of probabilities]. Paris: Bachelier.

7. For an excellent exposition of this topic, along with illustrations: Doron D. Swade (2011). Calculating engines: machines, mathematics, and misconceptions, in Flood R., Rice A., and Wilson R. (eds.) *Mathematics in Victorian Britain*. Oxford: Oxford University Press, Chapter 10.

8. John Stuart Mill (1843). *A System of Logic, Ratiocinative and Inductive*. Vol. 2, London: John Parker, p. 67.

9. Claude Bernard (1865). *Introduction à l'Étude de la Médecine Expérimentale*. Translated by H. C. Greene with an Introduction by L. J. Henderson in 1927 as *An Introduction to the Study of Experimental Medicine*. New York: Macmillan, p. 138. For more on the history of statistical methods used in clinical trials see: Herbert I. Weisberg (2011). Statistics and clinical trials: past, present and future. *Proceedings of the American Statistical Association*.

10. Gerd Gigerenzer Zeno Swijtink, Theodore Porter, Lorraine Daston, John Beatty, and Lorenz Kruger (1989). *The Empire of Chance: How Probability Changed Science and Everyday Life*. Cambridge: Cambridge University Press, p. 288.

11. Frank H. Knight (1921). *Risk, Uncertainty and Profit*. Cambridge: The Riverside Press.

12. John Maynard Keynes (1921). *A Treatise on Probability*. London: Macmillan.

13. William Byers (2011). *The Blind Spot: Science and the Crisis of Uncertainty*. Princeton, NJ: Princeton University Press, p. 114.

14. For a similar perspective by another philosophical heavyweight who recognized the role of ambiguity and of Keynes's insights: Alfred North Whitehead (1929). *Process and Reality*. New York: Macmillan, pp. 230–239.

15. The concept of evidence-based medicine refers to the development of recommendations derived from the best available empirical, usually in the form of the results of randomized clinical trials. See Gordon Guyatt (1992). Evidence-based medicine: a new approach to teaching the practice of medicine. *JAMA*, 268: 2420–2425; David L. Sackett (1996). Evidence based medicine: what it is and what it isn't. *British Medical Journal*, 312: 71–72.

16. Jerome Groopman and Pamela Hartzband (2011). *Your Medical Mind: How to Decide What is Right for You*. New York: Penguin, p. 212.

17. Kathryn Schulz (2010). *Being Wrong: Adventures in the Margin of Error*. New York: Harper Collins.

18. Walter Isaacson (2007) *Einstein: His Life and Universe*. New York: Simon & Schuster.
19. Herbert I. Weisberg (2010). *Bias and Causation: Models and Judgment for Valid Comparisons*. Hoboken, NJ: John Wiley & Sons, Inc. Preface.

CHAPTER 2: THE QUIET REVOLUTION

1. Jacob Bernoulli (1713). *Ars Conjectandi*. Basil: Thurnisiorum. Translated with an introduction and notes by Edith Dudley Sylla as *The Art of Conjecturing, together with Letter to a Friend on Sets in Court Tennis* (Baltimore: The Johns Hopkins University Press, 2006, p. 327). An earlier source for this quotation is a translation of Part IV of *Ars Conjectandi* by Bing Sung, which is available at http://cerebro.xu.edu/math/Sources/JakobBernoulli/ars_sung.pdf
2. Maurice G. Kendall (1970). Where shall the history of statistics begin?, in E. S. Pearson and M. G. Kendall (eds.) *Studies in the History of Statistics and Probability*. Darien, CT: Hafner, p. 46.
3. The question of whether (and when) mathematical findings should be regarded as more like a discovery or more like an invention has been widely discussed, especially in light of the "unreasonable effectiveness of mathematics." See, for example, Byers (2011) and Mario Livio (2009). *Is God a Mathematician?* New York: Simon & Schuster.
4. Nassim Nicholas Taleb (2010). *The Black Swan: The Impact of the Highly Improbable*, 2nd ed. New York: Random House.
5. Andrei Kolmogorov (1956). *Foundations of the Theory of Probability*, 2nd ed. New York: Chelsea.
6. Bertrand Russell (1913). On the notion of cause. *Proceedings of the Aristotelian Society*, 13: p. 1.
7. For an extensive exposition of the technical contributions of Galton and Pearson during the late 1800s, see Stephen M. Stigler (1986a). *The History of Statistics: The Measurement of Uncertainty before 1900*. Cambridge: Harvard University Press.
8. Francis Galton (1869). *Hereditary Genius*. London: Macmillan.
9. Francis Galton (1890). Kinship and correlation. *North American Review*, 150: p. 431.
10. Karl Pearson (1930). *The Life, Letters and Labours of Francis Galton*, Vol. 3A. London: Cambridge University Press, Chapter XIV.
11. In addition to his research on modern statistical theory and agricultural experimentation, Fisher was heavily involved in the creation of population genetics. Population genetics studies the changes in gene distributions resulting from various evolutionary processes. It was important in the development of the modern evolutionary synthesis. Fisher, Sewall Wright, and J. B. S. Haldane cofounded this new field.
12. The definitive, and rather candid, biography of Fisher was written by his daughter Joan Fisher Box, who is also the former wife of statistician George Box. J. F. Box (1978). *R. A. Fisher: The Life of a Scientist*. New York: John Wiley & Sons, Inc. Regrettably, this uniquely valuable resource is currently out of print and difficult to obtain.

13. In Fisher's case, I am referring mainly to the so-called "fiducial argument" that was never developed in a way that was accepted by other statisticians. In addition, his failure to accept the reality of the deleterious effects of tobacco smoking, despite enormous statistical evidence, was widely criticized.

14. The adoption of randomized experimentation in medical research was originally championed by Austin Bradford Hill (1897–1991), but took some time to overcome various practical and philosophical obstacles. See Harry M. Marks (1997). *The Progress of Experiment: Scientific and Therapeutic Reform in the United States, 1900–1999*. Cambridge: Cambridge University Press.

15. Philosopher Ian Hacking made this phrase famous as the title to his influential book Ian Hacking (1990). *The Taming of Chance*. Cambridge: Cambridge University Press.

16. The recently developed field of behavioral economics, especially the "heuristics and biases" subdiscipline, emphasizes particularly the common tendencies to make errors in properly applying the laws of probability. For an excellent summary by a founder of the field, see Daniel Kahneman (2011). *Thinking Fast and Slow*. New York: Farrar, Straus and Giroux. Other related books are Thomas Gilovich, Dale Griffin, and Daniel Kahneman (eds.) (2002). *Heuristics and Biases: The Psychology of Intuitive Judgment*. New York: Cambridge University Press; Leonard Mlodinow (2008). *The Drunkard's Walk: How Randomness Rules Our Lives*. New York: Vintage Books. See also Taleb (2010).

17. Alan Reifman (2012). *Hot Hand: The Statistics behind Sports' Greatest Streaks*. Dulles, VA: Potomac Books.

18. An extensive elaboration of Fisher's ideas about probability theory and its application to statistical methodology is presented in Chapters 9 and 10.

19. In the medical arena, the personalization of treatment has become an increasingly realistic objective, as genetic and other biomarkers are being examined for their relationships to effects of drugs. For a vision of the near future, Eric Topol (2012). *The Creative Destruction of Medicine: How the Digital Revolution will Create Better Health Care*. New York: Basic Books.

20. Herbert I. Weisberg (1974). *Short Term Cognitive Effects of Head Start Programs: A Report on the Third Year of Planned Variation—1971–72*. U. S. Department of Health, Education and Welfare.

21. *Head Start Impact Study Final Report*, Office of Planning, Research and Evaluation, Administration for Children and Families, U.S. Department of Health and Human Services, Washington, D.C., January, 2010.

22. *Third Grade Follow-Up to the Head Start Impact Study Final Report*, Office of Planning, Research and Evaluation, Administration for Children and Families, U.S. Department of Health and Human Services, Washington, D.C., October, 2012.

23. Richard Peto, R Gray, R Collins, K Wheatley, C Hennekens, K Jamrozik, C Warlow, B Hafner, E Thompson, S Norton, J Gilliland, and R Doll (1988). Randomized trial of prophylactic daily aspirin in British Male doctors. *British Medical Journal*, 296: 313–316; Steering Committee of the Physicians' Health Study Research Group (1989). Final report of the aspirin component of the ongoing Physicians' Health Study. *New England Journal of Medicine*, 321: 129–135.

24. U.S. Preventive Services Task Force (2009). Aspirin for the prevention of cardio-vascular disease: U.S. Preventive Services Task Force recommendation statement. *Annals of Internal Medicine*, 150: 396–404.
25. Antithrombotic Trialists' (ATT) Collaboration (2009). Aspirin in the primary and secondary prevention of vascular disease: collaborative meta-analysis of individual participant data from randomized trials. *Lancet*, 373: 1849–1860.

CHAPTER 3: A MATTER OF CHANCE

1. A great deal has been written about Pascal and Fermat, and especially about their famous correspondence of 1654. My historical dramatization is of course fictional, but the main facts are faithful to the historical record. See, for example, Florence N. David (1962). *Games, Gods and Gambling: A History of Probability and Statistical Ideas*. London: Charles Griffin & Company; Keith Devlin (2008). *The Unfinished Game: Pascal, Fermat and the Seventeenth-Century Letter that Made the World Modern*. New York: Basic Books; Peter L. Bernstein (1996). *Against the Gods: The Remarkable Story of Risk*. New York: John Wiley & Sons, Inc.
2. There have been many theories regarding exactly why mathematical probability began to develop so late and just when it did. Probably the most well-known and controversial account is by Ian Hacking (1975). *The Emergence of Probability*. Cambridge: Cambridge University Press (2nd edition, 2006). See also Gerd Gigerenzer, Zeno Swijtink, Theodore Porter, Lorraine Daston, John Beatty, and Lorenz Krüger. (1989). *The Empire of Chance: How Probability Changed Science and Everyday Life*. Cambridge: Cambridge University Press; James Franklin (2001). *The Science of Conjecture: Evidence and Probability before Pascal*. Baltimore: The Johns Hopkins University Press; and Lorraine Daston (1988). *Classical Probability in the Enlightenment*. Princeton, NJ: Princeton University Press.
3. An extensive discussion of "probabilism" is given by James Franklin (2001). *The Science of Conjecture: Evidence and Probability before Pascal*. Baltimore: The Johns Hopkins University Press, Chapter 4. See also Barbara J. Shapiro (1983). *Probability and Certainty in Seventeenth-Century England: A Study of the Relationships between Natural Science, Law, and Literature*. Princeton, NJ: Princeton University Press.
4. The quotation is from Edmund F. Byrne (1968). *Probability and Opinion*. The Hague: Martinus Nijhoff, p. 188.
5. James Franklin (2001). *The Science of Conjecture: Evidence and Probability before Pascal*. Baltimore: The Johns Hopkins University Press, p. 366.
6. James Franklin (2001). *The Science of Conjecture: Evidence and Probability before Pascal*. Baltimore: The Johns Hopkins University Press, p. 366.
7. James Franklin (2001). *The Science of Conjecture: Evidence and Probability before Pascal*. Baltimore: The Johns Hopkins University Press, p. 275.
8. James Franklin (2001). *The Science of Conjecture: Evidence and Probability before Pascal*. Baltimore: The Johns Hopkins University Press, Chapter 10.
9. Florence N. David (1962). *Games, Gods and Gambling: A History of Probability and Statistical Ideas*. London: Charles Griffin & Company.

10. The discussion here of Cardano's life is derived mainly from the delightful biography by mathematician Oystein Ore (1953). *Cardano, the Gambling Scholar*. Princeton, NJ: Princeton University Press; includes a translation from Latin by Sydney Henry Gould.

11. William Shakespeare, Henry IV, Part II, Act I, Scene 1, lines181–182.

12. Oystein Ore (1953). *Cardano, the Gambling Scholar*. Princeton, NJ: Princeton University Press, p. 148.

13. Oystein Ore (1953). *Cardano, the Gambling Scholar*. Princeton, NJ: Princeton University Press, p. 168.

14. A discussion of Galileo's contribution appears in Florence N. David (1962). *Games, Gods and Gambling: A History of Probability and Statistical Ideas*. London: Charles Griffin & Company, Chapter 6. The excerpts from Galileo's *Thoughts about Dice Games* appear in Appendix 2, which contains a translation by E. H. Thorne.

15. Luca Pacioli (1494). *Summa de arithmetica, geometrica, proportioni et proportionalita*, discussed in Florence N. David (1962). *Games, Gods and Gambling: A History of Probability and Statistical Ideas*. London: Charles Griffin & Company, Chapter 4.

16. Keith Devlin (2008). *The Unfinished Game: Pascal, Fermat and the Seventeenth-Century Letter that Made the World Modern*. New York: Basic Books, p. 63.

17. An excellent discussion of Pascal's philosophical perspective as it related to probability is given by James Franklin (2001). *The Science of Conjecture: Evidence and Probability before Pascal*. Baltimore: The Johns Hopkins University Press.

18. A translation of the relevant section of *Ars Cogitandi* by Richard J. Pulskamp can be found on http://cerebro.xu.edu/math/Sources/Arnauld/portroyal.pdf

19. A. W. F. Edwards (1983). Pascal's problem: the gambler's ruin. *International Statistical Review*, 51: 73–79; reproduced in Edwards (1987). *Pascal's Arithmetical Triangle: The Story of a Mathematical Idea*. Baltimore: The Johns Hopkins University Press, Appendix 2.

20. Florence N. David (1962). *Games, Gods and Gambling: A History of Probability and Statistical Ideas*. London: Charles Griffin & Company, p. 110.

21. Malcolm Gladwell (2008). *Outliers: The Story of Success*. New York: Little, Brown & Company.

22. There are numerous sources of biographical material on Huygens. I have relied primarily on Florence N. David (1962). *Games, Gods and Gambling: A History of Probability and Statistical Ideas*. London: Charles Griffin & Company, Chapter 11.

23. There are several available translations into English of Huygens's treatise. I have quoted from that in Florence N. David (1962). *Games, Gods and Gambling: A History of Probability and Statistical Ideas*. London: Charles Griffin & Company, Chapter 11. Two translations can be found on Richard J. Pulskamp's website: http://cerebro.xu.edu/math/Sources/Huygens.

24. The key axiom of probability can be stated in nonrigorous form as saying that for any two *mutually exclusive* events A and B, the probability that one or the other (or both) occurs equals the sum of the probabilities that each occurs individually. In mathematical form,

$$P(A \cup B) = P(A) + P(B).$$

CHAPTER 4: HARDLY TOUCHED UPON

1. Pierre de Montmort (1708). *Essay d'Analyse sur les Jeux de Hazard*, Paris. (2nd Edition, revised and augmented, and including letters between N. Bernoulli, Waldegrave, and Montmort, 1713).

2. See especially Ian Hacking (1975). *The Emergence of Probability*. Cambridge: Cambridge University Press, Chapter 2.

3. James Franklin (2001). *The Science of Conjecture: Evidence and Probability before Pascal*. Baltimore: The Johns Hopkins University Press, pp. 316–320.

4. Joseph Saveur (1679). Computation of the advantages of the banker in the game of Bassette. *Journal des Sçavans*. English translation by Richard J. Pulskamp available on his website: http://cerebro.xu.edu/math/Sources/Saveur.

5. Jacob Bernoulli (1685). *Problème proposé par M. Bernoulli*. [Problem proposed by Mr. Bernoulli], *Journal des Sçavans*. English translation by Richard J. Pulskamp available on his website: http://cerebro.xu.edu/math/Sources/JakobBernoulli.

6. Edith Dudley Sylla (2006). *The Art of Conjecturing, together with Letter to a Friend on Sets in Court Tennis*. Baltimore: The Johns Hopkins University Press, Introduction.

7. Strode's contribution is explained by Stephen M. Stigler (1999). *Statistics on the Table: The History of Statistical Concepts and Methods*. Cambridge, MA: Harvard University Press, Chapter 12. Stigler coined the phrase "dark ages of probability" to describe this period of apparent inactivity.

8. Biographical details about John Arbuthnot can be found at http://www-history.mcs.st-and.ac.uk/Biographies/Arbuthnot.html. A more complete biography—George A. Aitken (1892). *The Life and Works of John Arbuthnot*. Oxford: The Clarendon Press—is available on Google Books.

9. *Of the Laws of Chance*, which is basically a translation of Huygens's treatise is usually attributed to John Arbuthnot, physician, satirist, and occasional mathematician. There is little doubt that Arbuthnot wrote the Preface, but who really performed the translation remains a mystery.

10. David R. Bellhouse (1989). A manuscript on chance written by John Arbuthnot. *International Statistical Review*, 57: 255. The reference to Todhunter pertains to the authoritative classic early history of mathematical probability by Isaac Todhunter (1865). *A History of the Mathematical Theory of Probability: From the Time of Pascal to that of Laplace*. London: Macmillan. (Reprinted 1949, 1965 New York: Chelsea.)

11. David R. Bellhouse (1989). A manuscript on chance written by John Arbuthnot. *International Statistical Review*, 57: 257–258. Bellhouse may have discounted Gregory as the actual translator because he was under the impression that Arbuthnot did not know Gregory until he arrived at Oxford in 1694. However, there is evidence that Arbuthnot and Gregory may have been well acquainted in 1692, as Arbuthnot had studied with and befriended Gregory in Scotland prior to his emigration in 1691. See www.History.Mcs.st-andrews.ac.uk/Arbuthnot.html.

12. There have of course been a many biographies of Isaac Newton. I have relied primarily on James Gleick (2004). *Isaac Newton*. New York: Vintage Books.

13. The quotation is from a lecture delivered in July 1946, *Newton, the Man*, written by John Maynard Keynes, who had died two months before. It was read by

Keynes's brother Geoffrey Keynes. The text is available at: www-history.mcs.st-and.ac.uk/Extras/Keynes_Newton.html

14. Andrea A. Rusnock (2002). *Vital Accounts: Quantifying Health and Population in Eighteenth-Century England and France*. Cambridge: Cambridge University Press, Chapter 1.

15. Samuel Pepys (1663). *The Diary of Samuel Pepys,* vol. 3. Henry B. Wheatley (ed.) (1962). London: G. Bell & Sons.

16. Andrea A. Rusnock (2002). *Vital Accounts: Quantifying Health and Population in Eighteenth-Century England and France*. Cambridge: Cambridge University Press, Chapter 1. The text is available at http://cerebro.xu.edu/math/Sources/Graunt.

17. Andrea A. Rusnock (2002). *Vital Accounts: Quantifying Health and Population in Eighteenth-Century England and France*. Cambridge: Cambridge University Press is excellent as a source for information on how data tables were first created and utilized for scientific research.

18. John Graunt (1666). *Journal des Sçavans,* 1.

19. Andrea A. Rusnock (2002). *Vital Accounts: Quantifying Health and Population in Eighteenth-Century England and France*. Cambridge: Cambridge University Press, Chapter 1.

20. Jonathan Swift (1729). *A Modest Proposal.* Dublin: S. Harding. A Project Gutenberg eBook at: http://www.gutenberg.org/files/1080/1080-h/1080-h.htm

21. Information about Christiaan Huygens's correspondence related to probability, including translations of letters can be found at: http://cerebro.xu.edu/math/Sources/Huygens/

22. Biographical information about Johan de Witt, along with an extensive discussion of the actuarial analysis can be found in Anders Hald (2003). *History of Probability and Statistics before 1750*. Hoboken, NJ: John Wiley & Sons, Inc., Chapter 9.

23. Alexandre Dumas (1850). *La Tulipe Noire [The Black Tulip]*. Paris: Baudry. An English translation of the book published in 1904 by Little, Brown & Company is accessible on Google Books.

24. Edith Dudley Sylla (2006). *The Art of Conjecturing, together with Letter to a Friend on Sets in Court Tennis*. Baltimore: The Johns Hopkins University Press, Introduction.

25. Jacob Bernoulli (1686). *Journal des Sçavans.*

26. Much of this biographical information was taken from: www.encyclopedia.com/topic/Edmond_Halley.aspx. An additional source was: www. History.Mcs.st-andrews.ac.uk/Halley.html.

27. This quotation is attributed to the mathematician James Whitbread Glaisher (1848–1928) in: www.History. Mcs.st- andrews.ac.uk/Halley.html.

28. Edmond Halley (1693). "An estimate of the degrees of mortality of mankind...," *Philosophical Transactions,* 17: 596–610.

29. It is possible that Halley may have been influenced by Christiaan Huygens, whom he might have met on his visit to the Paris Observatory in 1680 and learned of the Dutch ideas about annuities. However, I am unaware of any evidence to support such a speculation.

30. James Franklin (2001). *The Science of Conjecture: Evidence and Probability before Pascal*. Baltimore: The Johns Hopkins University Press, pp. 234–235.

31. James Franklin (2001). *The Science of Conjecture: Evidence and Probability before Pascal*. Baltimore: The Johns Hopkins University Press, p. 224.

32. I have relied mainly on the biographical material on www. History. Mcs.st-andrews.ac.uk/Leibniz.html.

33. Gottfried W. Leibniz (1666). *Dissertatio de arte combinatoria, Sämtliche Schriften und Briefe* (Berlin: *Akademie Verlag*, 1923) A VI 1, p. 163; *Philosophische Schriften* (Gerhardt) Bd. IV S.30.

34. For a discussion of Medina's philosophy, see James Franklin (2001). *The Science of Conjecture: Evidence and Probability before Pascal*. Baltimore: The Johns Hopkins University Press, pp. 74–76.

35. James Franklin (2001). *The Science of Conjecture: Evidence and Probability before Pascal*. Baltimore: The Johns Hopkins University Press, p. 76.

36. Caramuel's remarkable career and personal exploits are chronicled in James Franklin (2001). *The Science of Conjecture: Evidence and Probability before Pascal*. Baltimore: The Johns Hopkins University Press, pp. 88–94.

37. A translation of the relevant section of *Ars Cogitandi* can be found on Richard J. Pulskamp's website: http://cerebro.xu.edu/math/Sources/Arnauld/portroyal.pdf

38. Edith Dudley Sylla (2006). *The Art of Conjecturing, together with Letter to a Friend on Sets in Court Tennis*. Baltimore: The Johns Hopkins University Press, pp. 24–28.

39. The general notion of drawing a parallel between inductive inference and gambling may well have been around for some time, even before the 1654 Pascal–Fermat correspondence. An interesting remark alluding to this notion is found in a text written by Roberval in 1647, which is quoted in James Franklin (2001). *The Science of Conjecture: Evidence and Probability before Pascal*. Baltimore: The Johns Hopkins University Press, p. 305.

40. Edith Dudley Sylla (2006). *The Art of Conjecturing, together with Letter to a Friend on Sets in Court Tennis*. Baltimore: The Johns Hopkins University Press, p. 37.

41. My source for the quotations from this Preface is http://cerebro.xu.edu/math/Sources/Arbuthnot/sources/preface.html

42. Edith Dudley Sylla (2006). *The Art of Conjecturing, together with Letter to a Friend on Sets in Court Tennis*. Baltimore: The Johns Hopkins University Press, pp. 316–317.

43. W. W. Rouse Ball (1888). *A Short Account of the History of Mathematics*. London: Macmillan, p. 77. Johann Bernoulli was extremely competitive and fractious in his dealings with others he perceived as rivals. He became involved in several bitter controversies over priority, including disputes with his brother Jacob and his son Daniel Bernoulli (1700–1782).

44. Stephen M. Stigler (1999). *Statistics on the Table: The History of Statistical Concepts and Methods*. Cambridge, MA: Harvard University Press, Chapter 13.

45. John Locke (1690). *An Essay Concerning Human Understanding*. London, Book IV, Chapter 14. See also Lorraine Daston (1988). *Classical Probability in the Enlightenment*. Princeton, NJ: Princeton University Press, pp. 193–194.

46. Stephen M. Stigler (1999). *Statistics on the Table: The History of Statistical Concepts and Methods*. Cambridge, MA: Harvard University Press, p. 254.

47. Anonymous (1699). A calculation of the credibility of human testimony. *Philosophical Transactions*, 21: 359–365. This work is now attributed to the Reverend George

Hooper; a discussion of the disputed authorship can be found in an article by A. I. Dale (1992). On the authorship of 'A calculation of the credibility of human testimony'. *Historia Mathematica*, 19: 414–417.

48. A. I. Dale (1992). On the authorship of 'A calculation of the credibility of human testimony'. *Historia Mathematica*, 19: 414–417.
49. http://royalsociety.org/uploadedFiles/Royal_Society_Content/about-us/fellowship/Fellows1660-2007.pdf
50. John Friesen (2003). Archibald Pitcairne, David Gregory and the Scottish origins of English Tory Newtonianism, 1688–1715. *History of Science*, 41: 163–191.
51. John Friesen (2003). Archibald Pitcairne, David Gregory and the Scottish origins of English Tory Newtonianism, 1688–1715. *History of Science*, 41: 191.

CHAPTER 5: A MATHEMATICIAN OF BASEL

1. My historical dramatization is of course fictional, but the main facts are faithful to the historical record.
2. English translations by Richard J. Pulskamp of extracts from three eulogies to Jacob Bernoulli delivered in November, 1705, are available on http://www.cs.xu.edu/math/Sources/. Bernard le Bovier Fontanelle was renowned for his many eulogies of famous men. See Charles B. Paul (1980). *Science and Immortality: The Éloges of the Paris Academy of Sciences (1699–1791)*. Berkeley: University of California Press.
3. Nicholas Bernoulli's *De Usu Artis Conjectandi in Jure* (The uses of the Art of Conjecturing in Law.) was submitted for his doctorate from the University of Basel, in 1709. Jacob's father and one of his brothers were named Nicholas. This Nicholas was the son and of Jacob's brother Nicholas. Jacob himself and his brother Johann also had sons named Nicholas. See Edith Dudley Sylla (2006). *The Art of Conjecturing, together with Letter to a Friend on Sets in Court Tennis*. Baltimore: The Johns Hopkins University Press, pp. 1–4.
4. The only complete English translation is by Edith Dudley Sylla (2006). *The Art of Conjecturing, together with Letter to a Friend on Sets in Court Tennis*. Baltimore: The Johns Hopkins University Press. All quotations from the *Ars Conjectandi* were from this source unless otherwise indicated.
5. Edith Dudley Sylla (2006). *The Art of Conjecturing, together with Letter to a Friend on Sets in Court Tennis*. Baltimore: The Johns Hopkins University Press, p. 134.
6. Edith Dudley Sylla (2006). *The Art of Conjecturing, together with Letter to a Friend on Sets in Court Tennis*. Baltimore: The Johns Hopkins University Press, p. 142.
7. Edith Dudley Sylla (2006). *The Art of Conjecturing, together with Letter to a Friend on Sets in Court Tennis*. Baltimore: The Johns Hopkins University Press, pp. 139–140.
8. Suppose that on each trial, there are b chances of success and c chances of failure. Today, we would formulate the problem as follows. What is the probability of obtaining exactly r successes in n independent "Bernoulli trials" with a success probability of p on each trial? Our p would correspond to Jacob's $b/(b + c)$. Bernoulli, however, was still thinking in terms of "chances" for and against success, not "probability" of success. Furthermore, he had in mind the *expectation* of winning

(obtaining exactly r successes in n trials), not the probability in our sense. However, he had arrived at the point of being able to abstract the expectation from a specific gamble, recognizing it as an inherent aspect of a generic event (exactly r successes in n trials) that could be calculated as a fraction between 0 and 1.

9. More generally, we can calculate combinations by first obtaining the number of permutations of r out of the n, and then dividing by the number of permutations of the r elements contained in each of the permutations. The resulting number of "combinations of n things taken r at a time" is now denoted by ^nC_r or $\binom{n}{r}$, and is also called the *binomial coefficient* because of their role in the algebraic expansion of expressions like $(a + b)^n$. For instance $(a + b)^3 = 1a^3 + 3a^2b + 3ab^2 + 1b^3$. The coefficients for the four terms in this expression (1,3,3,1) correspond to the values of $\binom{3}{3}$, $\binom{3}{2}$, $\binom{3}{1}$, $\binom{3}{0}$

10. Edwards (1987). *Pascal's Arithmetical Triangle: The Story of a Mathematical Idea.* Baltimore: The Johns Hopkins University Press.

11. Pierre Fermat (1679). *Opera Mathematica* (Samuel Fermat, Ed.).The mathematical works of Fermat that were known to Jacob Bernoulli were from this collection, edited by Fermat's son, Samuel. The complete collection of known works eventually was published by Tannery, P. and Henry, C. (eds.). *Oeuvres de Fermat.* Paris: Gauthier-Villars, 5 volumes, 1891–1922.

12. In his introduction to Part Two, Bernoulli acknowledged the prior work of several other writers on the subject of combinatorics, namely Frans van Schooten (Huygens's mentor), the great English mathematician John Wallis (1616–1703), the French mathematician and cleric Jean Prestet (1648–1690), and of course Gottfried Leibniz. Jacob's rather convoluted derivation of the general formula for calculating $\binom{n}{r}$ is one of the central results in Part Two of his book.

13. Edith Dudley Sylla (2006). *The Art of Conjecturing, together with Letter to a Friend on Sets in Court Tennis.* Baltimore: The Johns Hopkins University Press, pp. 193–194.

14. Edith Dudley Sylla (2006). *The Art of Conjecturing, together with Letter to a Friend on Sets in Court Tennis.* Baltimore: The Johns Hopkins University Press, p. 14.

15. Oystein Ore (1953). *Cardano, the Gambling Scholar.* Princeton, NJ: Princeton University Press, pp. 53–58. As a primary source, Ore refers to Henry Morley (1854). *The Life of Girolamo Cardano of Milan, Physician.* London: Chapman and Hall.

16. Edith Dudley Sylla (2006). *The Art of Conjecturing, together with Letter to a Friend on Sets in Court Tennis.* Baltimore: The Johns Hopkins University Press, pp. 197–201. The information about Proteus verses is found in Part Two of *Ars Conjectandi.* "Proteus verse" was coined by Julius Caesar Scaliger in *Poeticis libri, VII.* Geneva-Lyons, 1561.

17. Donald E. Knuth (2011). *The Art of Computer Programming,*Vol. 4A. Boston: Addison–Wesley.

18. Edith Dudley Sylla (2006). *The Art of Conjecturing, together with Letter to a Friend on Sets in Court Tennis.* Baltimore: The Johns Hopkins University Press, p. 193.

19. Edith Dudley Sylla (2006). *The Art of Conjecturing, together with Letter to a Friend on Sets in Court Tennis.* Baltimore: The Johns Hopkins University Press, p. 251.

20. Edith Dudley Sylla (2006). *The Art of Conjecturing, together with Letter to a Friend on Sets in Court Tennis.* Baltimore: The Johns Hopkins University Press, p. 305.

21. The quotations from Chapter 1 of Part IV are in Edith Dudley Sylla (2006). *The Art of Conjecturing, together with Letter to a Friend on Sets in Court Tennis.* Baltimore: The Johns Hopkins University Press, pp. 315–16.

22. The quotations from Chapter 2 of Part IV are in Edith Dudley Sylla (2006). *The Art of Conjecturing, together with Letter to a Friend on Sets in Court Tennis.* Baltimore: The Johns Hopkins University Press, pp. 317–321.

23. The quotations from Chapter 3 of Part IV are in Edith Dudley Sylla (2006). *The Art of Conjecturing, together with Letter to a Friend on Sets in Court Tennis.* Baltimore: The Johns Hopkins University Press, pp. 321–326.

24. The system proposed by Johann Lambert was intended to remedy this perceived shortcoming. See Glenn Shafer (1978). Non-additive probabilities in the work of Bernoulli and Lambert. *Archive for History of Exact Science,* 19: 309–370.

25. The quotations from Chapter 4 of Part IV are in Edith Dudley Sylla (2006). *The Art of Conjecturing, together with Letter to a Friend on Sets in Court Tennis.* Baltimore: The Johns Hopkins University Press, pp. 326–330.

26. Edith Dudley Sylla (2006). *The Art of Conjecturing, together with Letter to a Friend on Sets in Court Tennis.* Baltimore: The Johns Hopkins University Press, p. 329. The Latin word *fomitem* is translated by Sylla as "germ." This refers to germ in the sense of the root, or origin, and is unrelated to modern germ theory in medicine, which was not discovered until much later. The word *fomitem* was translated as "tinder" in the translation of Part IV of *Ars Conjectandi* by Bing Sung. See http://cerebro.xu.edu/math/Sources/JakobBernoulli/ars_sung.pdf.

27. Arthur P. Dempster (1966). Preface to the translation of Part IV of *Ars Conjectandi* by Bing Sung, Office of Naval Research Technical Report No. 2, Contract NR-042-097. It is available online at http://www.cs.xu.edu/math/Sources/JakobBernoulli/ars_sung.pdf

28. An English translation of the correspondence can be found at http://cerebro.xu.edu/math/Sources/JakobBernoulli/. For excerpts and extensive discussion of the letters, see Edith Dudley Sylla (2006). *The Art of Conjecturing, together with Letter to a Friend on Sets in Court Tennis.* Baltimore: The Johns Hopkins University Press, pp. 35–49.

29. Peter Harrison (2001). Curiosity, forbidden knowledge, and the reformation of natural philosophy in early modern England, *Isis,* 92: 278.

30. Edith Dudley Sylla (2006). *The Art of Conjecturing, together with Letter to a Friend on Sets in Court Tennis.* Baltimore: The Johns Hopkins University Press, pp. 329–330.

CHAPTER 6: A DEFECT OF CHARACTER

1. John Locke (1690). *An Essay Concerning Human Understanding.* London, Book IV, Chapter 14. See also Lorraine Daston (1988). *Classical Probability in the Enlightenment.* Princeton, NJ: Princeton University Press, pp. 193–194.

2. For the biographical information on de Moivre, I have relied primarily on David R. Bellhouse (2011). *Abraham De Moivre: Setting the Stage for Classical Probability and its Applications*, Boca Raton, FL: CRC Press. Bellhouse paints a somewhat more flattering portrait of de Moivre's personality and character than I have, and to be fair I would direct the interested reader to his comprehensive and scholarly biography. For another perspective, see Florence N. David (1962). *Games, Gods and Gambling: A History of Probability and Statistical Ideas*. London: Charles Griffin & Company, Chapter 15. A contemporaneous source is Matthew Maty (1755). Mémoire sur la vie & écrits de Mr. de Moivre. *Journal Britannique*, 18: 1–51. This has been translated in David R. Bellhouse and Christian Genest (2007). Maty's biography of Abraham de Moivre, translated, annotated and augmented. *Statistical Science*, 22: 109–136.

3. Helen M. Walker (1934). Abraham de Moivre. *Scripta Mathematica*, 2: 329. See also David Lasocki (1989). The life of Daniel de Moivre. *The Consort*, 45: 15–17. The quote is from a letter to Johann Bernoulli, dated December 2, 1707. De Moivre may have been exaggerating his financial plight, as he is known to have left £1600 invested in South Sea Annuities to his surviving family members. This was a very large sum at that time (David R. Bellhouse and Christian Genest (2007). Maty's biography of Abraham de Moivre, translated, annotated and augmented. *Statistical Science*, 22: 25).

4. David R. Bellhouse and Christian Genest (2007). Maty's biography of Abraham de Moivre, translated, annotated and augmented. *Statistical Science*, 22: 23–24.

5. Florence N. David (1962). *Games, Gods and Gambling: A History of Probability and Statistical Ideas*. London: Charles Griffin & Company, p. 163.

6. For a nice summary of this contretemps, see Florence N. David (1962). *Games, Gods and Gambling: A History of Probability and Statistical Ideas*. London: Charles Griffin & Company, Chapter 15.

7. Pierre de Montmort (1708). *Essay d'Analyse sur les Jeux de Hazard*, Paris.

8. Abraham de Moivre (1711). *De Mensura Sortis (On the Measurement of Chance).Philosophical Transactions*, 329. Translated by Bruce McClintock with a commentary by Anders Hald (1984). A. de Moivre: '*De Mensura Sortis*' or 'On the measurement of chance'. *International Statistical Review*, 52: 229–262.

9. Montmort (1713). *Essay d'Analyse sur les Jeux de Hazard* (2nd edition), Paris.

10. Florence N. David (1962). *Games, Gods and Gambling: A History of Probability and Statistical Ideas*. London: Charles Griffin & Company, p. 151. David notes that it was strange that the usually "sweet-tempered" Montmort would react so strongly to de Moivre's provocation. Perhaps this testifies to the lack of sensitivity and *savoir faire* that could get de Moivre into difficulties.

11. Brook Taylor was another well-known mathematician who is credited with several significant contributions to the infinitesimal calculus, most famously Taylor's Theorem and Taylor Series, although these were apparently discovered earlier by David Gregory's older brother James Gregory (1638–1675).

12. William Browne (1714). *Christiani Huygenii Libellus de Rationciniis in Ludo Aleae. Or, the value of all chances in games of fortune; cards, dice, wagers, lotteries &c, mathematically demonstrated.* London.

13. Abraham de Moivre (1718). *The Doctrine of Chances, or a Method of Calculating the Probability of Events in Play*, London.

14. A photocopy of the Stanford University Library's copy of Abraham de Moivre's *The Doctrine of Chances, or a Method of Calculating the Probability of Events in Play* is accessible at Google Books—books.google.com.

15. Helen Walker mentions that de Moivre expressed in his correspondence with Johann Bernoulli his dislike of David Gregory and other Scottish refugees [see Helen M. Walker (1934). Abraham de Moivre. *Scripta Mathematica*, 2: 323].

16. Florence N. David (1962). *Games, Gods and Gambling: A History of Probability and Statistical Ideas*. London: Charles Griffin & Company, p. 158. Translations by Richard J. Pulskamp of Montmort's correspondence with Nicholas Bernoulli, which were included in the second edition of Montmort's *Essay*, can be found at http://cerebro.xu.edu/math/Sources/Montmort.

17. Abraham de Moivre (1725). *Annuities upon Lives*, London. A photocopy of the original text is accessible at Google Books: books.google.com.

18. Abraham de Moivre (1738). *The Doctrine of Chances, or a Method of Calculating the Probability of Events in Play, Second Edition: Fuller, Clearer, and More Correct than the First*. London. A photocopy of the Bayer Staats Bibliotek's copy is accessible at Google Books—books.google.com.

19. A copy of this paper, written in 1733, was included in the Third Edition of *The Doctrine of Chances* (1756). It has been reproduced in Florence N. David (1962). *Games, Gods and Gambling: A History of Probability and Statistical Ideas*. London: Charles Griffin & Company, Appendix 5.

20. Jacob Bernoulli's name is sometimes rendered as Jakob in German publications, as James Bernoulli in English, and as Jacques Bernoulli in French.

21. The approximation improves as the number of trials increases, and to some extent as the probability on each trial is closer to 0.50. It may work sufficiently well even for sample sizes less than 20, depending on the situation in which it is being applied. However, with modern computing capabilities, it has become obsolete, since the exact values can be calculated.

22. W. W. Rouse Ball (1889). *A History of The Study of Mathematics at Cambridge*. Cambridge: The University Press, p. 205.

23. Biographical material can be found at: http://www-history.mcs.st-and.ac.uk/Biographies/Simpson.htm. Details on the interaction between Simpson and de Moivre can be found in David R. Bellhouse (2011). *Abraham De Moivre: Setting the Stage for Classical Probability and its Applications*, Boca Raton, FL: CRC Press, Chapter 13.

24. Thomas Simpson (1740). *The Nature and Laws of Chance*. London: Edward Cave.

25. Thomas Simpson (1742). *The Doctrine of Annuities and Reversion, Deduced from Evident and Evident Principles*. London: J. Nourse.

26. Abraham de Moivre (1743). *Annuities on Lives, Second Edition: Plainer, Fuller, and More Correct than the Former*. London: Woodfall.

27. Thomas Simpson (1743). *An Appendix, Containing Some Remarks on a Late Book on the Same Subject, with Answers to Some Personal and Malignant Representations in the Preface thereof.* London: J. Nourse.

28. Abraham de Moivre (1756). *The Doctrine of Chances, or a Method of Calculating the Probability of Events in Play, Third Edition: Fuller, Clearer, and More Correct than*

the Former. London: Millar. Reprinted: New York: Chelsea Publishing Company, 1967.

29. Helen M. Walker (1934). Abraham de Moivre. *Scripta Mathematica*, 2: 326. The quotation is attributed by Walker to an *Éloge* in the *Histoire de L'Académie Royale des Sciences* by Grandjean de Fouchy, 1754.

30. A summary of Newton's deplorable treatment of Leibniz can be found in many sources, including the biography of Newton by James Gleick.

31. Abraham de Moivre (1711). *De Mensura Sortis [On the Measurement of Chance]. Philosophical Transactions*, 329.

32. Abraham de Moivre (1718). *The Doctrine of Chances, or a Method of Calculating the Probability of Events in Play*, London.

33. Abraham de Moivre (1718). *The Doctrine of Chances, or a Method of Calculating the Probability of Events in Play*, London.

34. Abraham de Moivre (1718). *The Doctrine of Chances, or a Method of Calculating the Probability of Events in Play*, London.

35. Abraham de Moivre (1718). *The Doctrine of Chances, or a Method of Calculating the Probability of Events in Play*, London.

36. Abraham de Moivre (1718). *The Doctrine of Chances, or a Method of Calculating the Probability of Events in Play*, London.

CHAPTER 7: CLASSICAL PROBABILITY

1. A translation of Euler's letter can be found on Richard J. Pulskamp's website http://cerebro.xu.edu/math/Sources/Euler/. Euler is widely recognized as one of the greatest and most prolific mathematicians of all time. His work related to mathematical probability was substantial, but a rather limited aspect of his activity. Euler was the son of Paul Euler, who lived with Jacob Bernoulli while he was a student at the University of Basel. Leonhard studied under Johan Bernoulli, and was, later on, a colleague and friend of Johan Bernoulli's son, Daniel Bernoulli. Daniel was a famous mathematician and physicist, who made important contributions to the theory of risk, and to what would now be called epidemiology.

2. By far the most comprehensive information about the life and works of Thomas Bayes can be found in the biography Andrew I. Dale (2003). *Most Honourable Remembrance, The Life and Work of Thomas Bayes*, New York: Springer–Verlag.

3. James Gregory (1666–1731) was the younger brother of David Gregory (1661–1708), and the nephew of the eminent mathematician James Gregory (1638–1675). The Gregory family produced many eminent mathematicians and scientists through several generations. Several of these were named either James or David.

4. George Berkeley (1734). *The Analyst.* See www.maths.tcd.ie/pub/HistMath/People/Berkeley/Analyst/

5. A photocopy of the actual certificate that contained the nomination can be found in Andrew I. Dale (2003). *Most Honourable Remembrance, The Life and Work of Thomas Bayes*, New York: Springer–Verlag, p. 93.

6. Thomas Simpson (1755). A letter to the Right Honourable *George*, Earl of *Macclesfield*, President of the *Royal Society*, on the *Advantage* of taking the Mean of a Number of Observations in Practical Astronomy. *Philosophical Transactions*, 49: 82–93.

7. The relevant portion of this letter is quoted in Stigler (1986a), pp. 94–95.

8. A comprehensive discussion of Enlightenment associationist psychology and its relationship to ideas about probability can be found in Lorraine Daston (1988). *Classical Probability in the Enlightenment*. Princeton, NJ: Princeton University Press, Chapter 4.

9. David Hartley (1749). *Observations on Man, His Frame, His Duty, and His Expectations*, 2 Volumes. London: Richardson. For a synopsis of Hartley's medical and philosophical contributions, see Walter Langdon–Brown (1941). David Hartley: physician and philosopher (1705–1757). *Proceedings of the Royal Society of Medicine*, 34; 233–239. A photocopy of Hartley's *Observations* is accessible online at Google Books.

10. There is some disagreement about the true identity of Hartley's ingenious friend. Stigler leaned toward Nicholas Saunderson (1682–1739), offering a lighthearted Bayesian analysis in an entertaining essay: Stephen M. Stigler (1983). Who discovered Bayes' Theorem? *The American Statistician*, 37: 290–296. This article was reprinted in Stephen M. Stigler (1999). *Statistics on the Table: The History of Statistical Concepts and Methods*. Cambridge, MA: Harvard University Press, Chapter 15.

11. For biographical information on Richard Price, I have relied primarily on Carl B. Cone (1952). *Torchbearer of Freedom: The Influence of Richard Price on Eighteenth Century Thought*. Lexington, KY: University of Kentucky Press. For an extensive discussion of Price's philosophical ideas, see D. O. Thomas (1977). *The Honest Mind: The Thought and Work of Richard Price*. Oxford: Clarendon Press. A recent biographical sketch including some long-overdue recognition of Price's contributions and nice color graphics is by Martyn Hooper (2013). Richard Price, Bayes' Theorem, and God. *Significance*, 10: 36–39. Hooper is chairman of the Richard Price Society, founded in 2012: richardpricesociety.org.uk

12. Richard Price (1758). *A Review of the Principal Questions and Difficulties in Morals*. London: Millar.

13. Thomas Bayes (1764). An essay towards solving a problem in the doctrine of chances. *Philosophical Transactions*, 53:370–418. Bayes's essay has been reproduced in many places. It is available on Richard J. Pulskamp's website at http://cerebro.xu.edu/math/Sources/Bayes

14. Carl B. Cone (1952). *Torchbearer of Freedom: The Influence of Richard Price on Eighteenth Century Thought*. Lexington, KY: University of Kentucky Press, p. 40.

15. Richard Price (1769). *Observations on Reversionary Payments*, London: Cadell. A biography in which his actuarial work is featured was written by his nephew William Morgan, who served as president of the Equitable: William Morgan (1815). *Memoirs of the Life of The Rev. Richard Price, D.D., F.R.S.*, London: R. Hunter.

16. Richard Price (1776). *Observations on the Nature of Civil Liberty, the Principles of Government, and the Justice and Policy of the War with America,* London: Cadell. A photocopy is available on Google Books.

17. Richard Price (1777). *Additional Observations on the Nature and Value of Civil Liberty, and the War with America,* London: Cadell. A photocopy is available on Google Books.

18. In its usual form, Bayes's Theorem is expressed as

$$P(A|E) = \frac{P(E|A)P(A)}{P(E|A)P(A) + P(E|B)P(B)}.$$

19. Gerd Gigerenzer (2008). *Rationality for Mortals: How People Cope with Uncertainty.* Oxford: Oxford University Press.

20. Richard Price submitted Bayes' essay with a covering letter to John Canton, who was Secretary of the Royal Society, dated November 10, 1763. This letter, which was read on December 23, 1763, contained an extensive introduction to set the stage for the essay itself.

21. Joseph Butler (1736). *Analogy of Religion, Natural and Revealed, to the Constitution and Course of Nature.* London, Introduction.

22. David Hume (1739). *A Treatise of Human Nature.* London: John Noon, and (1748). *An Enquiry Concerning Human Understanding.* London.

23. Glenn Shafer (1978). Non-additive probabilities in the work of Bernoulli and Lambert. *Archive for History of Exact Science,* 19: 309–370. Thierry Martin (2011). J.–H. Lambert's theory of probable syllogisms. *International Journal of Approximate Reasoning,* 52: 144–152. Thierry Martin (2006). La logique probabiliste de Gabriel Cramer [The probabilistic logic of Gabriel Cramer]. *Mathematics and Social Sciences,* 44: 43–60.

24. Denis Diderot (1765?), *Probabilité* in d'Alembert and Diderot (eds.), *Encyclopédie, ou Dictionnaire raisonné des sciences, des arts, et des métiers,* 14:301–302. For a summary of the background and context of Diderot's interest in probability, see Jean Mayer (1991). Diderot et le calcul des probabilités dans l'Encyclopédie [Diderot and the calculus of probabilities in the Encyclopedia]. *Revue d'Histoire des Sciences.* 44: 375–391.

25. Lorraine Daston (1988). *Classical Probability in the Enlightenment.* Princeton, NJ: Princeton University Press, p. 318.

26. Marquis de Condorcet (1985). Essai sur l'application de l'analyse à la probabilité des décisions rendues à la pluralité des voix [Essay on the application of probability analysis to the decisions rendered by a plurality of votes]. Paris.

27. http://www-history.mcs.st-and.ac.uk/Biographies/Laplace.html.

28. Pierre-Simon Laplace (1774). Sur la probabilité des causes par les évènemens [On the probability of the causes given the events]. *Mémoires de Mathématique et de Physique,* 621–656. This was translated by Stephen Stigler (1986b). Memoir on the probability of the causes of events. *Statistical Science,* 1: 364–378.

29. Gillispie (1972). Probability and politics: Laplace, Condorcet, and Turgot. *Proceedings of the American Philosophical Society,* p. 14.

30. This quotation is from Napoleon's *Memoirs,* written while he was in exile in St. Helena, according to W. W. Rouse Ball (1888). *A Short Account of the History of Mathematics.* London: Macmillan, p. 346.

31. Pierre-Simon Laplace (1812). *Théorie Analytique des Probabilités*, Paris: Courcier.
32. The philosophical essay was published originally in 1795, was subsequently included as an introduction to the *TAP*, and republished separately as Pierre-Simon Laplace (1840). *Essai Philosophique sur les probabilies,* 6th ed. Paris: Courcier. It was translated by F.W. Truscott and F.L. Emory in 1902 as *A Philosphical Essay on Probabilities* and reprinted New York: Dover, 1951 and reproduced for publication by Rough Draft Printing in 2009.
33. Pierre-Simon Laplace (1795), p. 1.
34. Pierre-Simon Laplace (1795). *Essai Philosophique sur les probabilités. Paris: Courcier,* p. 4.
35. Pierre-Simon Laplace (1795), p. 6.
36. Pierre-Simon Laplace (1795), p. 10.
37. Pierre-Simon Laplace (1774).
38. Stephen M. Stigler (1986a). *The History of Statistics: The Measurement of Uncertainty before 1900.* Cambridge: Harvard University Press, pp. 122–131.
39. A recent book on the subject of Bayes's Theorem perpetuates this confusion by oversimplifying and misinterpreting the history and controversies surrounding its practical uses: Sharon Bertsch McGrayne (2011). *The Theory that would not Die: How Bayes' Rule Cracked the Enigma Code, Hunted Down Russian Submarines & Emerged Triumphant from Two Centuries of Controversy.* New Haven: Yale University Press.
40. Pierre-Simon Laplace (1795), p. 189.
41. David Hartley (1749). *Observations on Man, His Frame, His Duty, and His Expectations,* 2 Volumes. London: Richardson.
42. Stephen M. Stigler (1986a). *The History of Statistics: The Measurement of Uncertainty before 1900.* Cambridge: Harvard University Press, p. 132.
43. Richard Price (1768). *Four Dissertations.* London: Cadell. The 4th edition (1777) is available on Google Books. The footnote is contained in Dissertation IV: The importance of Christianity, the nature of historical evidence and miracles, pp. 395–398.
44. Carl B. Cone (1952). *Torchbearer of Freedom: The Influence of Richard Price on Eighteenth Century Thought.* Lexington, KY: University of Kentucky Press. pp. 58–59.
45. Gillispie (1972).

CHAPTER 8: BABEL

1. Leonard J. Savage (1954). *The Foundations of Statistics.* New York: John Wiley & Sons, Inc., p. 2.
2. Ian Hacking (1975). *The Emergence of Probability.* Cambridge: Cambridge University Press, pp. 90–91.
3. Edith Dudley Sylla (2006). *The Art of Conjecturing, together with Letter to a Friend on Sets in Court Tennis.* Baltimore: The Johns Hopkins University Press, p. 139.
4. Laplace (1795), p. 7.
5. Laplace (1795), Chapters 11–13.

6. Siméon Denis Poisson (1837). *Recherche sur la probabilité des jugements en matière criminelle et en matière civile, precédé des règles générale du calcul des probabilities* [Research on the probability of judgments in criminal and civil matters, preceded by general rules for the calculation of probabilities]. Paris: Bachelier.

7. John Stuart Mill (1843). *A System of Logic, Ratiocinative and Inductive*, vol. 2. London: John Parker, p. 67.

8. A wide variety of philosophical theories trying to pin down the precise meaning of probability have been offered. For an overview of the most prominent ones, see Henry Kyburg, Jr. and Mariam Thalos (eds.) (2003). *Probability is the Very Guide of Life: The Philosophical Uses of Chance.* Chicago: Open Court; Maria Carla Galavotti (2005). *Philosophical Introduction to Probability.* Palo Alto: CSLI Publications; Donald Gillies (2000). *Philosophical Thories of Probability.* New York: Routledge.

9. Robert Leslie Ellis (1849). On the foundations of the theory of probability. *Transactions of the Cambridge Philosophical Society,* 8: 1–6.

10. Antoine Augustin Cournot (1843). *Exposition de la Théorie des Chances et des Probabilités.* Paris: Hachette. For a summary of Cournot's views, see: Alain Desrosières (2006). From Cournot to public policy evaluation: paradoxes and controversies involving quantification. *Prisme,* 7: 1–42.

11. John Venn (1866). *The Logic of Chance.* London: Macmillan.

12. John Maynard Keynes (1921). *A Treatise on Probability.* London: Macmillan, p. 95.

13. All quotations from von Mises are taken from Richard von Mises (1928). *Probability, Statistics, and Truth.* New York: Dover, 1981. (Translated from the 1951 3rd edition of the German original by Hilda Geiringer.) The first edition appeared in 1928.

14. Hans Reichenbach (1949). *The Theory of Probability.* Berkeley: University of California Press, p. 150. This quotation can be found in Maria Carla Galavotti (2005). *Philosophical Introduction to Probability.* Palo Alto: CSLI Publications. An earlier German edition of Reichenbach's book was published in 1935.

15. Augustus de Morgan (1838). *An Essay on Probabilities, and on their Applications to Life, Contingencies, and Insurance Offices.* London: Longman.

16. Augustus De Morgan (1847). *Formal Logic, or, The Calculus of Inference, Necessary and Probable.* London: Taylor and Walton.

17. George Boole (1854). *An Investigation of the Laws of Thought, on which are Founded the Mathematical Theories of Logic and Probability.* London: Walton and Maberly. I discovered these "Boolean" quotations originally in Maria Carla Galavotti (2005). *Philosophical Introduction to Probability.* Palo Alto: CSLI Publications.

18. George Boole (1854). *An Investigation of the Laws of Thought, on which are Founded the Mathematical Theories of Logic and Probability.* London: Walton and Maberly, p. 250.

19. George Boole (1854). *An Investigation of the Laws of Thought, on which are Founded the Mathematical Theories of Logic and Probability.* London: Walton and Maberly, p. 258.

20. George Boole (1854). *An Investigation of the Laws of Thought, on which are Founded the Mathematical Theories of Logic and Probability.* London: Walton and Maberly, p. 386.

21. William Stanley Jevons (1873). *The Principles of Science.* London: Macmillan. Second edition, enlarged, 1877.

22. A nice summary of the statistical theories of William Stanley Jevons can be found in Maria Carla Galavotti (2005). *Philosophical Introduction to Probability*. Palo Alto: CSLI Publications, pp. 141–144.

23. For a broad overview of the logical theory and its main exponents, Maria Carla Galavotti (2005). *Philosophical Introduction to Probability*. Palo Alto: CSLI Publications, Chapter 6. See also: Gillies, Donald (2000). *Philosophical Theories of Probability*. New York: Routledge, Chapter 3.

24. The most influential of these was Rudolf Carnap (1891–1970). See Rudolf Carnap (1950). *Logical Foundations of Probability*. Chicago: University of Chicago Press.

25. C. D. Broad (1922). Review: *A Treatise on Probability* by J. M. Keynes. *Mind* (New Series), 3: 72–85.

26. John Maynard Keynes (1921). *A Treatise on Probability*. London: Macmillan, pp. 33–34.

27. John Maynard Keynes (1921). *A Treatise on Probability*. London: Macmillan, Chapter 4.

28. Frank Plumpton Ramsey (1926). Truth and probability in Paul Kegan and Richard Bevan Braithwaite (eds.) (1931) *The Foundations of Mathematics and other Logical Essays*. London: Routledge.

29. Bruno de Finetti (1937) *La prévision: ses lois logiques, ses sources subjectives, Annales de L'Institut Henri Poncaré* VII, 1–68. Translated as Foresight: Its Logical Laws, Its Subjective Sources in Henry Kyburg and Howard Smokler (eds.) (1964). *Studies in Subjective Probability*. New York: John Wiley & Sons, Inc., pp. 95–158.

30. Leonard J. Savage (1954). *The Foundations of Statistics*. New York: John Wiley & Sons, Inc.

31. Joseph Brent (1998). *Charles Sanders Peirce: A Life,* 2nd ed. Bloomington and Indianapolis: Indiana University Press. Louis Menant (2001). *The Metaphysical Club: A Story of Ideas in America*. New York: Farrar, Straus and Giroux.

32. T. S. Fiske (1988). The beginnings of the American Mathematical Society: reminiscences of Thomas Scott Fiske. *Historia Mathematica*, 1: 13–17.

33. Charles Sanders Peirce (1910). Notes on the doctrine of chances, in Charles Hartshorne and Paul Weiss (eds.) *Collected Works of Charles Sanders Peirce*. Cambridge: Harvard University Press, pp. 409–410.

34. Karl R. Popper (1959a). *The Logic of Scientific Discovery*. London: Routledge; and Karl R. Popper (1962). *Conjectures and Refutations*. London: Routledge.

35. Karl R. Popper (1959b). The Propensity interpretation of probability. *The British Journal for the Philosophy of Science*, 10: 25–42.

36. Karl R. Popper (1990). *A World of Propensities*. Bristol: Thoemmes.

CHAPTER 9: PROBABILITY AND REALITY

1. Daniel Ellsberg (1961). Risk, ambiguity, and the Savage axioms. *Quarterly Journal of Economics*, 75: 669.

2. Nassim Nicholas Taleb (2001). *Fooled by Randomness, The Hidden Role of Chance in Life and in the Markets*. New York: Random House; Nassim Nicholas Taleb

(2007). *The Black Swan: The Impact of the Highly Improbable*. New York: Random House.

3. Benoit Mandelbrot (1963). The variation of certain speculative prices. *Journal of Business*, 36: 394–419.

4. Arthur P. Dempster (1967). Upper and lower probabilities induced by a multi-valued mapping. *The Annals of Mathematical Statistics*, 38: 325–339; Glenn Shafer (1976). *A Mathematical Theory of Evidence*. Princeton, NJ: Princeton University Press; Arthur P. Dempster (2008). The Dempster–Shafer calculus for statisticians. *International Journal of Approximate Reasoning*, 48: 365–377.

5. Herbert I. Weisberg (1972). Upper and lower probability inferences from ordered multinomial data. *Journal of the American Statistical Association*, 67: 884–890.

6. Lofti A. Zadeh, (1978). Fuzzy sets as a basis for a theory of possibility. *Fuzzy Sets and Systems*, 1: 3–28.

7. Humberto R. Maturana and Francisco J. Varela, (1987). *The Tree of Knowledge: The Biological Roots of Human Understanding*. Boston: Shambhala Publications, p. 133.

8. Maturana and Varela (1987). *The Tree of Knowledge: The Biological Roots of Human Understanding*. Boston, MA: Shambhala Publications, pp. 136–137.

9. Ronald A. Fisher (1922). On the mathematical foundations of theoretical statistics. *Philosophical Transactions of the Royal Society of London. Series A*, 22: 312.

10. Ronald A. Fisher (1922). On the mathematical foundations of theoretical statistics. *Philosophical Transactions of the Royal Society of London. Series A*, 22: 313.

11. Ronald A. Fisher (1959a). Mathematical probability in the natural sciences. *Technometrics*, 1: 21–22.

12. Ronald A. Fisher (1959a). Mathematical probability in the natural sciences. *Technometrics*, 1: 22.

13. Ronald A. Fisher (1959a). Mathematical probability in the natural sciences. *Technometrics*, 1: 22.

14. Ronald A. Fisher (1959b). *Statistical Methods and Scientific Inference,* 2nd ed. Edinburgh: Oliver and Boyd, p. 32.

15. Ronald A. Fisher (1959b). *Statistical Methods and Scientific Inference,* 2nd ed. Edinburgh: Oliver and Boyd, pp. 32–33.

16. John Maynard Keynes (1922). Introduction to Hubert D. Henderson, *Supply and Demand*. New York: Harcourt, Brace and Company.

17. John Maynard Keynes (1921). *A Treatise on Probability*. London: Macmillan, p. 321.

18. John Maynard Keynes (1921). *A Treatise on Probability*. London: Macmillan, p. 71.

19. Ronald A. Fisher (1959a). Mathematical probability in the natural sciences. *Technometrics*, 1: 23.

20. Nate Silver (2012). *The Signal and the Noise: Why So Many Predictions Fail – But Some Don't*. New York: Penguin, p. 298.

21. Versions of this puzzle had been around for some time, but were not well known prior to the *Parade* column : Marilyn vos Savant, *Parade Magazine*, Sept. 9, 1990, 15. Follow-up articles appeared in the magazine on Dec. 2, 1990 and Feb. 17, 1991. See also: Steve Selvin (1975). Letter to the Editor: "A Problem in Probability," *The American Statistician*, 29: 67; and (1975). "On the Monty Hall Problem," *The American Statistician*, 29:134.

22. For an elaboration of the idea of the "protocol" and several interesting illustrative examples, see Joseph Y. Halpern, *Reasoning about Uncertainty*. Cambridge: MIT Press, 2003, p. 6.

23. Ronald A. Fisher (1959a). Mathematical probability in the natural sciences. *Technometrics*, 1: 23.

24. John Maynard Keynes (1921). *A Treatise on Probability*. London: Macmillan, p. 31. This passage is quoted and discussed in Ronald A. Fisher (1959b). *Statistical Methods and Scientific Inference*, 2nd ed. Edinburgh: Oliver and Boyd, pp. 44–45.

25. For an elaborate discussion of the two-envelope problem and the confusion engendered by it: Halpern (2003). *Reasoning about Uncertainty*. Cambridge: MIT Press, pp. 178–180.

CHAPTER 10: THE DECISION FACTORY

1. My historical dramatization is of course fictional, but the main facts are faithful to the historical record.

2. A highly informative biographical sketch of Gosset was written by Joan Fisher Box (1981). Gosset, Fisher, and the *t* distribution. *The American Statistician*, 35: 90–91. See also E. S. Pearson (1990). *"Student": A Statistical Biography of William Sealy Gosset*. Oxford: Clarendon Press.

3. See for example Herbert I. Weisberg (2010). *Bias and Causation: Models and Judgment for Valid Comparisons*. Hoboken, NJ: John Wiley & Sons, Inc.

4. Student (1908). The probable error of a mean. *Biometrika*, 6: 1–25; Student, Probable error of a correlation coefficient. *Biometrika*, 6: 302–310.

5. For the most complete exposition of this complicated subject, see Stephen M. Stigler (1986a). *The History of Statistics: The Measurement of Uncertainty before 1900*. Cambridge: Harvard University Press, Part 1, pp. 1–139.

6. Adolphe Quetelet (1835). *Sur l'homme et le développement de ses facultés, ou Essai de physique sociale*. Paris: Bachelier. Translated as *A Treatise on Man and the Development of his Faculties* (Edinburgh: Chambers, 1842). For modern perspectives on the contributions of Quetelet, see Stephen M. Stigler (1986a). *The History of Statistics: The Measurement of Uncertainty before 1900*. Cambridge: Harvard University Press, Chapter 5; Ian Hacking (1990). *The Taming of Chance*. Cambridge: Cambridge University Press. *The Taming of Chance*. Cambridge: Cambridge University Press, Chapter 13.

7. The probable error was a measure of the measurement precision. It was defined as the value of the error that would be exceeded (in absolute value) with probability 50%. For technical reasons, it was later replaced by the standard error, used exclusively today, which is exceeded with probability approximately 32%. See any standard introductory statistics textbook for details.

8. Ronald A. Fisher (1925). *Statistical Methods for Research Workers*, Edinburgh: Oliver and Boyd.

9. Joan Fisher Box (1978). *R. A. Fisher: The Life of a Scientist*. New York: John Wiley & Sons, Inc., p. 130.

10. The landmark in placing random selection on a firm theoretical footing was a paper by Neymen: Jerzy Neyman (1934). On the two different aspects of the representative method: the method of stratified sampling and the method of purposive selection. *Journal of the Royal Statistical Society*, 97: 558–625.

11. Rand Corporation (1955). *A Million Random Digits with 100,000 Normal Deviates*, New York: Free Press.

12. One of Fisher's earliest expositions was: Ronald A. Fisher (1926). The arrangement of field experiments. *Journal of Mining and Agriculture in Great Britain*, 33: 503–513. A decade later he summarized his extensive work on the subject in Ronald A. Fisher (1935a). *The Design of Experiments*, Edinburgh: Oliver and Boyd.

13. Karl Pearson (1900). On the criterion that a given system of deviations from the probable in the case of a correlated system of variables is such that it can be reasonably supposed to have arisen from random sampling. *Philosophical Magazine Series* 5, 50: 157–175.

14. For the details of Weldon's experiment, see: Zacariah Labby (2009). Weldon's dice, automated. *Chance*, 22: 6–13.

15. Ronald A. Fisher (1959b). *Statistical Methods and Scientific Inference*, 2nd ed. Edinburgh: Oliver and Boyd, pp. 103–104.

16. The definitive biography of Neyman is Constance Reid (1982). *Neyman from Life*. New York: Springer-Verlag. A succinct summary and insightful discussion of the relations between Fisher and Neyman, personal and technical, can be found in Erich L. Lehmann (2011). *Fisher, Neyman, and the Creation of Classical Statistics*. New York: Springer.

17. E. S. Pearson (1990). *"Student": A Statistical Biography of William Sealy Gosset*. Oxford: Clarendon Press, p. 77.

18. E. S. Pearson (1939). William Sealy Gosset: 'Student' as a statistician. *Biometrika*, 30: 210–250.

19. Arthur Conan Doyle (1890). *The Sign of Four*. London: Doubleday, p. 111.

20. E. S. Pearson (1939). William Sealy Gosset: 'Student' as a statistician. *Biometrika*, 30:. 77

21. Ronald A. Fisher (1935b). The logic of inductive inference. *Journal of the Royal Statistical Society*, 98: 54.

22. Jerzy Neyman (1961). Silver jubilee of my dispute with Fisher. *Journal of the Operations Research Society of Japan*, 3: 145–154.

23. Ronald A. Fisher (1959b). *Statistical Methods and Scientific Inference*, 2nd ed. Edinburgh: Oliver and Boyd, p. 101.

24. Herman Chernoff and Lincoln E. Moses (1959). *Elementary Decision Theory*. New York: John Wiley & Sons, Inc., p. 1.

25. Leonard J. Savage (1954). *The Foundations of Statistics*. New York: John Wiley & Sons, Inc., p. 4.

26. Leonard J. Savage (1954). *The Foundations of Statistics*. New York: John Wiley & Sons, Inc., p. 67.

27. Most prominent in this regard was the geophysicist Harold Jeffreys, who wrote an influential book—Harold Jeffreys (1939). *Theory of Probability*. Oxford: Clarendon Press.

CHAPTER 11: THE LOTTERY IN SCIENCE

1. Jorge Luis Borges (1941). La Loteria en Babilonia [The Lottery in Babylon] in *Ficciones* (1944). Buenos Aires: Editorial Sur; Translated by Anthony Bonner and published as *Ficciones* (1962). New York: Grove Press.
2. The dominance of technology in modern society and the resulting negative consequences have been forcefully delineated by Jacques Ellul (1964). *The Technological Society*. New York: Vintage Books; Neil Postman (1992). *Technopoly: The Surrender of Culture to Technology*. New York: Knopf.
3. John W. Tukey (1960). Conclusions vs. decisions. *Technometrics*, 2: 423–433.
4. John W. Tukey (1977). *Exploratory Data Analysis*. Reading, MA: Addison–Wesley.
5. John W. Tukey (1977). *Exploratory Data Analysis*. Reading, MA: Addison–Wesley, p. 3.
6. Recent research has begun to untangle the complex relationship between genetic predispositions and the efficacy of aspirin for prevention of cardiovascular events. Deepak Voora, Cyr D, Lucas J, Chi JT, Dungan J, McCaffrey TA, Katz R, Newby LK, Kraus WE, Becker RC, Ortel TL, and Ginsburg GS (2013). Aspirin exposure reveals novel genes associated with platelet function and cardiovascular events. *Journal of the American College of Cardiology*, 62(14):1267–1276.
7. For recent overviews of the Big Data revolution and its implications, see Eric Siegel (2013). Predictive Analytics: *The Power to Predict Who Will Click, Buy, Lie, or Die*. Hoboken, NJ: John Wiley & Sons, Inc. and Viktor Mayer–Schonberger and Kenneth Cukier (2013). *Big Data: A Revolution That Will Transform How We Live, Work, and Think*. Boston: Houghton Mifflin Harcourt.
8. George Boole (1854). *An Investigation of the Laws of Thought, on which are Founded the Mathematical Theories of Logic and Probability*. London: Walton and Maberly.
9. Paul E. Meehl (1954). *Clinical vs. Statistical Prediction*. Minneapolis: University of Minnesota Press, p. 119.
10. A classic compendium of major academic articles can be found in Thomas Gilovich, Dale Griffin, and Daniel Kahneman (eds.) (2002). *Heuristics and Biases: The Psychology of Intuitive Judgment*. New York: Cambridge University Press. See also Daniel Kahneman (2011). *Thinking Fast and Slow*. New York: Farrar, Straus and Giroux.
11. Daniel Kahneman (2011). *Thinking Fast and Slow*. New York: Farrar, Straus and Giroux, p. 8.
12. Daniel Kahneman (2011). *Thinking Fast and Slow*. New York: Farrar, Straus and Giroux, p. 77.
13. Nassim Nicholas Taleb (2007). *The Black Swan: The Impact of the Highly Improbable*. New York: Random House.
14. Philip E. Tetlock (2005). *Expert Political Judgment: How Good Is It? How Can We Know?* Princeton, NJ: Princeton University Press, pp. 117–118.
15. Arthur P. Dempster (1967). Upper and lower probabilities induced by a multivalued mapping. *The Annals of Mathematical Statistics*, 38: 325–339; Glenn Shafer (1976). *A Mathematical Theory of Evidence*. Princeton, NJ: Princeton University Press; Zadeh (1978), Arthur P. Dempster (2008). The Dempster–Shafer calculus for statisticians. *International Journal of Approximate Reasoning*, 48: 365–377.

16. Gary Klein (1998). *Sources of Power: How People Make Decisions*. Cambridge, MA: M.I.T. Press.

17. Herbert A. Simon (1992). What is an explanation of behavior? *Psychological Science*, 3: 150–161.

18. Daniel Kahneman and Gary Klein (2009). Conditions for intuitive expertise: A failure to disagree. *American Psychologist*, 64: 515–526.

19. Gigerenzer (2007). *Gut Feelings: The Intelligence of the Unconscious*. New York: Penguin and Gerd Gigerenzer (2008). *Rationality for Mortals: How People Cope with Uncertainty*. Oxford: Oxford University Press.

20. Gerd Gigerenzer (2008). *Rationality for Mortals: How People Cope with Uncertainty*. Oxford: Oxford University Press, p. 22.

21. Gerd Gigerenzer (2008). *Rationality for Mortals: How People Cope with Uncertainty*. Oxford: Oxford University Press, p. 19.

22. Malcolm Gladwell (2005). *Blink: The Power of Thinking without Thinking*. Boston: Little, Brown.

23. Frank H. Knight (1921). *Risk, Uncertainty and Profit*. Cambridge: The Riverside Press, p. 226.

24. Frank H. Knight (1921). *Risk, Uncertainty and Profit*. Cambridge: The Riverside Press, p. 227.

25. Antonio Damasio (1994). *Descartes' Error: Emotion, Reason, and the Human Brain*. New York: Penguin.

26. Antonio Damasio (1994). *Descartes' Error: Emotion, Reason, and the Human Brain*. New York: Penguin, p. 174.

27. Henry A. Kissinger (1994). *Diplomacy*. New York: Simon & Schuster.

28. William James (1890). *The Principles of Psychology*. Cambridge, MA: Harvard University Press, p. 462.

29. Schulz (2010). *Being Wrong: Adventures in the Margin of Error*. New York: Harper Collins, pp. 117–118.

30. Feng-Hsiung Hsu (2004). *Behind Deep Blue: Building the Computer that Defeated the World Chess Champion*. Princeton NJ, Princeton University Press; Kelly, John E. III and Hamm, Steven (2013). *Smart Machines: IBM's Watson and the Era of Cognitive Computing*. New York: Columbia University Press.

31. Daniel Kahneman (2011). *Thinking Fast and Slow*. New York: Farrar, Straus and Giroux, Chapter 14.

32. See, for example, Amos Tversky and Daniel Kahneman (1983). Extensional versus intuitive reasoning: the conjunction fallacy in probability judgment. *Psychological Review*, 90: 293–315.

33. Daniel Kahneman (2011). *Thinking Fast and Slow*. New York: Farrar, Straus and Giroux, Chapter 16.

34. Gerd Gigerenzer (2008). *Rationality for Mortals: How People Cope with Uncertainty*. Oxford: Oxford University Press, Chapter 12.

35. Daniel Kahneman (2011). *Thinking Fast and Slow*. New York: Farrar, Straus and Giroux, p. 167.

36. Daniel Ellsberg (1961). Risk, ambiguity, and the Savage axioms. *Quarterly Journal of Economics*, 75: 669

37. See Donald T. Campbell and David A. Kenny (1999). *A Primer on Regression Artifacts*. New York: The Guilford Press.

38. John P. A. Ioannidis (2005). Why most published research findings are false. *PloS Medicine*, 2: 696–701.

39. For a discussion of the need for routine replication and the obstacles that exist currently, see: Gary King (1995). Replication, replication. *Political Science and Politics*, 28: 443–499; John P. A. Ioannidis and Muin J. Khoury (2011). Improving validation practices in "omics" research. *Science*, 234: 1230–1232.

CHAPTER 12: TRUST BUT VERIFY

1. This rendition of the event is accurate to the best of my recollection, except for the actual date and weather conditions.

2. Jerry Cornfield (1912–1979) was a biostatistician who served in both academia and in government, and as president of the American Statistical Association in 1974. He is most famous for devising the standard methodology for analyzing case-control studies by using the odds ratio as a measure of relative risk: Jerome Cornfield (1951). A method of estimating comparative rates from clinical data: applications to cancer of the lung, breast and cervix. *Journal of the National Cancer Institute*, 11: 1269–1275.

3. Richard L. Kravitz, Naihua Duan, and Joel Braslow. (2004). Evidence-based medicine, heterogeneity of treatment effects, and the trouble with averages. *The Milbank Quarterly*, 4: 661–687.

4. Paul E. Meehl (1954). *Clinical vs. Statistical Prediction*. Minneapolis: University of Minnesota Press.

5. This phrase was a favorite of President Ronald Reagan (1911–2004) used by him to characterize his approach for dealing with the Soviet Union, and it later entered the popular vernacular.

6. Paul Tough (2012). *How Children Succeed: Grit, Curiosity, and the Hidden Power of Character*. Boston: Houghton Mifflin Harcourt, p. 140.

7. Claude Bernard (1865). *Introduction à l'Étude de la Médecine Expérimentale*. Translated by H. C. Greene with an Introduction by L. J. Henderson in 1927 as *An Introduction to the Study of Experimental Medicine*. New York: Macmillan, p. 32.

8. Claude Bernard (1865). *Introduction à l'Étude de la Médecine Expérimentale*. Translated by H. C. Greene with an Introduction by L. J. Henderson in 1927 as *An Introduction to the Study of Experimental Medicine*. New York: Macmillan, p. 40.

9. Claude Bernard (1865). *Introduction à l'Étude de la Médecine Expérimentale*. Translated by H. C. Greene with an Introduction by L. J. Henderson in 1927 as *An Introduction to the Study of Experimental Medicine*. New York: Macmillan, p. 92.

10. Alfred North Whitehead (1933). *Adventures of Ideas*. New York: Macmillan, p. 128.

11. Philip E. Tetlock (2005). *Expert Political Judgment: How Good Is It? How Can We Know?* Princeton, NJ: Princeton University Press.

12. Henry A. Kissinger (b. 1923) served as the U.S. National Security Advisor and Secretary of State during the administration of President Richard Nixon (1913–1994).

He was awarded the Nobel Peace Prize in 1973. Prior to his government posts, he had a distinguished academic career at Harvard University. His views were summarized in Henry Kissinger (1994). *Diplomacy*. New York: Simon & Schuster.

13. I have seen this quotation attributed to Krishnamurti in many places, but have been unable to locate an original source.

14. John P. A. Ioannidis (2005). Why most published research findings are false. *PloS Medicine*, 2: 696–701.

15. What I have in mind are various techniques that utilize the available data more efficiently and may provide an estimate of the variability of the hold-out estimate also. Such methods include N-fold cross-validation, bootstrap, and jackknife approaches.

16. Gary King (1995). Replication, replication. *Political Science and Politics*, 28: 443–499.

17. Viktor Mayer-Schonberger and Kenneth Cukier (2013). *Big Data: A Revolution That Will Transform How We Live, Work, and Think*. Boston: Houghton Mifflin Harcourt.

18. For this perceptive observation I am grateful to Michael B. Meyer (private communication).

19. Herbert I. Weisberg (2010). *Bias and Causation: Models and Judgment for Valid Comparisons*. Hoboken, NJ: John Wiley & Sons, Inc., p. 308.

20. Eric Topol (2012). *The Creative Destruction of Medicine: How the Digital Revolution will Create Better Health Care*. New York: Basic Books.

21. Tad Williams (1998). *Otherland Volume Two: River of Blue Fire*. New York: DAW Books, pp. 574–575.

22. For an extensive treatment of these topics, see, for example, Alain Desrosières (1998). *The Politics of Large Numbers*. Cambridge, MA: Harvard University Press. Translated by Camille Nash and Theodore M. Porter as *Trust in Numbers: The Pursuit of Objectivity in Science and Public Life* (Princeton, NJ: Princeton University Press, 1986).

APPENDIX: THE PASCAL–FERMAT CORRESPONDENCE OF 1654

1. Richard J. Pulskamp's translation of all the letters that have (so far) been discovered can be found at his website: http://cerebro.xu.edu/math/Sources/Problem_of_points/points.html and also in Appendix 4 of Florence N. David (1962). *Games, Gods and Gambling: A History of Probability and Statistical Ideas*. London: Charles Griffin & Company.

2. A comprehensive monograph on Pascal's *Treatise on the Arithmetical Triangle* has been published by A. W. F. Edwards (1987). *Pascal's Arithmetical Triangle: The Story of a Mathematical Idea*. Baltimore: The Johns Hopkins University Press. Richard J. Pulskamp's translation of Pascal's *Treatise* can be found on: http://cerebro.xu.edu/math/Sources/Pascal/Sources/arith_triangle.pdf.

BIBLIOGRAPHY

Aitken, George A. (1892). *The Life and Works of John Arbuthnot*. Oxford: The Clarendon Press.

Antithrombotic Trialists' (ATT) Collaboration (2009). Aspirin in the primary and secondary prevention of vascular disease: collaborative meta-analysis of individual participant data from randomized trials. *Lancet*, 373: 1849–1860.

Arbesman, Samuel (2012). *The Half-Life of Facts: Why Everything We Know Has an Expiration Date*. New York: Penguin.

Arbuthnot, John (1692). *Of the Laws of Chance*. London: Benjamin Motte.

Ball, W. W. Rouse (1888). *A Short Account of the History of Mathematics*. London: Macmillan.

Ball, W. W. Rouse (1889). *A History of the Study of Mathematics at Cambridge*. Cambridge: The University Press.

Bayes, Thomas (1764). An essay towards solving a problem in the doctrine of chances. *Philosophical Transactions of the Royal Society of London*, 53: 370–418.

Begley, C. Glenn and Ellis, Lee M. (2012). Raise standards for preclinical cancer research. *Nature*, 483: 531–533.

Bellhouse, David R. (1989). A manuscript on chance written by John Arbuthnot. *International Statistical Review*, 57: 249–259.

Bellhouse, David R. and Genest, Christian (2007). Maty's biography of Abraham de Moivre, translated, annotated and augmented. *Statistical Science*, 22: 109–136.

Bellhouse, David R. (2011). *Abraham De Moivre: Setting the Stage for Classical Probability and its Applications*. Boca Raton, FL: CRC Press.

Willful Ignorance: The Mismeasure of Uncertainty, First Edition. Herbert I. Weisberg.
© 2014 John Wiley & Sons, Inc. Published 2014 by John Wiley & Sons, Inc.

Berkeley, George (1734). *The Analyst*. London and Dublin: J. Tonson.

Bernard, Claude (1865). *Introduction à l'Étude de la Médecine Expérimentale*. Translated by H. C. Greene with an Introduction by L. J. Henderson in 1927 as *An Introduction to the Study of Experimental Medicine*. New York: Macmillan.

Bernoulli, Jacob (1685). Problème proposé par M. Bernoulli [Problem proposed by Mr. Bernoulli]. *Journal des Sçavans*, 314.

Bernoulli, Jacob (1686). *Journal des Sçavans*.

Bernoulli, Jacob (1713). *Ars Conjectandi*. Basel, Switzerland: Thurnisiorum. Translated with an introduction and notes by Edith Dudley Sylla in 2006 as *The Art of Conjecturing, together with Letter to a Friend on Sets in Court Tennis*. Baltimore: The Johns Hopkins University Press.

Bernoulli, Nicholas (1709). *De Usu Artis Conjectandi in Jure* [*The Uses of the Art of Conjecturing in Law*]. Basel, Switzerland.

Bernstein, Peter L. (1996). *Against the Gods: The Remarkable Story of Risk*. New York: John Wiley & Sons, Inc.

Boole, George (1854). *An Investigation of the Laws of Thought, on Which are Founded the Mathematical Theories of Logic and Probability*. London: Walton and Maberly.

Borges, Jorge Luis (1941). *La Loteria en Babilonia* [The Lottery in Babylon] in *Ficciones* (1944). Buenos Aires: Editorial Sur. Translated by Anthony Bonner and published as *Ficciones* (1962). New York: Grove Press.

Box, George E. P. and Draper, Norman (1987). *Empirical Model-Building and Response Surfaces*. New York: John Wiley & Sons, Inc.

Box, Joan Fisher (1978). *R. A. Fisher: The Life of a Scientist*. New York: John Wiley & Sons, Inc.

Box, Joan Fisher (1981). Gosset, Fisher, and the *t* distribution. *The American Statistician*, 35: 90–91.

Brent, Joseph (1998). *Charles Sanders Peirce: A Life*, 2nd ed. Bloomington and Indianapolis: Indiana University Press.

Broad, C. D. (1922). Review: a treatise on probability by J. M. Keynes. *Mind* (New Series), 3: 72–85.

Browne, William (1714). *Christiani Huygenii Libellus de Rationciniis in Ludo Aleae: Or, The Value of All Chances in Games of Fortune; Cards, Dice, Wagers, Lotteries &c, Mathematically Demonstrated*. London: T. Woodward.

Butler, Joseph (1736). *Analogy of Religion, Natural and Revealed, to the Constitution and Course of Nature*. London: J. and P. Knapton.

Byers, William (2011). *The Blind Spot: Science and the Crisis of Uncertainty*. Princeton, NJ: Princeton University Press.

Byrne, Edmund F. (1968). *Probability and Opinion*. The Hague, The Netherlands: Martinus Nijhoff.

Campbell, Donald T. and Kenny, David A. (1999). *A Primer on Regression Artifacts*. New York: The Guilford Press.

Cardano, Gerolamo (1563). *De Ludo Aleae* [*On Games of Chance*]. Translated by Sydney Henry Gould in Ore (1953).

Carnap, Rudolf (1950). *Logical Foundations of Probability*. Chicago, IL: University of Chicago Press.

Chatterjee, Samprit and Hadi, Ali S. (2012). *Regression Analysis by Example*, 4th edition. Hoboken, NJ: John Wiley & Sons, Inc.

Chernoff, Herman and Moses, Lincoln E. (1959). *Elementary Decision Theory*. New York: John Wiley & Sons, Inc.

Christakis, Nicholas A. (2013). Let's Shake Up the Social Sciences. *New York Times*, July 19, 2013.

Conan Doyle, Arthur (1890). *The Sign of Four*. London: Doubleday.

Condorcet, Marquis de (1785). *Essai sur l'application de l'analyse à la probabilité des décisions rendues à la pluralité des voix* [Essay on the application of probability analysis to the decisions rendered by a plurality of votes].Paris: Imprimerie Royale.

Cone, Carl B. (1952). *Torchbearer of Freedom: The Influence of Richard Price on Eighteenth Century Thought*. Lexington, KY: University of Kentucky Press.

Cornfield, Jerome (1951). A method of estimating comparative rates from clinical data: applications to cancer of the lung, breast and cervix. *Journal of the National Cancer Institute*, 11: 1269–1275.

Cournot, Antoine Augustin (1843). *Exposition de la Théorie des Chances et des Probabilités* [Exposition of the Theory of Chances and Probabilities]. Paris: Hachette.

Dale, Andrew I. (1992). On the authorship of 'A calculation of the credibility of human testimony.' *Historia Mathematica*, 19: 414–417.

Dale, Andrew I. (2003). *Most Honourable Remembrance: The Life and Work of Thomas Bayes*. New York: Springer-Verlag.

Damasio, Antonio (1994). *Descartes' Error: Emotion, Reason, and the Human Brain*. New York: Penguin.

Daston, Lorraine (1988).*Classical Probability in the Enlightenment*. Princeton, NJ: Princeton University Press.

David, Florence N. (1962). *Games, Gods and Gambling: A History of Probability and Statistical Ideas*. London: Charles Griffin & Company.

De Finetti, Bruno (1937). La prévision: ses lois logiques, ses sources subjectives [Foresight: its logical laws, its subjective sources]. *Annales de L'Institut Henri Poncaré*, VII: 1–68.

De Moivre, Abraham (1711). De Mensura Sortis [On the Measurement of Chance]. *Philosophical Transactions*, 29: 329–331.

De Moivre, Abraham (1718). *The Doctrine of Chances, or a Method of Calculating the Probability of Events in Play*. London: W. Pearson.

De Moivre, Abraham (1725). *Annuities upon Lives*. London: W. Pearson.

De Moivre, Abraham (1738). *The Doctrine of Chances, or a Method of Calculating the Probability of Events in Play*. Second Edition: Fuller, Clearer, and More Correct than the First. London: Woodfall.

De Moivre, Abraham (1743). *Annuities on Lives, Second Edition: Plainer, Fuller, and More Correct than the Former*. London: Woodfall.

De Moivre, Abraham (1756). *The Doctrine of Chances, or a Method of Calculating the Probability of Events in Play.* Third Edition: Fuller, Clearer, and More Correct than the Former. London: Millar. Reprinted in 1967, New York: Chelsea Publishing Company.

De Morgan, Augustus (1838). *An Essay on Probabilities, and on their Applications to Life, Contingencies, and Insurance Offices.* London: Longman.

De Morgan, Augustus (1847). *Formal Logic, or, The Calculus of Inference, Necessary and Probable.* London: Taylor and Walton.

Dempster, Arthur P. (1967). Upper and lower probabilities induced by a multivalued mapping. *The Annals of Mathematical Statistics*, 38: 325–339.

Dempster, Arthur P. (2008). The Dempster–Shafer calculus for statisticians. *International Journal of Approximate Reasoning*, 48: 365–377.

Desrosières, Alain (1998). *The Politics of Large Numbers*, translated by Camille Nash. Cambridge, MA: Harvard University Press.

Desrosières, Alain (2006). From Cournot to public policy evaluation: paradoxes and controversies involving quantification. *Prisme*, 7: 1–42.

Devlin, Keith (2008). *The Unfinished Game: Pascal, Fermat and the Seventeenth-Century Letter that Made the World Modern.* New York: Basic Books.

Diderot, Denis (1765) Probabilité. In: d'Alembert and Diderot (eds.), *Encyclopédie, ou Dictionnaire raisonné des sciences, des arts, et des métiers*, vol. 14, pp. 301–302.

Draper, Norman and Smith, Harry (1998). *Applied Regression Analysis*, 3rd edition. New York: John Wiley & Sons, Inc.

Dumas, Alexandre (1850). *La Tulipe Noire* [The Black Tulip]. Paris: Baudry.

Edwards, A. W. F. (1983). Pascal's problem: the gambler's ruin. *International Statistical Review*, 51: 73–79.

Edwards, A. W. F. (1987). *Pascal's Arithmetical Triangle: The Story of a Mathematical Idea.* Baltimore, MD: The Johns Hopkins University Press.

Ellis, Robert Leslie (1849). On the foundations of the theory of probability. *Transactions of the Cambridge Philosophical Society*, 8: 1–6.

Ellul, Jacques (1964). *The Technological Society.* New York: Vintage Books.

Ellsberg, Daniel (1961). Risk, ambiguity, and the Savage axioms. *Quarterly Journal of Economics*, 75: 643–669.

Fermat, Pierre (1679). *Opera Mathematica.* Paris: Gauthier-Villars edited by Samuel Fermat.

Fisher, Ronald A. (1922). On the mathematical foundations of theoretical statistics. *Philosophical Transactions of the Royal Society of London. Series A*, 22: 309–368.

Fisher, Ronald A. (1925). *Statistical Methods for Research Workers.* Edinburgh: Oliver and Boyd.

Fisher, Ronald A. (1926). The arrangement of field experiments. *Journal of Mining and Agriculture in Great Britain*, 33: 503–513.

Fisher, Ronald A. (1935a). *The Design of Experiments.* Edinburgh: Oliver and Boyd.

Fisher, Ronald A. (1935b). The logic of inductive inference. *Journal of the Royal Statistical Society*, 98:39–54.

Fisher, Ronald A. (1959a). Mathematical probability in the natural sciences. *Technometrics*, 1: 21–29.

Fisher, Ronald A. (1959b). *Statistical Methods and Scientific Inference*, 2nd edition. Edinburgh: Oliver and Boyd.

Fiske, T. S. (1988). The beginnings of the American Mathematical Society: reminiscences of Thomas Scott Fiske. *Historia Mathematica*, 1: 13–17.

Flood, R., Rice, A., and Wilson, R. (eds.) (2011). *Mathematics in Victorian Britain*. Oxford: Oxford University Press.

Franklin, James (2001). *The Science of Conjecture: Evidence and Probability before Pascal*. Baltimore, MD: The Johns Hopkins University Press.

Friesen, John (2003). Archibald Pitcairne, David Gregory and the Scottish origins of English Tory Newtonianism, 1688–1715. *History of Science*, 41: 163–191.

Galavotti, Maria Carla (2005). *Philosophical Introduction to Probability*. Palo Alto, CA: CSLI Publications.

Galton, Francis (1869). *Hereditary Genius*. London: Macmillan.

Galton, Francis (April, 1890). Kinship and correlation. *North American Review*, 150: 431.

Gigerenzer, Gerd Swijtink, Zeno, Porter, Theodore, Daston, Lorraine, Beatty, John, Krüger Lorenz (1989). *The Empire of Chance: How Probability Changed Science and Everyday Life*. Cambridge: Cambridge University Press.

Gigerenzer, Gerd (2007). *Gut Feelings: The Intelligence of the Unconscious*. New York: Penguin.

Gigerenzer, Gerd (2008). *Rationality for Mortals: How People Cope with Uncertainty*. Oxford: Oxford University Press.

Gillies, Donald (2000). *Philosophical Theories of Probability*. New York: Routledge.

Gillispie, Charles Coulston (1972). Probability and politics: Laplace, Condorcet, and Turgot. *Proceedings of the American Philosophical Society*, 16: 1–20.

Gilovich, Thomas, Griffin, Dale, and Kahneman, Daniel (eds.) (2002). *Heuristics and Biases: The Psychology of Intuitive Judgment*. New York: Cambridge University Press.

Gladwell, Malcolm (2005). *Blink: The Power of Thinking Without Thinking*. New York: Little, Brown & Company.

Gladwell, Malcolm (2008). *Outliers: The Story of Success*. New York: Little, Brown & Company.

Gleick, James (2004). *Isaac Newton*. New York: Vintage Books.

Gleick, James (2011). *The Information: A History, a Theory, a Flood*. New York: Pantheon Books.

Graunt, John (1666). *Journal des Sçavans*.

Greene, Brian (2005). *The Fabric of the Cosmos: Space, Time, and the Texture of Reality*. New York: Vintage Books.

Groopman, Jerome and Hartzband, Pamela (2011). *Your Medical Mind: How to Decide what is Right for You*. New York: Penguin.

Guyatt, Gordon (1992). Evidence-based medicine. A new approach to teaching the practice of medicine. *Journal of the American Medical Association*, 268: 2420–2425.

Hacking, Ian (1975). *The Emergence of Probability*. Cambridge: Cambridge University Press. (2nd edition, 2006).

Hacking, Ian (1990). *The Taming of Chance*. Cambridge: Cambridge University Press.

Hald, Anders (2003). *History of Probability and Statistics before 1750*. Hoboken, NJ: John Wiley & Sons, Inc.

Halley, Edmond (1693). An estimate of the degrees of mortality of mankind. *Philosophical Transactions*, 17: 596–610.

Halpern, Joseph Y. (2003). *Reasoning about Uncertainty*. Cambridge: MIT Press.

Harrison, Peter (2001). Curiosity, forbidden knowledge, and the reformation of natural philosophy in early modern England. *Isis*, 92: 265–290.

Hartley, David (1749). *Observations on Man, His Frame, His Duty, and His Expectations*, 2 Volumes. London: Richardson.

Hooper, George (1699). A calculation of the credibility of human testimony. *Philosophical Transactions*, 21: 359–365.

Hooper, Martyn (2013). Richard Price, Bayes' Theorem, and God. *Significance*, 10: 36–39.

Hsu, Feng-Hsiung (2004). *Behind Deep Blue: Building the Computer that Defeated the World Chess Champion*. Princeton, NJ: Princeton University Press.

Hume, David (1739). *A Treatise of Human Nature*. John Noon: London.

Hume, David (1748). *An Enquiry Concerning Human Understanding*. London: John Noon.

Ioannidis, John P. A. (2005). Why most published research findings are false. *PLOS Medicine*, 2: 696–701.

Ioannidis, John P. A. and Khoury, Muin J. (2011). Improving validation practices in "omics" research. *Science*, 234: 1230–1232.

Isaacson, Walter (2007). *Einstein: His Life and Universe*. New York: Simon & Schuster.

James, William (1890). *The Principles of Psychology*. Cambridge, MA: Harvard University Press.

Jeffreys, Harold (1939). *Theory of Probability*. Oxford: Clarendon Press.

Jevons, William Stanley (1873). *The Principles of Science*. London: Macmillan. (2nd edition, enlarged, 1877).

Johnson, Steven (2010). *Where Good Ideas Come From: The Natural History of Innovation*. New York: Penguin.

Kahneman, Daniel (2011). *Thinking, Fast and Slow*. New York: Farrar, Straus and Giroux.

Kahneman, Daniel and Klein, Gary (2009). Conditions for intuitive expertise: a failure to disagree. *American Psychologist*, 64: 515–526.

Kegan, Paul and Braithwaite, R. B. (eds.) (1931). *The Foundations of Mathematics and other Logical Essays*. London: Routledge.

Kelly, John E. III and Hamm, Steven (2013). *Smart Machines: IBM's Watson and the Era of Cognitive Computing*. New York: Columbia University Press.

Keynes, John Maynard (1921). *A Treatise on Probability*. London: Macmillan.

Keynes, John Maynard (1922). Introduction to Hubert D. Henderson, *Supply and Demand*. New York: Harcourt, Brace and Company.

King, Gary (1995). Replication, replication. *Political Science and Politics*, 28: 443–499.

Kissinger, Henry A. (1994). *Diplomacy*. New York: Simon & Schuster.

Klein, Gary (1998). *Sources of Power: How People Make Decisions*. Cambridge: MIT Press.

Knight, Frank H. (1921). *Risk, Uncertainty and Profit*. Cambridge: The Riverside Press.

Knuth, Donald E. (2011). *The Art of Computer Programming*, vol. 4A. Boston: Addison-Wesley.

Kolmogorov, Andrei (1956). *Foundations of the Theory of Probability*, 2nd edition. New York: Chelsea Publishing Company.

Kravitz, Richard L., DuanNaihua, and Braslow, Joel (2004). Evidence-based medicine, heterogeneity of treatment effects, and the trouble with averages. *The Milbank Quarterly*, 82: 661–687.

Kyburg, Henry Jr. and Smokler, Howard (eds.) (1964). *Studies in Subjective Probability*. New York: John Wiley & Sons, Inc.

Kyburg, Henry Jr. and Thalos, Mariam (eds.) (2003). *Probability is the Very Guide of Life: The Philosophical Uses of Chance*. Chicago, IL: Open Court.

Labby, Zacariah (2009). Weldon's dice, automated. *Chance*, 22: 6–13.

Langdon-Brown, Walter (1941). David Hartley: physician and philosopher (1705–1757). *Proceedings of the Royal Society of Medicine*, 34: 233–239.

Langer, Ellen J. (1989). *Mindfulness*. Reading, MA: Addison-Wesley.

Laplace, Pierre-Simon (1774). Sur la probabilité des causes par les évènemens [On the probability of the causes given the events]. *Mémoires de Mathématique et de Physique*, 6: 621–656.

Laplace, Pierre-Simon (1795). *Essai Philosophique sur les probabilités*. Paris: Courcier. Sixth edition in 1840. Translated by F. W. Truscott and F. L. Emory in 1902 as *A Philosphical Essay on Probabilities*, reprinted (1951), New York: Dover. Reproduced by Rough Draft Printing (2009).

Laplace, Pierre-Simon (1812). *Théorie Analytique des Probabilités* [Analytic Theory of Probabilities]. Paris: Courcier.

Lasocki, David (1989). The life of Daniel de Moivre. *The Consort*, 45: 15–17.

Lawson, Tony (2003). *Reorienting Economics*. London: Routledge.

Lehmann, Erich L. (2011). *Fisher, Neyman, and the Creation of Classical Statistics*. New York: Springer.

Lehrer, Jonah. (2010). The Truth Wears Off: Is There Something Wrong with the Scientific Method? *The New Yorker*, Dec 13, 2010. pp. 52–57

Leibniz, Gottfried W. (1666). *Dissertatio de arte combinatoria, Sämtliche Schriften und Briefe* (Berlin: Akademie Verlag, 1923) A VI 1, p. 163; *Philosophische Schriften* (Gerhardt) Bd. IV S.30.

Livio, Mario (2009). *Is God a Mathematician?* New York: Simon & Schuster.

Locke, John (1690). *An Essay Concerning Human Understanding*. London: Thomas Baffet.

Mandelbrot, Benoit (1963). The variation of certain speculative prices. *Journal of Business*, 36: 394–419.

Manzi, Jim (2012). *Uncontrolled: The Surprising Payoff of Trial-and-Error for Business, Politics, and Society*. New York: Basic Books.

Marks, Harry M. (1997). *The Progress of Experiment: Scientific and Therapeutic Reform in the United States, 1900–1999*. Cambridge: Cambridge University Press.

Martin, Thierry (2006). La logique probabiliste de Gabriel Cramer [The probabilistic logic of Gabriel Cramer]. *Mathematics and Social Sciences*, 44: 43–60.

Martin, Thierry (2011). J.-H. Lambert's theory of probable syllogisms. *International Journal of Approximate Reasoning*, 52: 144–152.

Maturana, Humberto R. and Varela, Francisco J. (1998). *The Tree of Knowledge: The Biological Roots of Human Understanding*. Boston, MA: Shambhala Publications.

Mayer, Jean (1991). Diderot et le calcul des probabilités dans l'encyclopédie [Diderot and the calculus of probabilities in the Encyclopedia]. *Revue d'Histoire des Sciences*, 44: 375–391.

Mayer-Schonberger, Viktor and Cukier, Kenneth (2013). *Big Data: A Revolution That Will Transform How We Live, Work, and Think*. Boston, MA: Houghton Mifflin Harcourt.

McClintock, Bruce A. (trans.) (1984). A. de Moivre: "De Mensura Sortis" or "On the Measurement of Chance" [with a commentary by Anders Hald]. *International Statistical Review*, 52: 229–262.

McGrayne, Sharon Bertsch (2011). *The Theory That Would Not Die: How Bayes' Rule Cracked the Enigma Code, Hunted Down Russian Submarines & Emerged Triumphant from Two Centuries of Controversy*. New Haven, CT: Yale University Press.

Meehl, Paul E. (1954). *Clinical vs. Statistical Prediction*. Minneapolis, MN: University of Minnesota Press.

Mill, John Stuart (1843). *A System of Logic, Ratiocinative and Inductive*, vol. 2. London: John Parker.

Mlodinow, Leonard (2008). *The Drunkard's Walk: How Randomness Rules our Lives*. New York: Vintage Books.

Montmort, Pierre (1708). *Essay d'Analyse sur les Jeux de Hazard*. Paris [2nd edition, revised and augmented, and including letters between N. Bernoulli, Waldegrave, and Montmort, 1713].

Morgan, William (1815). *Memoirs of the Life of the Rev. Richard Price, D.D., F.R.S.* London: R. Hunter.

Morley, Henry (1854). *The Life of Girolamo Cardano of Milan*, Physician. London: Chapman and Hall.

Neyman, Jerzy (1934). On the two different aspects of the representative method: the method of stratified sampling and the method of purposive selection. *Journal of the Royal Statistical Society*, 97: 558–625.

Neyman, Jerzy (1961). Silver jubilee of my dispute with Fisher. *Journal of the Operations Research Society of Japan*, 3: 145–154.

Ore, Oystein (1953). *Cardano, The Gambling Scholar*. Princeton, NJ: Princeton University Press.

Patterson, Scott (2010). *The Quants: How a New Breed of Math Whizzes Conquered Wall Street and Nearly Destroyed It*. New York: Random House.

Paul, Charles B. (1980). *Science and Immortality: The Éloges of the Paris Academy of Sciences (1699–1791)*. Berkeley: University of California Press.

Pearson, E. S. (1939). William Sealy Gosset: 'Student' as a statistician. *Biometrika*, 30: 210–250.

Pearson, E. S. (1990). *"Student": A Statistical Biography of William Sealy Gosset*. Oxford: Clarendon Press.

Pearson, E. S. and Kendall, M. G. (eds.) (1970). *Studies in the History of Statistics and Probability*. Darien, CT: Hafner.

Pearson, Karl (1900). On the criterion that a given system of deviations from the probable in the case of a correlated system of variables is such that it can be reasonably supposed to have arisen from random sampling. *Philosophical Magazine Series 5*, 50: 157–175.

Pearson, Karl (1930). *The Life, Letters and Labours of Francis Galton*. London: Cambridge University Press.

Peirce, Charles Sanders (1910). Notes on the doctrine of chances. In: Hartshorne, Charles and Weiss, Paul (eds.) (1932). *Collected Works of Charles Sanders Peirce*. Cambridge: Harvard University Press.

Pepys, Samuel (April 20, 1663). *The Diary of Samuel Pepys*, vol. 3, Wheatley, Henry B. (ed.) (1962). London: George Bell & Sons.

Peto, Richard, Gray, R., Collins, R., Wheatley, K., Hennekens, C., Jamrozik, K., Warlow, C., Hafner, B., Thompson, E., Norton, S., Gilliland, J., and Doll, R. (1988). Randomized trial of prophylactic daily aspirin in British male doctors. *British Medical Journal*, 296: 313–316.

Poisson, Siméon Denis (1837). *Recherche sur la probabilité des jugements en matière criminelle et en matière civile, precédé des règles générale du calcul des probabilités* [Research on the probability of judgments in criminal and civil matters, preceded by general rules for the calculation of probabilities]. Paris: Bachelier.

Popper, Karl R. (1959a). *The Logic of Scientific Discovery*. London: Routledge.

Popper, Karl R. (1959b). The propensity interpretation of probability. *The British Journal for the Philosophy of Science*, 10: 25–42.

Popper, Karl R. (1962). *Conjectures and Refutations*. London: Routledge.

Popper, Karl R. (1990). *A World of Propensities*. Bristol: Thoemmes.

Porter, Theodore M. (1986). *Trust in Numbers: The Pursuit of Objectivity in Science and Public Life*. Princeton, NJ: Princeton University Press.

Porter, Theodore M. (1995). *The Rise of Statistical Thinking 1820–1900*. Princeton, NJ: Princeton University Press.

Postman, Neil (1992). *Technopoly: The Surrender of Culture to Technology*. New York: Knopf.

Price, Richard (1758). *A Review of the Principal Questions and Difficulties in Morals*. London: Millar.

Price, Richard (1768). *Four Dissertations*. London: Cadell.

Price, Richard (1769). *Observations on Reversionary Payments*. London: Cadell.

Price, Richard (1776). *Observations on the Nature of Civil Liberty, the Principles of Government, and the Justice and Policy of the War with America*. London: Cadell.

Quetelet, Adolphe (1835). *Sur l'homme et le développement de ses facultés, ou Essai de physique sociale* [*A Treatise on Man and the Development of his Faculties*). Edinburgh: Chambers, 1842]. Paris: Bachelier.

Ramsey, Frank Plumpton (1926). Truth and probability. In: Kegan, Paul and Braithwaite, R. B. (eds.) (1931), *The Foundations of Mathematics and other Logical Essays*. London: Routledge.

Rand Corporation (1955). *A Million Random Digits with 100,000 Normal Deviates*. New York: Free Press.

Reichenbach, Hans (1949). *The Theory of Probability*. Berkeley, CA: University of California Press.

Reid, Constance (1982). *Neyman from Life*. New York: Springer-Verlag.

Reifman, Alan (2012). *Hot Hand: The Statistics Behind Sports' Greatest Streaks*. Dulles, VA: Potomac Books.

Rubin, Donald B. (1974). Estimating causal effects of treatments in randomized and non-randomized studies. *Journal of Educational Psychology*, 66: 688–701.

Rubin, Donald B. (2005). Causal inference using potential outcomes: design, modeling, decisions. *Journal of the American Statistical Association*, 100: 322–331.

Rusnock, Andrea A. (2002). *Vital Accounts: Quantifying Health and Population in Eighteenth-Century England and France*. Cambridge: Cambridge University Press.

Russell, Bertrand (1913). On the notion of cause. *Proceedings of the Aristotelian Society*, 13: 1–26.

Sackett, David L., Rosenberg, W. M., Gray, J. A., Haynes, R. B., Richardson, W. S. (1996). Evidence based medicine: what it is and what it isn't. *British Medical Journal*, 312: 71–72.

Salsburg, David (2001). *The Lady Tasting Tea: How Statistics Revolutionized Science in the Twentieth Century*. New York: Henry Holt and Company.

Savage, Leonard J. (1954). *The Foundations of Statistics*. New York: John Wiley & Sons, Inc.

Sauveur, Joseph (1679). Computation of the advantages of the banker in the game of Bassette. *Journal des Sçavans*. 44–52.

Schopenhauer, Arthur (1969). *The World as Will and Representation*. New York: Dover [Translated from the 1818 German original by E. F. J. Payne].

Schulz, Kathryn (2010). *Being Wrong: Adventures in the Margin of Error*. New York: Harper Collins.

Selvin, Steve (1975). Letter to the Editor: a problem in probability. *The American Statistician*, 29 (February): 67.

Selvin, Steve (1975). On the Monty Hall Problem. *The American Statistician*, 29 (August): 134.

Shafer, Glenn (1976). *A Mathematical Theory of Evidence*. Princeton, NJ: Princeton University Press.

Shafer, Glenn (1978). Non-additive probabilities in the work of Bernoulli and Lambert. *Archive for History of Exact Science*, 19: 309–370.

Shapiro, Barbara J. (1983). *Probability and Certainty in Seventeenth-Century England: A Study of the Relationships between Natural Science, Law, and Literature*. Princeton, NJ: Princeton University Press.

Siegel, Eric (2013). *Predictive Analytics: The Power to Predict Who Will Click, Buy, Lie, or Die*. Hoboken, NJ: John Wiley & Sons, Inc.

Silver, Nate (2012). *The Signal and the Noise: Why So Many Predictions Fail—But Some Don't*. New York: Penguin.

Simon, Herbert A. (1992). What is an explanation of behavior? *Psychological Science*, 3: 150–161.

Simpson, Thomas (1740). *The Nature and Laws of Chance*. London: Edward Cave.

Simpson, Thomas (1742). *The Doctrine of Annuities and Reversion, Deduced from Evident and Evident Principles*. London: J. Nourse.

Simpson, Thomas (1743). *An Appendix, Containing Some Remarks on a Late Book on the Same Subject, with Answers to Some Personal and Malignant Representations in the Preface Thereof*. London: J. Nourse.

Simpson, Thomas (1755). A Letter to the Right Honourable George, Earl of Macclesfield, President of the Royal Society, on the advantage of taking the mean of a number of observations in practical astronomy. *Philosophical Transactions*, 49: 82–93.

Steering Committee of the Physicians' Health Study Research Group (1989). Final report of the aspirin component of the ongoing Physicians' Health Study. *New England Journal of Medicine*, 321: 129–135.

Steiner, Christopher (2012). *Automate This: How Algorithms Came to Rule the World*. New York: Penguin.

Stigler, Stephen M. (1983). Who discovered Bayes' Theorem? *The American Statistician*, 37: 290–296.

Stigler, Stephen M. (1986a). *The History of Statistics: The Measurement of Uncertainty before 1900*. Cambridge, MA: Harvard University Press.

Stigler, Stephen M. (trans.) (1986b). Memoir on the probability of the causes of events. *Statistical Science*, 1: 364–378 [Translation of essay by Pierre-Simon Laplace, 1774].

Stigler, Stephen M. (1999). *Statistics on the Table: The History of Statistical Concepts and Methods*. Cambridge, MA: Harvard University Press.

Student (1908). The probable error of a mean. *Biometrika*, 6: 1–25.

Student (1908). Probable error of a correlation coefficient. *Biometrika*, 6: 302–310.

Sung, Bing (1966). Office of Naval Research Technical Report No. 2, Contract NR-042–097.

Swift, Jonathan (1729). *A Modest Proposal.* Dublin, Ireland: S. Harding.

Taleb, Nassim Nicholas (2001). *Fooled by Randomness. The Hidden Role of Chance in Life and in the Markets.* New York: Random House.

Taleb, Nassim Nicholas (2010). *The Black Swan: The Impact of the Highly Improbable,* 2nd edition. New York: Random House.

Tannery, P. and Henry, C. (eds.) (1891–1922). *Oeuvres de Fermat,* 5 volumes. Paris: Gauthier-Villars.

Tetlock, Philip E. (2005). *Expert Political Judgment: How Good Is It? How Can We Know?* Princeton, NJ: Princeton University Press.

Thomas, D. O. (1977). *The Honest Mind: The Thought and Work of Richard Price.* Oxford: Clarendon Press.

Todhunter, Isaac (1865). *A History of the Mathematical Theory of Probability: From the Time of Pascal to that of Laplace.* London: Macmillan [Reprinted in 1949 and 1965; New York: Chelsea Publishing Company].

Topol, Eric (2012). *The Creative Destruction of Medicine: How the Digital Revolution will Create Better Health Care.* New York: Basic Books.

Tough, Paul (2012). *How Children Succeed: Grit, Curiosity, and the Hidden Power of Character.* Boston, MA: Houghton Mifflin Harcourt.

Tukey, John W. (1960). Conclusions vs. decisions. *Technometrics,* 2: 423–433.

Tukey, John W. (1962). The future of data analysis. *Annals of Mathematical Statistics,* 1: 1–67.

Tukey, John W. (1977). *Exploratory Data Analysis.* Reading, MA: Addison-Wesley.

Tversky, Amos and Kahneman, Daniel (1983). Extensional versus intuitive reasoning: the conjunction fallacy in probability judgment. *Psychological Review,* 90: 293–315.

U.S. Department of Health and Human Services (January, 2010). *Head Start Impact Study Final Report.* Office of Planning, Research and Evaluation, Administration for Children and Families, Washington, D.C.

U.S. Department of Health and Human Services (October, 2012). *Third Grade Follow-Up to the Head Start Impact Study Final Report.* Office of Planning, Research and Evaluation, Administration for Children and Families, Washington, D.C.

U.S. Preventive Services Task Force (2009). Aspirin for the prevention of cardiovascular disease: U.S. Preventive Services Task Force recommendation statement. *Annals of Internal Medicine,* 150: 396–404.

Venn, John (1866). *The Logic of Chance.* London: Macmillan.

Von Mises, Richard (1928). *Probability, Statistics, and Truth.* New York: Dover, 1981 [Translated by Hilda Geiringer from the 3rd edition of the German original].

Voora, Deepak, Cyr, D., Lucas, J., Chi, J. T., Dungan, J., McCaffrey, T. A., Katz, R., Newby, L. K., Kraus, W. E., Becker, R. C., Ortel, T. L., Ginsburg, G. S. (2013). Aspirin exposure reveals novel genes associated with platelet function and cardiovascular events. *Journal of the American College of Cardiology,* 62: 1267–1276.

Vos Savant, Marilyn (1990). Ask Marilyn. *Parade Magazine*, September 9,1990, p. 15 [Follow-up articles appeared in the magazine on December 2, 1990 and February 17, 1991].

Walker, Helen M. (1934). Abraham de Moivre. *Scripta Mathematica*, 2: 316–333.

Weisberg Herbert I. (1972). Upper and lower probability inferences from ordered multinomial data. *Journal of the American Statistical Association*, 67: 884–890.

Weisberg, Herbert I. (1974). *Short Term Cognitive Effects of Head Start Programs: A Report on the Third Year of Planned Variation—1971–72*. U.S. Department of Health, Education and Welfare.

Weisberg, Herbert I. (2010). *Bias and Causation: Models and Judgment for Valid Comparisons*. Hoboken, NJ: John Wiley & Sons, Inc.

Weisberg, Herbert I. (2011). Statistics and clinical trials: past, present and future. *Proceedings of the American Statistical Association*.

Whitehead, Alfred North (1929). *Process and Reality*. New York: Macmillan.

Whitehead, Alfred North (1933). *Adventures of Ideas*. New York: Macmillan.

Williams, Tad (1998). *Otherland Volume Two: River of Blue Fire*. New York: DAW Books.

Young, Stanley S. and Karr, Alan (2011). Deming, data and observational studies: a process out of control and needing fixing. *Significance*, 8 (September): 116–120.

Zadeh, Lofti A. (1978). Fuzzy sets as a basis for a theory of possibility. *Fuzzy Sets and Systems*, 1: 3–28.

INDEX

Adams, John, 183
Additive property, 69, 168, 224, 312
Adolphe Quetelet, 4, 289, 316, 369
Aleatory contracts, 48
Annuities, 48, 90–94, 99, 145, 159, 163–164, 181–182, 204
Arbuthnot, John, 77–80, 87, 107–108, 157
Arnaud, Antoine, 61, 105, 117
Aspirin, 2, 13–14, 38–40, 315–319, 367
Astralagi, 49

Babbage, Charles, 4
Balzac, Honoré de, 369
Bauhuis, Bernard, 124
Bayes, Thomas, 173–197, 206–212, 218, 236, 244
    essay, 174–184, 197, 206, 211–214
    postulate, 193, 307
    scholium, 206, 208
Bayes's Theorem, 173–179, 184–193, 207–209, 218, 231, 244–246, 307–308, 337
Behavioral economics, 320
Belief functions, xiv, 254, 323
Bernoulli, Jacob, 22–30, 64, 71–80, 89, 94–95, 103, 106–108, 114–149,
154–160, 165–168, 190–196, 201–203, 206, 208, 213–215, 219–220, 230–235, 241, 245, 253, 258–264, 281–282, 284, 295, 323, 331–332, 336, 357
Ars Conjectandi, 106, 108, 116–125, 154–158, 165–167, 195, 220, 230, 235
axioms of prudent behavior, 130–131, 139
correspondence with G. Leibniz, 142–146
eulogies, 71, 116, 154
Golden Theorem, 106, 122, 141–142, 158, 160
metaphorical lottery, 120, 139
mixed argument, 131–133, 148
pure argument, 131–133
Bernoulli, Johann, 27, 76, 80, 106, 109, 115–117, 142, 154, 158, 164, 194
Bernoulli, Nicholas, 117, 155, 158, 160
Bias, 5, 32, 178, 287, 291–293, 310, 320–344, 351, 358, 362
Big Data, 37, 353
Bills of Mortality, 82–85, 95, 98, 108, 145
Biometrika, 297–299
Bonaparte, Napoléon, 199–200

Willful Ignorance: The Mismeasure of Uncertainty, First Edition. Herbert I. Weisberg.
© 2014 John Wiley & Sons, Inc. Published 2014 by John Wiley & Sons, Inc.

Boole, George, 229–234, 320
   Investigation of the Laws of Thought, 229, 320
Borges, Jorge Luis, v, 313, 370
Broad, C. D., 233
Browne, William, 156
Butler, Joseph, 191–192

Caesar, Julius, 191
Caramuel y Lobkowitz, Juan, 74, 103–105, 128
Carcavi, Pierre, 41–42, 65–66
Cardano, Gerolamo, 51–56
   De Ludo Aleae, 52
   general rule of wagering, 54, 57
   Scaliger fiasco, 124
Cassini, Giovanni, 96
Central Limit Theorem, 159, 201
Chess, 52–53, 58, 324, 331, 352, 355, 370
Cheyne, George, 153–154
Clinical trial, 2, 39–40, 226, 308, 346, 360
Colson, John, 162
Combinatorics, 50, 76, 103, 108, 122–126, 135, 138, 150, 154
Collective, 223–228, 276
Conditional probability, 169, 187, 206, 244, 270–273, 375
Condorcet, Marquis de, 196–199, 212, 216
Confidence interval, 4, 301
Confounding, 287, 291, 293, 310
Conjunction fallacy, 334, 367
Continental Congress, 183
Cournot, Antoine Augustin, 221
Craig, John, 108
Cramer, Gabriel, 194
Cromwell, Oliver, 86–87

D'Alembert, Jean le Rond, 195–198, 205, 236, 238
Damasio, Antonio, 328–329
   somatic markers, 328
Darwin, Charles, 27–28, 290
Daston, Lorraine, 195
De Bessy, Bernard Frenicle, 73
De Finetti, Bruno, 243–246
   exchangeability, 244–245
   Bayesian statistics, 246
De Medina, Bartolomé, 103–104, 128

De Moivre, Abraham, 112, 117, 150–170, 175, 178, 181, 190–194, 201–207, 213–215, 220, 245, 258
   De Mensura Sortis, 165–166
   Annuities upon Lives, 159, 163
   The Doctrine of Chances, 166–170
De Morgan, Augustus, 228–230
De Witt, Johann, 88, 91–94, 99–100, 146
Decision theory, 47, 247, 300, 348
Declaration of Independence, 183
Decline effect, 1, 343–344, 347
Dempster, Arthur, xv, 141, 254, 323
Descartes, René, 24, 41, 65, 86, 102, 328, 331
Dewey, John, 248
Dickens, Charles, 369
Diderot, Denis, 195–196
Dublin Society, 87
Dumas, Alexandre, 94
Dutch Book, 242

Eames, John, 180
Edict of Nantes, 150
Einstein, Albert, xii, 17, 247, 250, 257, 281
   Theory of General Relativity, 17, 250
Ellis, Robert Leslie, 219–220, 223, 228–229
Ellsberg, Daniel, 253, 338
   Ellsberg Paradox, 338
   Pentagon Papers, 253
Equitable Society, 181
Errors of measurement, 176–178, 201, 288–289
Euler, Leonhard, 171
Evidence-based, 2, 5, 13, 31, 318, 351, 365
Expectation
   archaic sense, 48–49, 53, 329, 373–385
   in Huygens's Treatise, 67–70, 93, 119–121, 126, 137–141, 149, 166–169, 171, 214, 329
   in problem of the points, 376–384
   mathematical, 59–60, 67–70, 75, 89–95, 101, 119–121
Extrinsic argument, 46, 129

Factorial design, 293
Fermat, Pierre, 19, 22–23, 42–43, 47, 52, 56–69, 72, 86, 120–123, 170, 205, 230, 238, 259, 368, 373–384

Fisher, Ronald A., v, xi–xii, 29–31, 35–36, 257–261, 265–267, 270–277, 284, 288, 290–305, 309, 313–316, 327, 345, 348, 351, 370
  disputes with J. Neyman, 35, 298–305
  hypothetical infinite population, 257–260
  inductive reasoning, 303–304
  randomized experiments, 291–294, 309–311
  recognizability, 36, 261, 263, 272, 274, 277, 327, 350
  relevant subsets, 261, 274, 277, 291, 344, 351
  Statistical Methods for Research Workers, 290
Flamsteed, John, 95, 97
Fontanelle, Bernard, 116
Forster, E. M., 233
Franklin, Benjamin, 182–183, 212
Franklin, James, xvii, 104
French Academy of Sciences, 65, 116, 197, 199–200
Friesen, John, 113
Fundamental probability set, 49, 54–55, 63
Fuzzy logic, xiv, 254

Galilei, Galileo, 55–56, 63, 76
Galton, Francis, 27–29, 284, 302, 312, 340–342
  correlation coefficient, 28–29
  regression to the mean, 340–342
Gambler's ruin problem, 62, 66
Gauss, Carl Friedrich, 288
Gigerenzer, Gerd, 187, 325–327, 337
Gladwell, Malcolm, 64, 327
Gombaud, Antoine (a.k.a. Chevalier de Méré), 42, 64
Gossett, W. S. (a.k.a. Student), 285–290, 296, 299–300
Graunt, John, 82–89, 97–98, 101, 145, 358
  bills of mortality, 82–85, 95, 98, 145
  estimation of population of London, 84
  invention of data, 82
  life table, 85–86, 98
Gregory, David, 77–80, 97, 108–109, 112–113, 153, 157, 174
Gregory, James (brother of David Gregory), 174
Gregory, James (uncle of David Gregory), 77
Guinness Brewery, 285–287

Hacking, Ian, 215
Halley, Edmond, 95–100, 111–112, 146, 153–156, 159, 182
  Breslau mortality data and analysis, 97–100, 111, 146, 159, 182
Hardy, G. H., 233
Hartley, David, 178–179, 192, 212
  associationist psychology, 178
Hawking, Stephen, 162
Head Start, 2, 38, 315
Hermann, Jacob, 116–117
Heuristics and biases, 320–326, 330–336, 340, 342, 351
Hevelius, Johannes, 96
Hobbes, Thomas, 86, 102
Homme moyen, 288
Hooke, Robert, 96
Hooper, George, 110–112
Howard, John, 182
Hudde, Johan, 73, 88, 91–94, 99
Hume, David, 182, 192–194, 212, 244
Huygens, Christiaan, 65–81, 88–93, 96, 99, 102–103, 107, 115–5, 119–120, 128, 150, 155–157, 166, 197, 219
  De Ratiociniis in Ludo Aleae, 66
Huygens, Ludwig, 65, 89

Ignorance fallacy, 34–35
Induction, 43, 189, 191–192, 196, 202–204, 212, 243, 307
Inside information, 34, 270, 276–277
Insufficient reason, 191, 208–211, 218, 231–233, 236–238, 307
Intrinsic arguments, 46, 129
Inverse probability, 179, 186, 190–191, 199, 206–212, 218, 231–233, 244, 305. *See also* Bayes's Theorem
Ioannidis, John, 342–344, 347, 359

James. William, 248
Jansen, Cornelius, 105
Jansenism, 61, 105
Jefferson, Thomas, 183
Jeopardy (the TV game), 331
Jevons, William Stanley, 232–233

Kahneman, Daniel, 320–325, 337–338, 342, 353

Keynes, John Maynard, v, 7–9, 12, 81, 105, 191, 221–222, 233–241, 245, 253–254, 260–265, 275, 279, 282, 308, 323, 335, 338, 351, 369
   A Treatise on Probability, 7, 233–234, 240
   principle of indifference (see also insufficient reason), 191, 238–239
   weight of evidence, 263–264
Klein, Gary, 323–325, 329
Knight, Frank, 6–9, 12, 253, 323, 327–328, 338
Kolmogorov, Andrei, 26, 233
Kolmogorov Axioms, 26, 233

Lagrange, Joseph, 199–200
Lambert, Johann Heinrich, 194–195, 254
Langer, Ellen, 16
Laplace, Pierre-Simon, 30–31, 150, 173–175, 194–222, 228, 230–232, 236, 239, 244–247, 258, 261, 279–282, 288, 307, 348, 369
   Analytical Theory of Probabilities, 200–202
   Central Limit Theorem, 201
   insufficient reason, 208–211
   inverse probability, 174, 198–199
   Philosophical Essay on Probabilities, 202, 211
   probability of causes, 198–199, 208
   Rule of Succession, 218, 232
Law of large numbers, 33, 141, 148, 159, 190, 206, 220, 245
Leibniz, Gottfried Wilhelm, 19, 21, 24, 71, 74, 79, 81, 97, 102–103, 106, 114–116, 142–146, 154, 164
   correspondence with Jacob Bernoulli, 142–146
   dispute with Isaac Newton, 154, 164
L'Hôpital, Marquis de, 106, 142
Linda Problem, 334–336
Locke, John, 109–110, 147
   An Essay Concerning Human Understanding, 109
Louis XIV, 65, 75, 150

Main effects, 37–38, 316–319, 350–351, 363, 365–366
   main-effect fallacy, 38, 316–317
Malebranche, Nicolas, 102
Mandelbrot, Benoit, 254
Maturana, Humberto, 255
Maty, Matthew, 153

Meehl, Paul, 320, 322, 351, 356
Mendel, Gregor, 247
Mersenne, Marin, 41
Mill, John Stuart, 4, 216, 231
Mindfulness, 15–17, 35, 216, 368–371
Montmort, Pierre, 71–72, 77, 112, 117, 154–159, 165–166
Monty Hall Problem, 267–270, 277–281, 332
Moore, G. E., 233
Moral certainty, 94, 128–129, 139–141, 206, 284–297
Moray, Robert, 88
Morellet, Abbé, 212
Mylon, Claude, 65–66

Narrative fallacy, 34–35, 319, 334
Neumann, Caspar, 97–98, 146
Newton, Isaac, 19–24, 71, 77–82, 91, 96–97, 102, 109–112, 153–156, 164–165, 173–175, 180, 198, 203, 250, 312
   dispute with Gottfried Leibniz, 145, 164
   Principia Mathematica, 96, 109
Neyman, Jerzy, 30–31, 35, 298–306, 351
   disputes with R. A. Fisher, 35, 298–305
   inductive behavior, 303–304
Neyman–Pearson theory, 31, 300–302, 305–306
Nicole, Pierre, 61, 117
Normal distribution, 160, 201
Null hypothesis, 294, 296, 299–306, 358
Nye, Stephen, 112

Odds, 8, 49–53, 64, 95, 98–102, 111, 138, 145, 149, 166–171, 177–179, 191, 211, 224, 242, 295, 306, 370–376, 382
   in Shakespeare's plays, 53
Optimistic bias, 342
Ore, Oystein, 54, 168
Outliers, 64, 248, 289

Pacioli, Luca, 58
Paine, Thomas, 183
Paris Observatory, 96, 200
Pascal, Blaise, 19, 22–23, 41–43, 47, 52, 56–67, 69, 72–74, 76, 86, 105, 120–123, 128, 170, 230, 259, 368, 373–385
   Treatise on the Arithmetical Triangle, 73, 76, 122, 377

Pascal-Fermat correspondence, 22, 43, 52, 63, 65, 67, 72, 373–385
Pascal's Wager, 61, 105
Pearson, Egon (E. S.), 30, 299–306, 358
Pearson, Karl, 27–31, 111–112, 284, 287, 294–296, 298–299, 309, 312
   invention of Chi-Squared test, 294–296, 309, 342
   on authorship of 1699 paper on probability, 111
Peirce, Benjamin, 248
Peirce, Charles Sanders (C. S.), 248–249, 251–252, 312, 316
   propensity theory of probability, 248–252
   tychism, 249
Pepys, Samuel, 83
Petty, William, 84–88, 97–98
Philosophes, 195–196, 212
Pitcairne, Archibald, 77, 153–154
Poisson, Siméon-Denis, 4–5, 216, 219–220, 222, 228, 231, 245
Popper, Karl, 250–251, 312
   falsifiability, 251
   propensity interpretation, 250–251, 316
Port-Royal *Logic*, 61, 82, 105, 117, 134
Positivism, 26, 355
Power (statistical), 301–302, 363
Prestet, Jean, 125, 150
Price, Richard, 174, 179–185, 189–193, 206, 212
   Bayes's Essay, 174, 180, 189–191
   Four Dissertations, 181, 212
   Observations on Civil Liberty and the War in America, 183
   Observations on Reversionary Payments, 184
Priestley, Joseph, 182, 212
Probabilism, 46, 62, 102–105, 128
Probable error, 289
Probability distribution, 33, 93, 160, 177, 191, 201, 218, 244, 246, 246, 279, 287, 292, 294, 300, 303, 306–308
Problem of the points, 21, 57, 60, 376–380
Proteus verses, 124, 133
Protocol, 269–270, 277–279, 280–281, 332
   Monty Hall game, 270, 277–279, 281, 332
   Two Envelope game, 279, 281, 332
Purposive sampling, 291–294

Quantum theory, 247, 250–252, 261, 276, 312
Queen Elizabeth II, 291
Quincy, Josiah, 183

Ramsey, Frank P., 240–243, 245, 305–306
Random number tables, 292
Random variable, 176–177, 201, 245
Randomization, 225, 291, 293–294, 310
Randomness, 28, 31–32, 34–35, 147, 203, 224–226, 247, 252, 254, 294, 313, 319, 368–369
Reference class, 7, 137, 225, 227–228, 231, 259, 261–276, 318, 327, 333, 339, 341–344, 349
Reichenbach, Hans, 222, 226–228
Reign of Terror, 200
Recognition primed decision-making (RPD), 324–327
Regression to the mean, 339–344
Replication, 17, 309, 343–345, 359–364
Representativeness fallacy, 332–336
Robartes, Francis, 155, 165
Roberval, Gilles, 65–66, 382, 384
Rothamsted experimental station, 284, 290, 298
Roulette, 32, 276, 292
Royal Observatory, 97
Royal Society, 65, 84, 87–88, 96–97, 109–110, 112, 153, 174–176, 178, 180–181, 184, 197, 290
   Philosophical Transactions, 112, 153–155, 161, 165, 174, 176, 181
Russell, Bertrand, 26, 233–234
Russell, John, 284
Russian Revolution, 298

Salisbury, John of, 101
Sampling frame, 262, 292
Sauveur, Joseph, 74–75, 106, 126
Savage, Leonard (Jimmie), 246–247, 276, 306–307
Scaliger, Julius Caesar, 124
Schulz, Kathryn, 17, 330–331, 336
Scientific Revolution, 19, 31
Shafer, Glenn, 254, 323
Shakespeare, William, 53, 102
Silver, Nate, 266
Simon, Herbert, 324
Simpson, Thomas, 162–163, 175–179, 190
Slaughter's Coffee House, 152, 159

Smith, Adam, 182
Spiegel, Elizabeth, 352
Stanhope, Philip, 175
Statistical significance, 4, 294–299, 301, 304, 309–311, 343–345, 347–348, 358–365, 370
Strachey, Lytton, 233
Stratton, F. J. M., 288, 290
Strode, Thomas, 76
Swift, Jonathan, 77, 87–88

Taleb, Nassim Nicholas, 25, 253–254, 322
Tartaglia, Nicolas, 58–59
Taylor, Brook, 156
Tough, Paul, 352
Tower of Babel, 213–214
Trinitarianism, 112
Tukey, John W., 3, 314–317, 362
    exploratory data analysis, 314–315
Turgot, A. R. J., 197, 212
Tversky, Amos, 320
Twain, Mark, 369
Two Envelope Problem, 277–279, 281, 332
Tychism, 249

U. S. Coast Survey, 248

Van Schooten, Frans, 65–67, 69, 71, 91
Varela, Francisco, 255
Venn, John, 221–223, 229, 231
    The Logic of Chance, 221
Von Mises, Richard, 222–228, 276–277
Vos Savant, Marilyn, 267

Waller, Richard, 97
Wallis, John, 96, 125
Washington, George, 184
Weldon, Frank, 295–296
Whitehead, Alfred North, 233–234, 355
Williams, Tad, 368
Willful ignorance, xi–xiv, 12, 15, 23–24, 90, 137, 176, 246, 258, 301, 304, 319, 327, 332, 348, 350, 367, 369, 371
Wittgenstein, Ludwig, 240
Wollstonecraft, Mary, 181

Yates, Frank, 292

Zadeh, Lofti, 252, 323

Printed and bound by CPI Group (UK) Ltd, Croydon, CR0 4YY

27/10/2024

14580263-0001
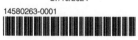